Diagnosis and Treatment of
Spinal Cord Injuries

Diagnosis and Treatment of Spinal Cord Injuries

Editor: Carson Diaz

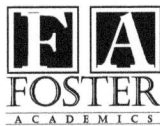

FOSTER
ACADEMICS

www.fosteracademics.com

www.fosteracademics.com

FA
FOSTER
ACADEMICS

Cataloging-in-Publication Data

Diagnosis and treatment of spinal cord injuries / edited by Carson Diaz.
    p. cm.
Includes bibliographical references and index.
ISBN 978-1-63242-734-2
1. Spinal cord--Wounds and injuries. 2. Spinal cord--Wounds and injuries--Diagnosis.
3. Spinal cord--Wounds and injuries--Treatment. I. Diaz, Carson.
RD594.3 .D53 2019
617.482 044--dc23

Foster Academics,
118-35 Queens Blvd., Suite 400,
Forest Hills, NY 11375, USA

ISBN 978-1-63242-734-2 (Hardback)

Contents

Preface

This book was inspired by the evolution of our times; to answer the curiosity of inquisitive minds. Many developments have occurred across the globe in the recent past which has transformed the progress in the field.

Spinal cord injuries refer to the damage to the spinal cord caused as a result of accidents, falls, gunshots, infections, tumors, etc. This may lead to temporary or permanent changes in the functioning of the spinal cord. Loss of autonomic function, muscle function and sensation is common in spinal cord injuries. The damage to the spinal cord can be divided into primary and secondary injury. Injury can also be complete or incomplete based on the degree of loss of sensation. A radiographic evaluation using a MRI, CT or X-ray scan can evaluate the degree of damage to the spinal column and the location of the trauma. Pre-hospitalization care aimed at basic life support and prevention of further injury, initial care aimed at adequate breathing and cardiovascular function, spinal motion restriction and repeated neurological assessments are part of the first line of care. After this stage, patients require extended treatments in intensive care units and specialized units. The degree of functional recovery and autonomy achieved in activities of daily living after treatment depends on the level and severity of the injury. The objective of this book is to give a general view of the different diagnostic and treatment strategies of spinal cord injuries. It brings forth some of the most innovative concepts and elucidates the unexplored aspects of spinal cord injuries. It is a vital tool for all researching and studying this domain.

This book was developed from a mere concept to drafts to chapters and finally compiled together as a complete text to benefit the readers across all nations. To ensure the quality of the content we instilled two significant steps in our procedure. The first was to appoint an editorial team that would verify the data and statistics provided in the book and also select the most appropriate and valuable contributions from the plentiful contributions we received from authors worldwide. The next step was to appoint an expert of the topic as the Editor-in-Chief, who would head the project and finally make the necessary amendments and modifications to make the text reader-friendly. I was then commissioned to examine all the material to present the topics in the most comprehensible and productive format.

I would like to take this opportunity to thank all the contributing authors who were supportive enough to contribute their time and knowledge to this project. I also wish to convey my regards to my family who have been extremely supportive during the entire project.

Editor

Non-invasive Brain Stimulation to Characterize and Alter Motor Function after Spinal Cord Injury

Aaron Z. Bailey, Hunter J. Fassett, Tea Lulic,
Jenin El Sayes and Aimee J. Nelson

Abstract

Advances in transcranial magnetic stimulation (TMS) now permit the precise assessment of circuitry in human motor cortices that contribute to movement. Further, TMS approaches are used to promote neural plasticity within cortical and spinal circuitry in an attempt to create short-term changes in motor control. This review is focused on the application of TMS techniques in the study of characterizing and promoting neural plasticity within individuals presenting with chronic spinal cord injury. We review TMS research performed in individuals with SCI and consider new opportunities for the use of TMS approaches to promote neural plasticity for improving motor recovery.

Keywords: spinal cord injury, motor recovery, noninvasive brain stimulation, transcranial magnetic stimulation, neural plasticity

1. Introduction

Noninvasive brain stimulation (NIBS) approaches are used to both characterize and modify neural activity within the targeted cortices and the spinal cord. These approaches are, therefore, well-suited for understanding and attempting to improve functional recovery following spinal cord injury. There is, however, a gap in our present understanding of how the cortical physiology is altered in individuals with spinal cord injury (SCI). In this review, we focus on the characterization of motor cortical circuitry in individuals with SCI using transcranial magnetic stimulation (TMS). This basic knowledge is essential to developing therapies that aim to induce long-term changes in neural circuits that participate in motor control. NIBS approaches are also capable of inducing short-term plasticity within motor cortical neural circuits and may be combined with other techniques to promote greater functional changes in individuals with SCI. Therefore, the second goal of this review is to survey the literature that has utilized NIBS approaches for promoting neural plasticity within the motor system in individuals with SCI. We subsequently explore new opportunities for the use of NIBS to characterize and promote neural plasticity in SCI for improving motor recovery.

2. Noninvasive brain stimulation to characterize motor function

NIBS provides an opportunity to assess the neural circuitry within motor cortical areas as well as the excitatory and inhibitory influences on neural output to specific muscles. These circuits may originate within the motor cortex (intracortical) and/or operate between cortical areas (intercortical) or hemispheres (interhemispheric). Following SCI, the excitability of the motor cortex and the corresponding cortical circuits may be altered, and these changes may be, in part, related to the functional reorganization of the central nervous system. TMS techniques offer the opportunity to characterize alterations in cortical circuits following SCI and are described following. Importantly, these techniques are ideal for monitoring changes that accompany motor recovery in SCI populations.

2.1. Motor-evoked potentials (MEPs)

TMS delivered over the motor cortex trans-synaptically activates corticospinal neurons that ultimately give rise to a motor-evoked potential (MEP) recorded in the target muscle. The amplitude of the MEP represents the overall corticospinal excitability including contributions from the upper and lower motorneurons and the functional integrity of the corticospinal path [1]. The MEP amplitude may be modulated by factors such as action planning [2, 3], pharmaceuticals [4], or neuromuscular diseases [5–7]. The evaluation of MEP amplitude is a commonly used method to quantify changes in excitability within the descending motor pathways following experimental manipulation [8] or during the process of recovery [9]. The MEP latency provides an additional source of neurophysiological information and represents the conduction time for descending signals originating within the motor cortex to travel to the muscle effector, a measure that serves a diagnostic purpose for a number of disease states [10].

Following SCI, MEP amplitude and latency are often altered. When using TMS to assess muscles caudal to the spinal lesion level, smaller amplitude and longer latency MEPs are reported [11, 12]. This is thought to be due to the structural damage to descending corticospinal fibers including fewer intact axons and significant demyelination surrounding the lesion [13]. In individuals with SCI, such decrements in MEP amplitude may be lessened by introducing low level active contraction in the muscle of interest [14]. However, voluntary control of a muscle is not necessarily indicative of corticospinal connectivity to that particular muscle since MEPs may be elicited in muscles not under volitional control in individuals with SCI [15].

The origin of MEPs is complex, as pyramidal tract neurons are influenced directly and indirectly (trans-synaptically) in response to cortical stimulation. Additionally, MEPs depend on spinal motorneuron excitability and are influenced by cortical areas outside of motor cortex such as the premotor and supplementary motor areas [8]. As such, the ambiguity in the origin of the MEP creates challenges in its interpretation. Nonetheless, MEP characteristics have a value for assessing motor recovery following SCI such that both MEP amplitude and latency, in the acute stage of injury, predict the recovery of ambulation and hand function [10].

2.2. Motor threshold (MT)

MT is defined as the minimal stimulation intensity that elicits a MEP in a target muscle. MT can be assessed in two ways. Resting motor threshold (RMT) is often obtained by finding the lowest stimulation intensity that produces a MEP of at least 50 µV in 5 out of 10 consecutive trials, while the target muscle is relaxed [16, 17]. Furthermore, motor threshold can be determined while the participant maintains low levels of muscle contraction (i.e., active motor threshold or AMT). AMT is commonly defined as the lowest stimulation intensity to elicit MEPs of at least 200 µV in 5 out of 10 consecutive trials, while the participant maintains a contraction corresponding to 10–15% of their maximum [16]. RMT represents the resting membrane excitability throughout the efferent system at both cortical and spinal levels [18]. During this resting state, spinal motorneurons require a number of descending volleys from the cortex to summate in order to produce a MEP. This requirement for greater corticospinal summation at rest has been speculated to be due to glutamatergic synaptic activity [18]. Pharmacological studies have shown that AMT and RMT depend on the axon membrane excitability, specifically on voltage-gated sodium channel activity [19]. Application of various drugs that block the action of these channels such as carbamazepine and lamotrigine increase the required stimulation intensity to elicit RMT and AMT (see Paulus et al. 2008 for review) [18]. Despite the fact that pharmacological studies have not been able to isolate changes in RMT without a simultaneous change in AMT [18], differences in levels of synaptic excitability have been inferred from studies of MT latency, where RMT is seen to have a longer latency than AMT [20]. By maintaining a small contraction, low levels of synaptic firing are sustained and are thought to be more reliant on levels of excitability at the axonal membrane.[18].

Individuals with SCI may demonstrate increases in RMT and AMT. Davey et al. [11] found that RMT and AMT were higher for muscles below the level of injury whereas muscles innervated by fibers rostral to the injury had thresholds similar to the uninjured control group. Other research has shown that alterations following SCI are more prevalent when examining AMT [21, 22]. Bailey et al. [22] demonstrated increased AMT elicited from the flexor carpi radialis muscle of the forearm in participants with chronic cervical SCI. They suggested that this increase in AMT without a corresponding increase in RMT may be due to abnormalities in regulation of membrane excitability via voltage-gated ion channels. Collectively, the published data suggest that RMT may or may not be altered while AMT is increased in SCI participants. However, it has been established that changes in both RMT and AMT are dependent on the location of the target muscle relative to the level of the lesion. Further, changes in MT in chronic SCI are likely to differ depending on the severity and location of injury.

2.3. Motor cortical maps

The motor cortex is somatotopically organized in that cortical representations of the muscles are found in relatively predictable locations in the medial–lateral direction [23]. The extent of cortical territory occupied by a given muscle representation is thought to correspond to the amount of dexterity and fine motor control needed by the corresponding muscle such that larger representations exist for small distal muscles of the hand while smaller representations are present for larger proximal muscles of the arm and shoulder [12]. Most cortical muscle representations correspond to effectors of the contralateral limb although some degrees of ipsilateral projections have been found in proximal upper limb muscles in uninjured individuals [24]. Motor cortical maps can be obtained by delivering TMS pulses at suprathreshold intensities using a spatial grid aligned with the precentral gyrus and recording MEPs from target muscles [25]. Motor cortical maps are typically evaluated by quantifying the area, volume, and center of gravity for the representation of each muscle of interest. Map area and volume scale linearly with increasing TMS intensity and are considered a reliable method to evaluate cortical organization [26].

Studies of motor maps following SCI revealed enlarged representations of the most proximally spared muscles that tended to shift into cortical territory corresponding to the muscles below the level of injury [27, 28]. Takeover of de-innervated territory was supported by findings in which the representation of the extensor digitorum communis muscle was shifted anterolaterally (into the hand region) following incomplete cervical SCI [21, 29]. Brouwer and Hopkins-Fosseel [12] quantified motor maps in SCI participants for a variety of contracted upper arm muscles and found that proximal muscles were represented to a greater extent than distal hand muscles, and there was an extensive overlap of different muscle representations when compared to uninjured participants. This overlap may be beneficial for organization as the neurons projecting to single muscles are not focally distributed and may act to minimize complete functional losses following neurological injury. Cortical reorganization following SCI occurs rapidly as evident by the changes in the shape and location of biceps brachii motor cortical maps only 6–17 days following SCI [29]. More recently, a study using neuroimaging techniques demonstrated that representations of the tongue were significantly shifted in their location within motor cortex in participants with cervical SCI compared to uninjured participants [30]. Collectively, the motor cortical maps indicate that the reorganization of motor cortex somatotopy takes place following SCI, suggesting that plasticity may compensate for the loss of neuronal communication between the cortex and the muscles of the body. Although the mechanisms for such reorganization are unknown in humans, it may be speculated that changes in cortical organization are shaped through GABA mediated lateral inhibitory circuits [31].

A number of practical considerations are important for cortical mapping studies using TMS. Mapping protocols require many grid points with approximately 3–10 pulses delivered to each point to capture cortical organization with appropriate resolution. This may require a number of hours to generate a motor map if a large number of points are used [26]. Furthermore, heightened motor thresholds commonly accompany SCI, requiring higher stimulation intensities to elicit MEPs, and this may impact the comfort of the participant and increase the likelihood of coil heating.

2.4. Short-interval intracortical inhibition (SICI)

SICI is an inhibitory circuit within the motor cortex that is comprised of low-threshold GABAergic interneurons [18] and can be evaluated using paired-pulse TMS. By delivering an initial subthreshold conditioning stimulus (CS) approximately 1–5 ms prior to a suprathreshold test stimulus (TS) to the motor cortex, the resulting MEP is reduced when compared to MEPs produced when the TS is applied alone [32]. The subthreshold CS is typically set at an intensity of 70–90% of AMT, showing that the MEP modulation is of cortical origin as no descending volleys to the muscles are produced at these intensities [32]. The mechanism of inhibition involves presynaptic inhibition as inhibitory postsynaptic potentials are generated on neurons upstream of the corticospinal output neurons [18]. $GABA_A$ receptors are implicated in SICI since The delivery of Lorazepam or Diazepam ($GABA_A$ Receptor agonist) reduces SICI [33, 34].

It is well documented that SICI is reduced in individuals with SCI. One case report examined SICI in the relaxed extensor digitorum communis muscle using various interstimulus intervals and a single CS intensity [35]. This method was also used elsewhere in the relaxed first dorsal interosseous muscle [36]. Both cases demonstrated a reduction in SICI when compared to controls [35, 36]. However, the aforementioned studies used a single CS and TS intensity, making interpretation difficult, as the required stimulator output to produce MEPs in SCI participants is typically greater relative to able-bodied individuals. Roy et al. [37] explored SICI in SCI participants by measuring recruitment curves whereby CS intensities were altered from 60 to 110% AMT. They recorded responses from both tibialis anterior in the lower leg and the first dorsal interosseous muscle of the hand during contraction of each muscle. The results indicated a reduction of SICI responses in SCI participants compared to controls, although both retained a U-shaped recruitment curve. Individuals with SCI were seen to have a smaller range of CS intensities eliciting inhibition of the MEP when compared to the recruitment curves of uninjured individuals [37]. Therefore, recruitment characteristics of SICI appear to be unchanged following SCI while the overall amount of inhibition is reduced. The authors speculate that this may be due to spinal inhibitory mechanisms, or to reductions in GABAergic activity following cortical reorganization that occurs with SCI. Mi et al. [38] examined SICI in chronic cervical SCI. Similar to the results found by Roy et al. [37], the authors identified a smaller range of CS intensities to elicit SICI in the flexor carpi radialis muscle of the forearm compared to controls. In this case, significant inhibition of the TS-evoked response was only seen at 90% AMT in SCI compared to the wider range of 70, 80, and 90% AMT in controls [38]. This may reflect the reduced excitability of corticospinal neurons following SCI as the pattern of recruitment is maintained, while the range of inhibition is reduced. Therefore, impairment in GABAergic circuitry mediating SICI in the motor cortex has been established following lesion to the spinal cord.

2.5. Long-interval intracortical inhibition (LICI)

LICI represents intracortical circuitry that acts to modulate MEPs and can be observed via paired-pulse TMS to the motor cortex. The inhibitory pathways involved in LICI can be probed by delivering a suprathreshold CS before a subsequent suprathreshold TS with an interval between 50 and 200 ms to the motor cortex [39, 40]. This produces two MEPs; however, the amplitude of the second MEP is reduced (i.e., inhibited) compared to the MEP evoked by delivery of the single TS pulse. Similar to SICI, the interneuron interactions leading to MEP inhibition are mediated by GABA as seen in pharmacological studies [41, 42]. The longer interstimulus intervals leading to the inhibition are due to $GABA_B$ receptor activity which has been confirmed in studies using $GABA_B$ receptor agonists such as baclofen to increase the inhibitory response [43].

Limited research has examined alterations in LICI after SCI. Barry et al. [43] compared LICI in SCI versus uninjured controls in the resting and active muscle states to examine the effects of $GABA_B$ agonist Baclofen. They examined the first dorsal interosseous muscle of the hand, which showed a decrease in LICI in the active state in the control group as well as in SCI individuals that were taking Baclofen. However, SCI participants not medicated with Baclofen did not show a reduction in LICI during active contraction. This finding suggests abnormal $GABA_B$ receptor activity following SCI as the MEP responses continue to be further inhibited with increasing tonic efferent activity introduced by sustained muscle contraction. Interestingly, this decrease in LICI associated with muscle contraction appears to be rectified by the application of Baclofen, normalizing the inhibitory response in SCI to that of the control group. Another study examined the recruitment of the LICI circuitry in the active muscle state by applying CS intensities at 10% increments from 90 to 130% AMT to capture the pattern of $GABA_B$ mediated response in SCI [38]. An increase in LICI was observed in SCI participants at higher CS intensities (120 and 130% AMT), while the uninjured group did not show any LICI with increasing CS intensity. The authors attributed the increase in inhibition to Baclofen, which as a $GABA_B$ agonist may return LICI circuitry to its normative state.

2.6. Intracortical facilitation (ICF)

ICF can be observed within motor cortex, demonstrating the presence of excitatory circuits impacting the descending corticospinal output. ICF is elicited by delivering a subthreshold TMS pulse over the motor representation of a muscle followed by a suprathreshold TS after an interval of 7–20 ms [32]. This paired-pulse TMS method elicits a net facilitation of the MEP as seen by increased response amplitudes when compared to MEPs evoked from the single TS [33]. Pharmacological approaches reveal that ICF is the net effect of both inhibitory and excitatory contributions. Application of $GABA_A$ receptor agonists such as Diazepam result in decreased ICF, showing an influence of GABAergic inhibition onto corticospinal output neurons [44]. This demonstrates that although ICF is affected by GABAergic activity [44], there is a large excitatory component resulting in net facilitation. Thus, it is speculated that that NMDA receptors play a role in the facilitation observed in ICF [45]. These receptors respond to glutamate when nearby AMPA receptors are active to excite postsynaptic neurons. The role of NMDA receptor activity in ICF is supported by the finding that the application of NMDA receptor antagonists also causes a decrease in facilitation, implicating their role in the physiology of ICF [45].

A single case study examined ICF in a participant with cervical myelopathy using a CS intensity of 80% RMT and TS intensity of 120% RMT at a number of different interstimulus intervals. ICF was only observed when the interstimulus interval was 10 ms [35]. Further research with larger sample sizes and control groups should examine alterations in ICF in individuals with SCI. Collection of recruitment curves for ICF may provide a more comprehensive view of excitatory mechanisms contributing to corticospinal output following SCI.

2.7. Short and long latency afferent inhibition (SAI/LAI)

SAI demonstrates the influence of a peripherally evoked afferent volley on the MEP and is observed when an electrical stimulus applied to a peripheral nerve is followed by a single suprathreshold TMS pulse to the motor cortex. The temporal interval between the peripheral and cortical stimulation corresponds to the conduction time for the afferent volley to reach the somatosensory cortex. This timing causes the afferent information to arrive shortly before the suprathreshold TMS pulse, which is subsequently inhibited compared to the MEP evoked by the TS pulse delivered alone. This circuit is commonly studied in intrinsic muscles of the hand where the interstimulus interval is roughly 18–21 ms [46, 47]. The exact mechanisms underpinning this pathway remains unclear, although pharmacological intervention using drugs such as Scopolamine (cholinergic antagonist) or Diazepam indicate that SAI is mediated by both cholinergic and GABAergic circuits [48, 49]. LAI is another example of sensory modulation to cortical pathways involved in MEP generation. The method of eliciting LAI is similar to that of SAI with the exception of a longer interstimulus interval of ~100–200 ms [46, 50]. LAI is speculated to modulate corticospinal output by exclusively GABAergic systems, particularly those mediated by $GABA_B$ receptors [49]. The modulation of MEPs induced by sensory input suggests that SAI and LAI provide insight into sensorimotor integration [51].

The literature surrounding afferent regulation of the motor cortex following SCI is minimal. Roy et al. [14] stimulated the common peroneal nerve at the ankle to modify MEPs elicited from tibialis anterior using interstimulus intervals ranging from 30 to 80 ms. Results indicated an inhibition of MEPs from tibialis anterior when the internal between the TS pulse and the peripheral electrical stimulation corresponded to the latency of the afferent volley from the common peroneal nerve. However, this effect was reduced in the SCI group. The decrease in SAI relative to controls is expected in this population, as the transmission of afferent information from the periphery to the cortex is largely dependent on spinal mechanisms that are likely to be affected by damage to the spinal cord. Further, a recent study examined SAI within the flexor carpi radialis muscle in cervical SCI participants and found that, compared to uninjured controls SAI was reduced when the muscle was in the active and resting state [22]. The authors speculated that this impairment in SAI circuitry is due to plasticity effects in the processing and/or transmission of the information within the cortex as well as reductions in afferent transmission to the cortex. Thus, literature regarding sensory modulation of motor output suggests that afferent integration is impaired following SCI.

2.8. Cortical silent period (CSP)

The CSP represents descending inhibitory signals during active contraction of the muscle. When maintaining a constant level of muscle contraction, stimulation of the motor cortex at suprathreshold intensities produces a CSP in the active contralateral muscle. The duration of the CSP may provide some indication of functional ability. For example, the ability to modulate muscle activity following large descending efferent volleys may impact motor tasks involving fine motor control where small, precise movements are required. The CSP is commonly ~200 ms in duration and is impacted by both cortical and spinal factors. Initial inhibition (~50–75 ms) is attributed to the refractory period of efferent fibers within the spinal cord following suprathreshold TMS, while the remaining duration is thought to originate from the cortex [52–54]. This effect is physiologically mediated by multiple GABAergic systems as treatment with pharmaceuticals that reduce synaptic clearance of GABA increase CSP durations [42, 55]. At the receptor level, $GABA_A$ appears to modulate the CSP at lower TMS intensities as benzodiazepines increase the CSP duration [52]. However, at high TMS stimulation intensities, treatment with benzodiazepines shortens the CSP [56]. The latter finding suggests that $GABA_A$ activity suppresses the effects of $GABA_B$ receptors when such inputs are presented to the motor cortex [56].

The CSP duration appears to be altered in SCI. Shimizu et al. [36] investigated the CSP in three individuals with cervical SCI. In all participants, there was no observable CSP in the foot muscle, and in two individuals, the CSP was additionally absent in the hand muscles. The loss of this silent period suggests that there may have been reorganization at the level of the cortex or hyper excitability of the cortex as GABA systems are suppressed [36]. Barry et al. [43] examined the GABA system involved in producing the CSP in intrinsic hand muscles of chronic, incomplete SCI groups that either were or were not taking Baclofen. Baclofen did not alter the CSP in SCI, and all SCI participants displayed a longer CSP duration than age-matched uninjured controls [43]. Another study examined the CSP, while generating motor maps of forearm extensor muscles and reported an inverse relationship between the duration of the CSP and the amount of spinal cord atrophy via inspection of MRI images [21]. Therefore, when increases in the CSP are observed in SCI, it is likely due to intact inhibitory corticospinal projections to the muscle although spinal modulation of inhibitory circuits is impaired.

2.9. Inter-hemispheric inhibition (IHI)

IHI is a circuit that results from the extensive interconnectivity between the two cerebral hemispheres via the corpus callosum. The integrity of this cross-communication can be assessed by paired-pulse TMS over the motor cortices. By providing a suprathreshold CS over the motor representation of a muscle in one hemisphere followed by a suprathreshold TS over the homologous motor representation in the opposite hemisphere, inhibition of the MEP in response to the CS is observed [57, 58]. This suppression occurs at interstimulus intervals of 10 and 40 ms [57]. Modulation of MEP amplitude with IHI is mediated via GABAergic systems as application of $GABA_B$ agonist Baclofen induces an increase in inhibition at both paired-pulse intervals [59].

IHI in SCI has not been studied extensively. One report used an interstimulus interval of 10 ms for probing IHI in cervical SCI and found that there was neither enhancement nor suppression of the MEP when the participants were at rest or maintaining a contraction at a level that corresponded to either 30 or 70% MVC [60]. The authors speculate that the lack of change in IHI may be due to interactions with other circuitry that has been affected by injury such as SICI. One challenge in measuring IHI in the SCI population is that a MEP must be obtained with amplitude that is large enough to observe suppression following modulation from the opposite hemisphere. Decreased muscle responses are well established in SCI, making it difficult to elicit a MEP that is large enough to be modulated by the CS of the opposite hemisphere. Therefore, the IHI protocol may need to be adapted for the SCI population.

2.10. Summary

Please refer to **Table 1** for a summary of the previous findings. Changes in motor cortical excitability and circuitry follow SCI and yield alterations in corticospinal output. The available information regarding changes in cortical circuitry for motor output in SCI is limited, making a comprehensive view of neurophysiological rehabilitation difficult in this population. Thus, further studies should identify and quantify aberrant motor cortical circuits in SCI.

Measure	Source	Classification	Muscle tested	Response
Motor-evoked potentials	Davey et al. [11]	Tetraplegic	Thenar Muscles (APB)	↓Amplitude
	Brouwer and Hopkins-Rosseel [12]	Tetraplegic	Biceps, Triceps,	↓ Amplitude (no MEP response in most SCI subjects)
	Roy et al. [37]	Para/Tetraplegic	Deltoid	↓Amplitude
	Roy et al. [14]	Para/Tetraplegic	TA, FDI	↓Amplitude, ↑ MEP duration
	Edwards et al. [15]	Tetraplegic	TA, FDI	=No change in amplitude
			Biceps, ECR, FCR, APB	
Motor threshold	Davey et al. [11]	Tetraplegic	Biceps, Thenar Muscles	No change in biceps (above injury level), ↑ AMT in APB (below injury level)
	Freund et al. [21]	Tetraplegic	EDC	
	Bailey et al. [22]	Tetraplegic	FCR	
	Saturno et al. [35]	Tetraplegic	EDC	↑ AMT (associated with amount of spinal cord atrophy)
				No change in RMT, ↑ AMT
				↑ RMT
Motor maps	Levy et al. [27]	Tetraplegic	Biceps, Deltoid	↑ Map area, latency, and amplitude of response inversely related in SCI
	Cohen et al. [28]	Paraplegic	TA, External Oblique	
	Freund et al. [21]	Tetraplegic	EDC	↑ Map area of obliques (above injury), no responses from TA (below injury)
	Streletz et al. [29]	Acute Tetraplegic	Biceps, APB	
	Brouwer and Hopins-Rosseel [12]	Tetraplegic	Biceps, Triceps, Deltoid	CoG shifted posteriorly
	Mikulis et al. [30]	Tetraplegic		

Measure	Source	Classification	Muscle tested	Response
			Wrist extensors, Tongue	↑ Map area of Biceps, Bicep map shifted laterally
				↓ Map volumes, No change in area
				No change in activation volume, peak response site shifted medially for tongue*
Short-interval intracortical inhibition	Saturno et al. [35]	Ischemic Myelopathy	EDC	↓ SICI
	Shimizu et al. [36]	Myelopathy	FDI, FHB	↓SICI in FDI
	Roy et al. [37]	Tetraplegic	TA, FDI	↓ magnitude of active SICI, similar recruitment with increasing CS intensity
	Mi et al. [38]	Para/Tetraplegic Tetraplegic	FDI	No change in magnitude, reduced range of intensities showing SICI
Long-interval intracortical inhibition	Barry et al. [43]	Tetraplegic	FDI	no change with baclofen, ↑ active LICI without baclofen
	Mi et al. [38]	Tetraplegic	FDI	↑ active LICI
Intracortical facilitation	Saturno et al. [35]	Ischemic Myelopathy	EDC	No change
Short-latency afferent inhibition	Roy et al. [14]	Tetraplegia	TA	↓ SAI (absent)
	Bailey et al. [22]	Tetraplegia	FCR	↓ active and resting SAI
Cortical silent period	Shimizu et al. [36]	Tetraplegic	FDI, FHB	↓ CSP duration
	Barry et al. [43]	Tetraplegic	FDI	↑ CSP duration, correlated with spinal atrophy
	Freund et al. [21]	Tetraplegic	EDC	↑ CSP duration
Interhemispheric inhibition	Bunday and Perez [60]	Tetraplegic	FDI	No change

Table 1. Cortical circuitry in spinal cord injury.

3. NIBS to induce plasticity in individuals with SCI

NIBS provide an opportunity to modulate the neural circuits that are altered following SCI and have the potential to improve motor function. There are several NIBS protocols that have been used to promote plasticity with the two main forms including repetitive TMS (rTMS), and transcranial direct current stimulation (tDCS). RTMS and tDCS protocols are each founded in the principle of homosynaptic plasticity, while TMS and tDCS protocols paired with peripheral nerve stimulation have effects based on spike-timing dependent plasticity (STDP). Homosynaptic plasticity refers to plasticity occurring at a single synapse that is undergoing stimulation [61, 62]. STDP refers to plasticity induced by timing two stimuli, typically a cortical and a peripheral stimulus, to activate both the presynaptic and postsynaptic neurons coincidentally. These protocols are able to produce effects that resemble long-term potentiation (LTP) or long-term depression (LTD) of synaptic connectivity. Typically, activation of the presynaptic neuron prior to the postsynaptic neuron lends to the generation of LTP while LTD occurs when the postsynaptic neuron is activated first [61]. STDP can be timed such that the two stimuli coincide at different levels of the central nervous system to create either spinal or cortical plasticity. We provide an overview of the literature that has used NIBS approaches to promote plasticity in the motor system in individuals with SCI.

3.1. Repetitive TMS (rTMS)

RTMS is thought to induce homosynaptic plasticity within the target cortex. RTMS may increase or decrease cortical activity via alterations in the activity of glutamatergic NMDA receptors [63]. The frequency, intensity, and duration of rTMS determine whether the plasticity effect is LTD or LTP-like [63, 64]. Typically, rTMS delivered over motor cortex at a frequency of <1 Hz results in LTD-like effects while frequencies >5 Hz yield LTP-like effects [63]. In SCI, the primary focus of rTMS is to modulate descending projections and strengthen the intact corticospinal connections.

In a study by Belci et al. [65], rTMS was applied over the motor cortex for five consecutive days using a protocol that included doublets of TMS delivered at a frequency of 10 Hz with each doublet being separated by 10 s for a total 720 stimuli. Following real rTMS, measures of CSP were reduced. Further, motor and sensory function, determined by the assessment of motor and sensory function by the American Spinal Injury Association (ASIA), was improved, as was performance in the timed peg-board task. Further, the sensory perceptual threshold to an electrical stimulus was reduced suggesting alterations within the somatosensory cortex. These measures remained improved for 2 weeks post-intervention while sham rTMS revealed no benefit [65]. Ellaway et al. [66] delivered real versus sham rTMS via 2 s trains of 5 Hz stimulation separated by 8 s for a total of 15 min over the motor cortex in individuals with SCI. The real and sham interventions were performed over 5 consecutive days. Measurements of the ASIA score, active research arm test (ARAT) which includes testing grasp, grip, pinch and gross movement, electrical stimulation perceptual threshold, MEPs, AMT, and CSP were assessed before and following intervention. Results revealed that AMT was increased and ARAT improved following rTMS compared to the sham intervention, without changes in other measures. Another study delivered real versus sham high-frequency (20 Hz) rTMS over 15 consecutive days to assess improvement in lower limb function [67]. Measurements included lower extremities motor score (LEMS), modified Ashworth scale (MAS), walking index for SCI, ten-meter walking test, step length, cadence assessment, and a timed up and go (TUG) test. At the cessation of the rTMS intervention, LEMS improved, MAS score was reduced, gait was altered (i.e., increased velocity, cadence, step length) and an improvement was observed in TUG without changes in the walking index. Effects returned to baseline 2 weeks following the last intervention [67]. Finally, an rTMS protocol consisting of 4 pulse trains (quadropulse) delivered at a frequency of 250–500 Hz with an inter-train interval of 5–6 s (250–360/day) for either 1 or 5 consecutive days (i.e., ~1000–1440 pulses per day) was delivered to individuals with SCI [68]. Hand dexterity, MEPs, and spinal excitability were measured. After a single session of rTMS, there was no change in hand dexterity although MEPs increased and spinal excitability decreased. Further, after 5 consecutive days of rTMS there was a 10% increase in hand dexterity. These data indicate that rTMS delivered over consecutive days is more effective than single session at promoting motor improvements [68].

3.2. Transcranial direct current stimulation (TDCS)

TDCS is a neuromodulating technique that utilizes homosynaptic plasticity, similar to rTMS. However, unlike rTMS, tDCS does not produce neuronal action potentials since the static field produced by tDCS does not produce the rapid depolarization of neurons [69]. TDCS modifies spontaneous neuronal excitability by either creating tonic depolarization or hyperpolarization [69]. The direction of current flow appears to determine whether the protocol results in LTD or LTP-like effects; anodal tDCS results in neuron depolarization (LTP) while cathodal tDCS results in neuron hyperpolarization (LTD) [69, 70]. There exists one study that has shown evidence for promoting plasticity in individuals with SCI using tDCS. Murray et al. [71] delivered anodal tDCS for 20 min once per week over 3 weeks at varying intensities; 1, 2 mA and sham. Measurements of MEP amplitude, sensory threshold, and muscle strength were performed before and after intervention. MEP amplitude was significantly increased after delivery of 2 mA anodal tDCS but not 1 mA or sham conditions. Sensory threshold was significantly reduced after both 2 and 1 mA but not sham stimulation. No protocol was effective at changing muscle strength [71]. It is evident that the extent of research in tDCS aimed at altering motor function in individuals with SCI is limited. However, early results show that tDCS may be an effective tool to alter corticospinal excitability and improve motor function.

3.3. Paired associative stimulation (PAS) and spinal associative stimulation (SAS)

PAS is a plasticity inducing protocol that utilizes STDP to alter cortical or spinal function. Traditionally, PAS involves timing peripheral electrical nerve stimulation with a TMS pulse over the motor cortex. When these two stimuli are timed to arrive in the cortex at approximately the same time, the protocol is known as PAS and when they are timed to coincide at the level of the spinal cord, the technique is known as spinal associative stimulation (SAS). PAS delivered at an ISI of 25 ms and targeting motor cortex has been effective at increasing MEP amplitude in uninjured individuals [72], while PAS delivered at an ISI of 20 ms has been effective at altering spinal excitability by increasing the amplitude of the spinal H-reflex [73]. There have been three studies performed in SCI where PAS or variations of PAS have been used to induce cortical and/or spinal plasticity promoting functional recovery.

Roy et al. [14] assessed corticospinal excitability in the lower limb before and following PAS delivered at an interval to promote near coincident activation within the motor cortex (i.e., the N20 latency of somatosensory-evoked potential +6 ms). The protocol included 120 pairs of peripheral afferent stimuli and TMS pulses at a frequency of 0.2 Hz [14]. MEPs were measured during tonic 20% contraction (active MEPs) and at rest (resting MEPs). Results indicated significant increases to resting but no change to active MEPs [14]. Bunday and Perez [74] tested the SAS protocol in individuals with SCI and delivered 100 pairs of stimuli at a frequency of 0.1 Hz and timed the ISI such that the TMS efferent volley and the PNS antidromic efferent volley arrived at the corticospinal-motorneuronal synapse at the C7 spinal level nearly simultaneously. Measurements of MEPs, spinal F-waves, voluntary motor output, and manual dexterity were performed post-intervention. Results showed increases in MEPs, no change in F-waves, and increases to both maximum voluntary EMG/force and a reduction in the time to complete the 9-hole pegboard task [74]. Finally, Yamaguchi et al. [75] paired peripheral nerve stimulation with anodal tDCS. During a 20 min, 1 mA anodal tDCS protocol peripheral electrical stimulation trains consisting of 10 pulses delivered at a frequency of 100 Hz were delivered every 2 s. Measurements of reciprocal inhibition from the tibialis anterior and ankle movement were assessed after stimulation. Results indicate reduced reciprocal inhibition, and increased ankle movements following the combination of peripheral electrical stimulation and anodal tDCS [75].

3.4. Summary

Please refer to **Table 2** for a summary of the previous findings. Collectively these studies reveal promising indications that rTMS, TCDS, and PAS approaches can modulate cortical function leading to short-term improvements in the motor system in individuals with SCI. Although, these results are not always unanimous, (i.e., differential effects on MEPs and CSP), they may relate to the specific protocol parameters as existing studies in SCI have utilized variable stimulation parameters. Further research should determine the most effective protocol at yielding changes to neural physiology and improvements in motor function in individuals with SCI. NIBS combined with other techniques might be a promising new avenue for research for the ultimate goal of creating long-term functional improvements.

Intervention	Source	Parameters	Classification	Response
rTMS	Belci et al. [65] Ellaway et al. [66] Benito et al. [67] Alexeeva et al. [68]	- Doublets of TMS delivered at a frequency of 10 Hz - 10 s between doublets - 360 doublets delivered - 90% RMT intensity - 5 consecutive days - trains of TMS delivered at a frequency of 5 HZ over 2 s - 8 s between trains - 15 min of stimulation - 5 consecutive days - TMS delivered at frequ	Incomplete tetraplegic Incomplete tetraplegic Incomplete para/ tetraplegic Incomplete para /tetraplegic	*Physiological* - improved sensory and motor scores on ASIA *Behavioral* - improved time for pegboard task *Physiological* - improved AMT *Behavioral* - improved active reach arm test *Behavioral* - improved lower

Intervention	Source	Parameters	Classification	Response
		ency of 20 Hz		extremities motor score
		- 15 consecutive days		- improved modified ashworth scale
		- 4 pulses of TMS delivered in trains at a freq uency of 250–500 Hz		- improved gait mechanics
		- 5–6 s between trains		- improved time up and go
		- 250–360 pulses delivered		*Physiological*
		- 1–5 consecutive days		- increased motor-evoked potentials
				- reduced spinal excitability
tDCS	Murray et al. [71]	- Anodal tDCS at 1 or 2 mA	Incomplete tetraplegic	*Physiological*
		- 20 min protocol		- increased motor-evoked potentials
		- once per week for 3 consecutive weeks		- reduced sensory threshold
PAS/SAS	Roy et al. [37] Bunday and Perez [74] Yamaguchi et al. [75]	- ISI of N20 + 6 ms for stimuli to arrive in M1	Incomplete para /tetraplegic Incomplete tetraplegic Incomplete para /tetraplegic	*Physiological* - increased resting motor-evoked potentials
		- 120 pairs of peripheral stimulation and TMS delivered at a frequency of 0.2 Hz		*Physiological* - increased motor-evoked potentials
		- ISI for stimuli to arrive at the C7 spinal level		- increased maximum voluntary EMG activity
		- 100 pairs of peripheral stimulation and TMS delivered at a frequency of 0.1 Hz		*Behavioral*
		- pairing of peripheral nerve stimulation with anodal tDCS		- increased maximum voluntary force production
		- 1 mA tDCS delivered over 20 min		- reduced time to complete 9-hole pegboard task
		- peripheral stimulation was trains of 10 stimuli delivered at a		

Intervention	Source	Parameters	Classification	Response
		frequency of 100 Hz with 2 s between trains		*Physiological* - reduced reciprocal inhibition *Behavioral* - increased ankle movements

Table 2. Summary of NIBS to promote plasticity in SCI.

4. Coupling NIBS with movement protocols

A primary goal of motor Training is to improve functional ability by repeated exposure to a particular task, such as treadmill training to improve walking ability. In clinical populations, motor training can promote plastic changes in unaffected motor networks by increasing the efficacy of synaptic transmission [76]. Therefore, there is an opportunity to promote neural plasticity via motor training in intact cortical and spinal motor circuitry in individuals with SCI.

4.1. Pairing NIBS with motor training

Previous studies have shown that motor training can influence corticospinal excitability. In participants with SCI, locomotor resistance training using Lokomat facilitates spinal reflexes at 20 and 80 ms in the soleus muscle and improves gait quality as assessed by LEMS, walking index for SCI and velocity [77], as well as MEP amplitudes in tibialis anterior [78]. Treadmill training in SCI participants for ~2 months (5 sessions per week for 1 h) increases MEP amplitudes in tibialis anterior, increases manual muscle strength in ankle dorsiflexors as measured by 11-point manual muscle strength score, and increases the duration of the CSP [79]. Although motor training alone promotes motor recovery, the functional outcomes are often limited and patients still exhibit substantial motor impairments.

Motor training and NIBS are each, independently effective at promoting plasticity in SCI participants. Therefore, the combination of the two may lead to plasticity effects that exceed their individual components. Few studies have tested the effects of pairing NIBS with motor training to facilitate functional motor recovery. Gomes-Osman et al. [80] evaluated upper limb function in SCI participants. They delivered 10 Hz rTMS (800 pulses at 80% RMT) with repetitive task practice involving 30 s of practice with the 9-hole pegboard task. The results revealed a decrease in the time to complete the Jebsen Taylor test following real and sham rTMS paired with repetitive task practice. However, the effects were larger following real versus sham rTMS paired with repetitive task practice. Measures of RMT and AMT were unchanged [80]. Alexeeva et al. [68] combined rTMS with motor training in SCI participants. Participants experienced 5 consecutive days of each intervention: rTMS, motor training, and rTMS + motor training. A washout period of at least 4 weeks elapsed between each intervention. RTMS consisted of 4-pulse trains with a ~0.2–1.5 Hz train delivery rate at an intensity set to 80–90% RMT (i.e., quadropulse rTMS). Motor training consisted of hand tasks in participants 1 and 2 (10 tasks performed 10 times each: grasp and release, hand pronation and supination, isometric and concentric contractions of the wrist, thumb, and interphalangeal joints) and locomotor training in participant 3 (walking on a treadmill at a self-selected pace for 30 min with belt speed ≥0.05 m/s). In participant 1 and 2, "rTMS" and "motor training" improved 9-hole pegboard task performance and increased MEP amplitudes without changing SICI, ICF, or CSP. The combined intervention led to the greatest improvements in 9-hole pegboard task. In participant 3, the largest improvements in treadmill walking speeds were seen following the combined interventions as well [68]. Collectively, studies pairing NIBS with motor training reveal that larger functional gains may be induced compared to the effects of NIBS or motor training delivered in isolation.

4.2. Pairing NIBS with aerobic exercise

Using aerobic exercise to prime the brain prior to NIBS may also lead to larger changes in corticospinal excitability. Regular physical activity and aerobic exercise promote plasticity by increasing levels of growth factors including brain-derived neurotrophic factor (BDNF) and insulin-like growth factor (IGF-1) [81, 82]. Further, aerobic exercise can modify plasticity [83] via increases in cerebral blood flow [84] and angiogenesis [85]. Rojas Vega et al. [86] investigated the effects of aerobic exercise on BDNF and IGF-1 serum concentrations in SCI participants. The SCI participants completed an aerobic exercise session on a hand-bike that included a 10-min warm-up followed by a timed trial over a distance of 42 km. Blood samples were collected before, after the warm-up, and immediately following aerobic exercise. The warm-up resulted in a 1.5-fold increase in BDNF concentration, although no significant differences were seen between pre- and post-aerobic exercise measures. Additionally, IGF-1 concentrations were increased following both the warm-up and aerobic exercise [86] suggesting that aerobic exercise has the ability to prime the central nervous system for neuroplastic changes. This has been supported by recent evidence that aerobic exercise, such as cycling, is able to prime the brain prior to NIBS in healthy participants [87, 88]. In uninjured individuals, priming the cortex with aerobic exercise prior to PAS enhances the plasticity effect relative to PAS alone as measured by increases in the MEP recruitment curve slope [87]. Additionally, recent evidence suggests that individuals who exercise regularly are more prone to motor cortex plasticity following PAS relative to sedentary/low physically active individuals. Those who exercise regularly had increased MEP amplitudes and steeper input/output recruitment curves after intervention, while no significant changes were seen in sedentary/low physically active individuals [89].

4.3. Summary

There are challenges for future research focused on combining NIBS with aerobic exercise or motor training. For example, one consideration involves timing the delivery of NIBS with respect to aerobic exercise and/or motor training. Thus far, NIBS has been delivered simultaneously [80] or in advance of [68] motor training yet their combined effect may be influenced by their order of delivery [90]. In addition, the outcome of pairing protocols may be dependent on parameters of NIBS, aerobic exercise, or motor training, such as intensity and number of sessions; multiple sessions may be needed to induce any significant changes in motor function [91]. Therefore, pairing NIBS with aerobic exercise and/or motor training has the potential to drive neuroplastic changes in SCI participants that may exceed the functional gains achieved by a singular intervention, but further investigation is required.

5. New opportunities for NIBS to promote motor recovery in SCI

Motor recovery in SCI participants via NIBS and paired protocols are promising. However, other forms of NIBS including theta burst stimulation (TBS), rapid rate paired associative stimulation (rPAS), or transspinal direct current stimulation (ts-CCS) have the potential to induce plasticity and promote motor recovery and have yet to be explored in SCI.

TBS is a form of rTMS at low intensity that delivers continuous (cTBS) or intermittent (iTBS) high-frequency pulses inducing homosynaptic plasticity in the stimulated area. TBS effects depend on corticospinal output depend on the nature of stimulation. iTBS over motor cortex increases the amplitude of MEPs [92, 93], while cTBS over motor cortex decreases the amplitude of MEPs [92, 94], although this pattern is not always observed [95–97]. In participants with stroke, iTBS improves hand function [98] and increases MEP amplitudes [98, 99]. In addition, applying multiple sessions of cTBS in participants with amyotrophic lateral sclerosis decrease MEP amplitudes and increase RMT [100]. Although it has yet to be tested, TBS over motor cortex representation of the affected muscle in SCI may have the potential to modulate intracortical (i.e., SICI, ICF) and corticospinal circuitry (i.e., MEP amplitude). Hence, TBS, like rTMS, may be a suitable tool to influence synaptic interactions by strengthening the residual connections [92] and therefore increase motor output from the affected muscle. Further, by modulating plasticity within the cortex, indirect changes in the spinal circuitry may occur. Hence, TBS may provide an alternate method to induce plasticity in the cortex that may lead to motor recovery in SCI participants.

RPAS is based on the principles of STDP and involves pairing 5 Hz rTMS with peripheral nerve stimulation at a specific interstimulus interval [101]. Unlike PAS, which requires ~30 min to deliver, rPAS provides a particularly fast method (i.e., ~3–4 min for 600 pulses) to induce increases in corticospinal excitability. RPAS over the motor cortex increases MEP amplitudes and reduces SAI [101–104] in uninjured individuals. However, rPAS has yet to be investigated in clinical populations presenting with motor impairments. In rPAS, the pairing of TMS with nerve stimuli activates both, afferent and efferent pathways. Recently, it has been speculated that reorganization in the cortex following afferent stimulation may be crucial in neurorehabilitation of the hand [105]. Since rPAS is highly efficient in increasing corticospinal excitability in healthy adults for prolonged periods of time, it may provide a useful tool to promote sensory-motor coupling [102] in SCI participants.

Another promising NIBS technique involves the delivery of 40 min of constant current stimulation to the spinal cord [106]. Long-lasting transspinal constant current stimulation (ts-

CCS) alters cortical, corticospinal, and spinal plasticity in uninjured participants. Knikou et al. [106] found that both cathodal tsCCS and anodal tsCCS decreased afferent-mediated MEP facilitation, increased MEP amplitudes, and decreased transspinal-evoked potentials (TEPs) of knee flexors. Further, cathodal tsCCS increased TMS-mediated tibialis anterior flexor reflex facilitation, while anodal tsCCS decreased TMS-mediated TA flexor reflex facilitation and decreased post-activation depression of TEPs for the soleus H-reflex. This technique provides a way to directly stimulate the spinal cord, changing the synaptic efficacy between descending motor axons and spinal motorneurons, cortical interneurons and descending motor axons and Ia afferents and motorneurons [106]. While more research is required to determine the efficacy of this tool at modulating changes in the cortex and spinal cord to promote motor recovery in clinical populations, it may have the potential to improve voluntary motor function in SCI participants.

Author details

Aaron Z. Bailey, Hunter J. Fassett, Tea Lulic, Jenin El Sayes and Aimee J. Nelson*

*Address all correspondence to: nelsonaj@mcmaster.ca

Department of Kinesiology, McMaster University, Hamilton, Ontario, Canada

References

[1] Siebner HR, Rothwell J. Transcranial magnetic stimulation: new insights into representational cortical plasticity. Exp Brain Res 2003;148:1–16. doi:10.1007/s00221-002-1234-2

[2] Duque J, Labruna L, Verset S, Olivier E, Ivry RB. Dissociating the role of prefrontal and premotor cortices in controlling inhibitory mechanisms during motor preparation. J Neurosci 2012;32:806–16. doi:10.1523/JNEUROSCI.4299-12.2012

[3] Sinclair C, Hammond GR. Excitatory and inhibitory processes in primary motor cortex during the foreperiod of a warned reaction time task are unrelated to response expectancy. Exp Brain Res 2009;194:103–13. doi:10.1007/s00221-008-1684-2

[4] Ziemann U. TMS and drugs. Clin Neurophysiol 2004;115:1717–29. doi:10.1016/j.clinph.2004.03.006.

[5] Bütefisch CM, Netz J, Wessling M, Seitz RJ, Hömberg V. Remote changes in cortical excitability after stroke. Brain 2003;126:470–81.

[6] Neva JL, Lakhani B, Brown KE, Wadden KP, Mang CS, Ledwell NHM, et al. Multiple measures of corticospinal excitability are associated with clinical features of multiple sclerosis. Behav Brain Res 2016;297:187–95. doi:10.1016/j.bbr.2015.10.015

[7] Vucic S, Ziemann U, Eisen A, Hallett M, Kiernan MC. Transcranial magnetic stimulation and amyotrophic lateral sclerosis: pathophysiological insights. J Neurol Neurosurg Psychiatr 2013;84:1161–70. doi:10.1136/jnnp-2012-304019

[8] Bestmann S, Krakauer JW. The uses and interpretations of the motor-evoked potential for understanding behaviour. Exp Brain Res 2015;233:679–89. doi:10.1007/s00221-014-4183-7

[9] Grover HJ, Thornton R, Lutchman LN, Blake JC. Using transcranial magnetic stimulation to evaluate the motor pathways after an intraoperative spinal cord injury and to predict the recovery of intraoperative transcranial electrical motor evoked potentials: a case report. J Clin Neurophysiol 2015;1. doi:10.1097/WNP.0000000000000200

[10] Curt A, Keck ME, Dietz V. Functional outcome following spinal cord injury: significance of motor-evoked potentials and ASIA scores. Arch Phys Med Rehabil 1998;79:81–6.

[11] Davey NJ, Smith HC, Savic G, Maskill DW, Ellaway PH, Frankel HL. Comparison of input–output patterns in the corticospinal system of normal subjects and incomplete spinal cord injured patients. Exp Brain Res 1999;127:382–90.

[12] Brouwer B, Hopkins-Rosseel DH. Motor cortical mapping of proximal upper extremity muscles following spinal cord injury. Spinal Cord 1997;35:205–12.

[13] Smith HC, Savic G, Frankel HL, Ellaway PH, Maskill DW, Jamous MA, et al. Corticospinal function studied over time following incomplete spinal cord injury. Spinal Cord 2000;38:292–300.

[14] Roy FD, Yang JF, Gorassini MA, Roy FD, Yang JF, Gorassini MA. Afferent regulation of leg motor cortex excitability after incomplete spinal cord injury. J Neurophysiol 2010;103:2222–33. doi:10.1152/jn.00903.2009

[15] Edwards DJ, Cortes M, Thickbroom GW, Rykman A, Pascual-Leone A, Volpe BT. Preserved corticospinal conduction without voluntary movement after spinal cord injury. Spinal Cord 2013;51:765–7. doi:10.1038/sc.2013.74

[16] Rossini PM, Burke D, Chen R, Cohen LG, Daskalakis Z, Di Iorio R, et al. Non-invasive electrical and magnetic stimulation of the brain, spinal cord, roots and peripheral nerves: basic principles and procedures for routine clinical and research application. An updated report from an I.F.C.N. Committee. Clin Neurophysiol 2015;126:1071–107. doi:10.1016/j.clinph.2015.02.001

[17] Rothwell JC, Hallett M, Berardelli A. Magnetic stimulation: motor evoked potentials. Electroencephalogr Clin Neurophysiol Suppl 1999;52:9–103.

[18] Paulus W, Classen J, Cohen LG, Large CH, Di Lazzaro V, Nitsche M, et al. State of the art: pharmacologic effects on cortical excitability measures tested by transcranial magnetic stimulation. Brain Stimul 2008;1:151–63. doi:10.1016/j.brs.2008.06.002

[19] Hodgkin AL, Huxley AF. A quantitative description of membrane current and its application to conduction and excitation in nerve. J Physiol (Lond) 1952;117:500–44. doi:10.1111/(ISSN)1469-7793

[20] Day BL, Dressler D, Maertens de Noordhout A, Marsden CD, Nakashima K, Rothwell JC, et al. Electric and magnetic stimulation of human motor cortex: surface EMG and single motor unit responses. J Physiol (Lond) 1989;412:449–73. doi:10.1111/(ISSN)1469-7793

[21] Freund P, Thompson AJ, Rothwell J, Craggs M, Bestmann S. Corticomotor representation to a human forearm muscle changes following cervical spinal cord injury. Eur J Neurosci 2011;34:1839–46. doi:10.1111/j.1460-9568.2011.07895.x

[22] Bailey AZ, Mi YP, Nelson AJ. Short-latency afferent inhibition in chronic spinal cord injury. Transl Neurosci 2015;6:1–9. doi:10.1515/tnsci-2015-0025

[23] Penfield W, Boldrey E. Somatic motor and sensory representation in the cerebral cortex of man as studied by electrical stimulation. Brain J Neurol 1937;60:389–443. doi:10.1093/brain/60.4.389

[24] Raineteau O, Schwab ME. Plasticity of motor systems after incomplete spinal cord injury. Nat Rev Neurosci 2001;2:263–73. doi:10.1038/35067570

[25] Romero JR, Ramirez DM, Aglio LS, Gugino LD. Brain mapping using transcranial magnetic stimulation. Neurosurg Clin N Am 2011;22:141–52–vii. doi:10.1016/j.nec.2010.11.002

[26] van de Ruit M, Grey MJ. The TMS Map Scales with Increased Stimulation Intensity and Muscle Activation. Brain Topogr 2016;29:56–66. doi:10.1007/s10548-015-0447-1

[27] Levy WJ, Amassian VE, Traad M, Cadwell J. Focal magnetic coil stimulation reveals motor cortical system reorganized in humans after traumatic quadriplegia. Brain Res 1990;510:130–4

[28] Cohen LG, Roth BJ, Wassermann EM, Topka H, Fuhr P, Schultz J, et al. Magnetic stimulation of the human cerebral cortex, an indicator of reorganization in motor pathways in certain pathological conditions. J Clin Neurophysiol 1991;8:56–65.

[29] Streletz LJ, Belevich JK, Jones SM, Bhushan A, Shah SH, Herbison GJ. Transcranial magnetic stimulation: cortical motor maps in acute spinal cord injury. Brain Topogr 1995;7:245–50.

[30] Mikulis DJ, Jurkiewicz MT, McIlroy WE, Staines WR, Rickards L, Kalsi-Ryan S, et al. Adaptation in the motor cortex following cervical spinal cord injury. Neurology 2002;58:794–801.

[31] DeFelipe J, Conley M, Jones EG. Long-range focal collateralization of axons arising from corticocortical cells in monkey sensory-motor cortex. J Neurosci 1986;6:3749–66.

[32] Kujirai T, Caramia MD, Rothwell JC, Day BL, Thompson PD, Ferbert A, et al. Corticocortical inhibition in human motor cortex. J Physiol (Lond) 1993;471:501–19. doi:10.1111/(ISSN)1469-7793

[33] Ziemann U, Lönnecker S, Steinhoff BJ, Paulus W. Effects of antiepileptic drugs on motor cortex excitability in humans: a transcranial magnetic stimulation study. Ann Neurol 1996;40:367–78. doi:10.1002/ana.410400306

[34] Ilić TV, Meintzschel F, Cleff U, Ruge D, Kessler KR, Ziemann U. Short-interval paired-pulse inhibition and facilitation of human motor cortex: the dimension of stimulus intensity. J Physiol (Lond) 2002;545:153–67.

[35] Saturno E, Bonato C, Miniussi C, Lazzaro V, Callea L. Motor cortex changes in spinal cord injury: a TMS study. Neurol Res 2008;30:1084–5. doi:10.1179/174313208X332968

[36] Shimizu T, Hino T, Komori T, Hirai S. Loss of the muscle silent period evoked by transcranial magnetic stimulation of the motor cortex in patients with cervical cord lesions. Neurosci Lett 2000;286:199–202.

[37] Roy FD, Zewdie ET, Gorassini MA. Short-interval intracortical inhibition with incomplete spinal cord injury. Clin Neurophysiol 2011;122:1387–95. doi:10.1016/j.clinph.2010.11.020

[38] Mi YP, Bailey AZ, Nelson AJ. Short- and long-intracortical inhibition in incomplete spinal cord injury. Can J Neurol Sci 2016;43:183–91. doi:10.1017/cjn.2015.310

[39] Valls-Solé J, Pascual-Leone A, Wassermann EM, Hallett M. Human motor evoked responses to paired transcranial magnetic stimuli. Electroencephalogr Clin Neurophysiol 1992;85:355–64.

[40] Wassermann EM, Samii A, Mercuri B, Ikoma K, Oddo D, Grill SE, et al. Responses to paired transcranial magnetic stimuli in resting, active, and recently activated muscles. Exp Brain Res 1996;109:158–63.

[41] McDonnell MN, Orekhov Y, Ziemann U. The role of GABA(B) receptors in intracortical inhibition in the human motor cortex. Exp Brain Res 2006;173:86–93. doi:10.1007/s00221-006-0365-2

[42] Werhahn KJ, Kunesch E, Noachtar S, Benecke R, Classen J. Differential effects on motorcortical inhibition induced by blockade of GABA uptake in humans. J Physiol (Lond) 1999;517 (Pt 2):591–7. doi:10.1111/j.1469-7793.1999.0591t.x

[43] Barry MD, Bunday KL, Chen R, Perez MA. Selective effects of baclofen on use-dependent modulation of GABAB inhibition after tetraplegia. J Neurosci 2013;33:12898–907. doi:10.1523/JNEUROSCI.1552-13.2013

[44] Mohammadi B, Krampfl K, Petri S, Bogdanova D, Kossev A, Bufler J, et al. Selective and nonselective benzodiazepine agonists have different effects on motor cortex excitability. Muscle Nerve 2006;33:778–84. doi:10.1002/mus.20531

[45] Schwenkreis P, Witscher K, Janssen F, Addo A, Dertwinkel R, Zenz M, et al. Influence of the N-methyl-D-aspartate antagonist memantine on human motor cortex excitability. Neurosci Lett 1999;270:137–40.

[46] Chen R, Corwell B, Hallett M. Modulation of motor cortex excitability by median nerve and digit stimulation. Exp Brain Res 1999;129:77–86.

[47] Hirashima F, Yokota T. Influence of peripheral nerve stimulation on human motor cortical excitability in patients with ventrolateral thalamic lesion. Arch Neurol 1997;54:619–24.

[48] Di Lazzaro V, Pilato F, Dileone M, Tonali PA, Ziemann U. Dissociated effects of diazepam and lorazepam on short-latency afferent inhibition. J Physiol (Lond) 2005;569:315–23. doi:10.1113/jphysiol.2005.092155

[49] Di Lazzaro V, Oliviero A, Profice P, Pennisi MA, Di Giovanni S, Zito G, et al. Muscarinic receptor blockade has differential effects on the excitability of intracortical circuits in the human motor cortex. Exp Brain Res 2000;135:455–61.

[50] Sailer A, Molnar GF, Cunic DI, Chen R. Effects of peripheral sensory input on cortical inhibition in humans. J Physiol (Lond) 2002;544:617–29.

[51] Tokimura H, Di Lazzaro V, Tokimura Y, Oliviero A, Profice P, Insola A, Mazzone P, Tonali P, Rothwell JC. Short latency inhibition of human hand motor cortex by somatosensory input from the hand. J Physiol 2000;523:503–13.

[52] Kimiskidis VK, Papagiannopoulos S, Sotirakoglou K, Kazis DA, Kazis A, Mills KR. Silent period to transcranial magnetic stimulation: construction and properties of stimulus-response curves in healthy volunteers. Exp Brain Res 2005;163:21–31. doi: 10.1007/s00221-004-2134-4

[53] Fuhr P, Agostino R, Hallett M. Spinal motor neuron excitability during the silent period after cortical stimulation. Electroencephalogr Clin Neurophysiol 1991;81:257–62.

[54] Ziemann U, Netz J, Szelényi A, Hömberg V. Spinal and supraspinal mechanisms contribute to the silent period in the contracting soleus muscle after transcranial magnetic stimulation of human motor cortex. Neurosci Lett 1993;156:167–71.

[55] Pierantozzi M, Marciani MG, Palmieri MG, Brusa L, Galati S, Caramia MD, et al. Effect of Vigabatrin on motor responses to transcranial magnetic stimulation: an effective tool to investigate in vivo GABAergic cortical inhibition in humans. Brain Res 2004;1028:1–8. doi:10.1016/j.brainres.2004.06.009

[56] Inghilleri M, Berardelli A, Marchetti P, Manfredi M. Effects of diazepam, baclofen and thiopental on the silent period evoked by transcranial magnetic stimulation in humans. Exp Brain Res 1996;109:467–72.

[57] Ferbert A, Priori A, Rothwell JC, Day BL, Colebatch JG, Marsden CD. Interhemispheric inhibition of the human motor cortex. J Physiol (Lond) 1992;453:525–46. doi:10.1111/(ISSN)1469-7793

[58] Daskalakis ZJ, Christensen BK, Fitzgerald PB, Roshan L, Chen R. The mechanisms of interhemispheric inhibition in the human motor cortex. J Physiol (Lond) 2002;543:317–26. doi:10.1113/jphysiol.2002.017673

[59] Kukaswadia S, Wagle-Shukla A, Morgante F, Gunraj C, Chen R. Interactions between long latency afferent inhibition and interhemispheric inhibitions in the human motor cortex. J Physiol (Lond) 2005;563:915–24. doi:10.1113/jphysiol.2004.080010

[60] Bunday KL, Perez MA. Impaired crossed facilitation of the corticospinal pathway after cervical spinal cord injury. J Neurophysiol 2012;107:2901–11. doi:10.1152/jn.00850.2011

[61] Chistiakova M, Bannon NM, Bazhenov M, Volgushev M. Heterosynaptic plasticity: multiple mechanisms and multiple roles. Neuroscientist 2014;20:483–98. doi:10.1177/1073858414529829

[62] Tazoe T, Perez MA. Effects of repetitive transcranial magnetic stimulation on recovery of function after spinal cord injury. Arch Phys Med Rehabil 2015;96:S145–55. doi:10.1016/j.apmr.2014.07.418

[63] Ridding MC, Ziemann U. Determinants of the induction of cortical plasticity by non-invasive brain stimulation in healthy subjects. J Physiol (Lond) 2010;588:2291–304. doi:10.1113/jphysiol.2010.190314

[64] Pell GS, Roth Y, Zangen A. Modulation of cortical excitability induced by repetitive transcranial magnetic stimulation: influence of timing and geometrical parameters and underlying mechanisms. Prog Neurobiol 2011;93:59–98. doi:10.1016/j.pneurobio.2010.10.003

[65] Belci M, Catley M, Husain M, Frankel HL, Davey NJ. Magnetic brain stimulation can improve clinical outcome in incomplete spinal cord injured patients. Spinal Cord 2004;42:417–9. doi:10.1038/sj.sc.3101613

[66] Ellaway PH, Maksimovic R, Craggs MD, Mathias CJ, Gall A, Balasubramaniam AV, et al. Action of 5Hz repetitive transcranial magnetic stimulation on sensory, motor and autonomic function in human spinal cord injury. Clin Neurophysiol 2011;122:2452–61. doi:10.1016/j.clinph.2011.04.022

[67] Benito J, Kumru H, Murillo N, Costa U, Medina J, Tormos JM, et al. Motor and gait improvement in patients with incomplete spinal cord injury induced by high-frequency repetitive transcranial magnetic stimulation. Top Spinal Cord Inj Rehabil 2012;18:106–12. doi:10.1310/sci1802-106

[68] Alexeeva N, Calancie B. Efficacy of QuadroPulse rTMS for improving motor function after spinal cord injury: three case studies. J Spinal Cord Med 2016;39:50–7. doi: 10.1179/2045772314Y.0000000279

[69] Nitsche MA, Cohen LG, Wassermann EM, Priori A, Lang N, Antal A, et al. Transcranial direct current stimulation: state of the art 2008. Brain Stimul 2008;1:206–23. doi: 10.1016/j.brs.2008.06.004

[70] Kuo H-I, Paulus W, Batsikadze G, Jamil A, Kuo M-F, Nitsche MA. Chronic enhancement of serotonin facilitates excitatory transcranial direct current stimulation-induced neuroplasticity. Neuropsychopharmacology 2015. doi:10.1038/npp.2015.270

[71] Murray LM, Edwards DJ, Ruffini G, Labar D, Stampas A, Pascual-leone A, et al. Intensity dependent effects of transcranial direct current stimulation on corticospinal excitability in chronic spinal cord injury. Arch Phys Med Rehabil 2015;96:S114–21. doi:10.1016/j.apmr.2014.11.004

[72] Player MJ, Taylor JL, Alonzo A, Loo CK. Paired associative stimulation increases motor cortex excitability more effectively than theta-burst stimulation. Clin Neurophysiol 2012;123:2220–6. doi:10.1016/j.clinph.2012.03.081

[73] Lamy J-C, Russmann H, Shamim EA, Meunier S, Hallett M. Paired associative stimulation induces change in presynaptic inhibition of Ia terminals in wrist flexors in humans. J Neurophysiol 2010;104:755–64. doi:10.1152/jn.00761.2009

[74] Bunday KL, Perez MA. Motor recovery after spinal cord injury enhanced by strengthening corticospinal synaptic transmission. Curr Biol 2012;22:2355–61. doi:10.1016/j.cub.2012.10.046

[75] Yamaguchi T, Fujiwara T, Tsai Y-A, Tang S-C, Kawakami M, Mizuno K, et al. The effects of anodal transcranial direct current stimulation and patterned electrical stimulation on spinal inhibitory interneurons and motor function in patients with spinal cord injury. Exp Brain Res 2016:1–10. doi:10.1007/s00221-016-4561-4

[76] Rioult-Pedotti MS, Friedman D, Hess G, Donoghue JP. Strengthening of horizontal cortical connections following skill learning. Nat Neurosci 1998;1:230–4. doi: 10.1038/678

[77] Benito Penalva J, Opisso E, Medina J, Corrons M, Kumru H, Vidal J, et al. H reflex modulation by transcranial magnetic stimulation in spinal cord injury subjects after gait training with electromechanical systems. Spinal Cord 2010;48:400–6. doi: 10.1038/sc.2009.151

[78] Chisholm AE, Peters S, Borich MR, Boyd LA, Lam T. Short-term cortical plasticity associated with feedback-error learning after locomotor training in a patient with incomplete spinal cord injury. Phys Ther 2015;95:257–66. doi:10.2522/ptj.20130522

[79] Thomas SL, Gorassini MA. Increases in corticospinal tract function by treadmill training after incomplete spinal cord injury. J Neurophysiol 2005;94:2844–55. doi: 10.1152/jn.00532.2005

[80] Gomes-Osman J, Field-Fote EC. Improvements in hand function in adults with chronic tetraplegia following a multiday 10-Hz repetitive transcranial magnetic stimulation intervention combined with repetitive task practice. J Neurol Phys Ther 2015;39:23–30. doi:10.1097/NPT.0000000000000062

[81] Cotman CW, Berchtold NC, Christie L-A. Exercise builds brain health: key roles of growth factor cascades and inflammation. Trends Neurosci 2007;30:464–72. doi: 10.1016/j.tins.2007.06.011

[82] Colcombe SJ, Kramer AF, Erickson KI, Scalf P, McAuley E, Cohen NJ, et al. Cardiovascular fitness, cortical plasticity, and aging. Proc Natl Acad Sci USA 2004;101:3316–21. doi:10.1073/pnas.0400266101

[83] Kramer AF, Erickson KI. Capitalizing on cortical plasticity: influence of physical activity on cognition and brain function. Trends Cogn Sci (Regul Ed) 2007;11:342–8. doi:10.1016/j.tics.2007.06.009

[84] Xiong J, Ma L, Wang B, Narayana S, Duff EP, Egan GF, et al. Long-term motor training induced changes in regional cerebral blood flow in both task and resting states. NeuroImage 2009;45:75–82. doi:10.1016/j.neuroimage.2008.11.016

[85] Swain RA, Harris AB, Wiener EC, Dutka MV, Morris HD, Theien BE, et al. Prolonged exercise induces angiogenesis and increases cerebral blood volume in primary motor cortex of the rat. Neuroscience 2003;117:1037–46.

[86] Rojas Vega S, Abel T, Lindschulten R, Hollmann W, Bloch W, Strüder HK. Impact of exercise on neuroplasticity-related proteins in spinal cord injured humans. Neuroscience 2008;153:1064–70. doi:10.1016/j.neuroscience.2008.03.037

[87] Mang CS, Campbell KL, Ross CJD, Boyd LA. Promoting neuroplasticity for motor rehabilitation after stroke: considering the effects of aerobic exercise and genetic variation on brain-derived neurotrophic factor. Phys Ther 2013;93:1707–16. doi: 10.2522/ptj.20130053

[88] McDonnell MN, Buckley JD, Opie GM, Ridding MC, Semmler JG. A single bout of aerobic exercise promotes motor cortical neuroplasticity. J Appl Physiol 2013;114:1174–82. doi:10.1152/japplphysiol.01378.2012

[89] Cirillo J, Lavender AP, Ridding MC, Semmler JG. Motor cortex plasticity induced by paired associative stimulation is enhanced in physically active individuals. J Physiol (Lond) 2009;587:5831–42. doi:10.1113/jphysiol.2009.181834

[90] Bolognini N, Pascual-leone A, Fregni F. Using non-invasive brain stimulation to augment motor training-induced plasticity. J Neuroeng Rehabil 2009;6:8. doi: 10.1186/1743-0003-6-8

[91] Froc DJ, Chapman CA, Trepel C, Racine RJ. Long-term depression and depotentiation in the sensorimotor cortex of the freely moving rat. J Neurosci 2000;20:438–45.

[92] Huang Y-Z, Edwards MJ, Rounis E, Bhatia KP, Rothwell JC. Theta burst stimulation of the human motor cortex. Neuron 2005;45:201–6. doi:10.1016/j.neuron.2004.12.033

[93] Zafar N, Paulus W, Sommer M. Comparative assessment of best conventional with best theta burst repetitive transcranial magnetic stimulation protocols on human motor cortex excitability. Clin Neurophysiol 2008;119:1393–9. doi:10.1016/j.clinph.2008.02.006

[94] Wu SW, Shahana N, Huddleston DA, Gilbert DL. Effects of 30Hz θ burst transcranial magnetic stimulation on the primary motor cortex. J Neurosci Methods 2012;208:161–4. doi:10.1016/j.jneumeth.2012.05.014

[95] Gentner R, Wankerl K, Reinsberger C, Zeller D, Classen J. Depression of human corticospinal excitability induced by magnetic theta-burst stimulation: evidence of rapid polarity-reversing metaplasticity. Cereb Cortex 2008;18:2046–53. doi:10.1093/cercor/bhm239

[96] Hamada M, Murase N, Hasan A, Balaratnam M, Rothwell JC. The role of interneuron networks in driving human motor cortical plasticity. Cereb Cortex 2013;23:1593–605. doi:10.1093/cercor/bhs147

[97] López-Alonso V, Cheeran B, Río-Rodríguez D, Fernández-Del-Olmo M. Inter-individual variability in response to non-invasive brain stimulation paradigms. Brain Stimul 2014;7:372–80. doi:10.1016/j.brs.2014.02.004

[98] Talelli P, Greenwood RJ, Rothwell JC. Exploring Theta Burst Stimulation as an intervention to improve motor recovery in chronic stroke. Clin Neurophysiol 2007;118:333–42. doi:10.1016/j.clinph.2006.10.014

[99] Di Lazzaro V, Pilato F, Dileone M, Profice P, Capone F, Ranieri F, et al. Modulating cortical excitability in acute stroke: a repetitive TMS study. Clin Neurophysiol 2008;119:715–23. doi:10.1016/j.clinph.2007.11.049

[100] Munneke MAM, Rongen JJ, Overeem S, Schelhaas HJ, Zwarts MJ, Stegeman DF. Cumulative effect of 5 daily sessions of θ burst stimulation on corticospinal excitability in amyotrophic lateral sclerosis. Muscle Nerve 2013;48:733–8. doi:10.1002/mus.23818

[101] Quartarone A, Rizzo V, Bagnato S, Morgante F, Sant'Angelo A, Girlanda P, et al. Rapid-rate paired associative stimulation of the median nerve and motor cortex can produce long-lasting changes in motor cortical excitability in humans. J Physiol (Lond) 2006;575:657–70. doi:10.1113/jphysiol.2006.114025

[102] Naro A, Russo M, AbdelKader M, Manganotti P, Genovesi V, Marino M, et al. A local signature of LTP-like plasticity induced by repetitive paired associative stimulation. Brain Topogr 2015;28:238–49. doi:10.1007/s10548-014-0396-0

[103] Tsang P, Bailey AZ, Nelson AJ. Rapid-rate paired associative stimulation over the primary somatosensory cortex. Plos One 2015;10:e0120731. doi:10.1371/journal.pone. 0120731

[104] Morgante F, Quartarone A, Ricciardi L, Arena MG, Rizzo V, Sant'Angelo A, et al. Impairment of sensory-motor plasticity in mild Alzheimer's disease. Brain Stimul 2013;6:62–6. doi:10.1016/j.brs.2012.01.010

[105] Conforto AB, Kaelin-Lang A, Cohen LG. Increase in hand muscle strength of stroke patients after somatosensory stimulation. Ann Neurol 2002;51:122–5. doi:10.1002/ana. 10070

[106] Knikou M, Dixon L, Santora D, Ibrahim MM. Transspinal constant-current long-lasting stimulation: a new method to induce cortical and corticospinal plasticity. J Neurophysiol 2015;114:1486–99. doi:10.1152/jn.00449.2015

2

Emerging Techniques for Assessment of Sensorimotor Impairments after Spinal Cord Injury

Filipe Barroso, Diego Torricelli and Juan C. Moreno

Abstract

Gait function can be altered after incomplete spinal cord (iSCI) lesions. Muscular weakness, co-activation of antagonist muscles, and altered muscle mechanics are likely to provoke abnormal gait and postural movements. Functional scales are available for assessment of functional walking in SCI patients, such as walking index for spinal cord injury (WISCI II), timed up and go (TUG) test, 10-meter walk test (10MWT), and 6-minute walk test (6MWT). Novel metrics for a more detailed comprehension of neuromuscular control in terms of degree of voluntary motor control have been recently proposed. This section describes novel techniques based on muscle synergy and frequency domain analysis of electromyographic signals. Such techniques are illustrated as potential tools for assessment of motor function after SCI with experimental data and a case study describing a diagnostic scenario. This chapter presents a discussion of the current status of the emerging metrics for assessment of sensorimotor impairments. Conclusions are given with respect to the availability of enriched information about neuromuscular behavior between functional tasks (walking and pedalling) and the potential relevance of these new techniques to improve the efficacy of treatment to improve locomotion after iSCI.

Keywords: Rehabilitation, spinal cord injury, walking, functional scales

1. Introduction

Gait function can be altered after incomplete spinal cord (iSCI) lesions. Muscular weakness, co-activation of antagonist muscles, and altered muscle mechanics are likely to provoke abnormal gait and postural movements. Human walking involves the coordination of several muscles and its correct activation. One of the main goals of treatment after SCI is to recover the ability to walk again. The assessment of the neurorehabilitation process has traditionally been done based on the qualitative methods (classic clinical scales) or subjective assessment from physiotherapists (based on clinical gaze) [1]. Traditional techniques are prone to low reliability and, as a consequence, may result in inadequate or costly interventions. More importantly, clinical tests focused on behavioral outcomes provide little information about the underlying differences between healthy and impaired nervous system [1]. It is becoming more and more clear that a more profound understanding of impairments may be crucial not only to prescribe effective treatments to individual patients but also to gather comparative results and evidence that are needed to develop novel therapies. Thus, motor neurorehabilitation should be informed by more reliable and repeatable metrics that allow a quantitative assessment of motor control performance and recovery.

Gait analysis is broadly known as means to adequately assess and follow-up patients and supports a clinical decision on the best treatment [2]. Clinical gait analysis involves a variety of techniques including kinematic or joint motion measurements; kinetic or joint torque assessment, electromyographic (EMG) measurements, and video analysis. Measures derived from gait analysis provide a detailed and quantitative description. This might further be used to extract important information to select a task-oriented approach that might enhance therapeutic response, which cannot be provided by clinical evaluation alone [2]. Instrumented clinical gait analysis, despite its objectivity, is not straightforward in practice. Thus, more concise indexes of gait function are to be developed to assess the changes in gait function over time and evaluate interventions.

Most widely used functional scales for gait rehabilitation in SCI patients are walking index for spinal cord injury (WISCI II), timed up and go (TUG) test, 10-meter walk test (10MWT), and 6-minute walk test (6MWT). As mentioned above, to achieve adequate treatment, it is crucial to investigate not only the functional effect but also the mechanisms underlying the impaired function. Recently, the use of quantitative metrics based on electromyography and biomechanical features is bringing a new insight into the motor recovery mechanisms and performance outcomes after neural damage. EMG features provide useful information concerning brain motor control strategies [3]. Muscle activation patterns and muscle synergies have been proposed as a potential technique to measure motor recovery following therapeutic interventions [4]. Muscle synergies, understood as groups of co-activated muscles that are responsible for task execution in different conditions, can explain the way that central nervous system (CNS) solves control of multiple muscles and degrees of freedom by means of a smaller number of neural parameters [5]. This brings a more comprehensive understanding of the underlying motor strategies responsible for impaired locomotion.

The aim of this chapter is to present the emerging indexes based on EMG and biomechanical data to support therapeutic interventions in SCI patients who are commonly affected with spastic paresis and require targeted relearning and activation of a residual motor function. Novel metrics based on computational methods, such as muscle coherence and muscle synergy analysis, are presented as tools for a more detailed comprehension of neuromuscular control in terms of degree of voluntary motor control. Conclusions are given with respect to the availability of enriched information about neuromuscular behavior between functional tasks (walking and pedalling) and the potential relevance of these new techniques to improve the efficacy of treatment to improve locomotion after iSCI.

2. Sensorimotor impairments after SCI

The spinal lesion leads to sensorimotor impairments in both upper and lower extremities. Ambulation results limited due to the sensory and proprioceptive impairments and muscle spasticity, commonly found even in subjects that reach a sufficient level of ambulation. The mechanisms involved in muscle spasticity are related to the lesion in the CNS that leads to changes in the excitability of spinal reflexes and loss of supraspinal drive. This results in abnormal muscle function and leads to altered mechanical muscle properties. In addition to this, proprioceptive and sensory impairment lead to altered or loss afferent feedback to the CNS, which in turn progressively affects motor control and leads to unstable, non-physiological gait. In particular, symptoms such as muscular weakness, co-activation of antagonist muscles, and altered muscle mechanics provoke abnormal gait and postural movements.

The relationship between hypertonia and gait function is still not clear controversial [6]. The difficulty to classify iSCI subjects as spastic or not is a well-known problem [7]. Spasticity in SCI patients is mostly associated (clinically) with the presence of flexor and extensor spasms triggered by cutaneous stimulation. In practice, it is important to determine whether an impaired gait is mainly caused by disabling paresis but also altered afferent feedback to the CNS. Novel metrics to assess motor control based on detailed EMG analysis are required to complement and optimize interventions that focus on the clinical signs of spasticity, such as exaggerated reflexes and muscle tone (e.g., medication).

3. Clinical assessment of walking ability after SCI

The main goal of clinical assessments is to quantify the motor recovery by observing and measuring the functional changes that occur in the patient after the injury. This is normally done by scales, which quantify the patient's residual functions under a wide spectrum, and therefore support scientifically the clinical practice in making effective choice on the treatment, studying cost-benefit of the rehabilitation process and quantifying objectively the degree of incapacity or handicap. Nevertheless, the sensitivity and reliability of current scales are still limited. For instance, the score assignment still relies on a strong subjective component, which causes high intra and inter-rater variability, even when the scale is carried out by experienced examiners [8]. In addition, scales often have similar content and purpose, which makes difficult to decide which of the available tests are superior and should be used as outcome measures. Therefore, there is a need to incorporate new and more objective methods to assess of motor recovery into the existing panorama. In the following, we present and briefly describe the main measures used in clinical settings to evaluate the functional recovery after SCI.

3.1. ASIA impairment scale (AIS)

This scale [9] provides a correct assessment of the severity of the SCI and can assess the developmental stage of the lesion. The evaluation is mainly based on motor exploration and includes complementary tests for sensory and muscle assessment. Ten muscles are evaluated (covering upper and lower limbs) to get muscle balance score between 0 and 5. The sensory examination measures superficial and deep sensitivity on a scale of 0–2 in 28 sensitive key points (for example, the big toe to C6 or armpit for L2). The sum of the motor and sensory scores reflects the global degree of impairment. According to international standards established by the American Association of SCI AIS, this can be classified into five levels, ranging between complete lesion (A, sensory but not motor function is preserved below the neurological level and includes the sacral segments S4–S5) and normality (E, the sensorimotor functions are completely preserved).

3.2. Walking index for spinal cord injury (WISCI II)

This index [10] specifically measures the functionality of walking and aims to quantify the secondary physical limitations in SCI. A recent study on functional measures of gait in people with SCI [11] showed how previous scales (e.g., 10 m and timed up and go, TUG) were unable to discriminate the improvement in function of patients who needed assistive devices during walking, such as walker or crutches. These data suggest that the WISCII scale serves as a valid tool for measuring changes in locomotion and effectiveness of treatment after SCI when technical help or the assistance of an external person is required to realize gait function. The scoring method is based on visual observation of the patient's ability during walking over at least 10 m. Walking ability is classified in this index, from the level with the most severe disabilities (0), to less severe disability (20). Within this range, the patient is classified according to the use of devices, braces, and physical assistance of one or two people.

3.3. Timed up and go (TUG) test

Originally developed to study the balance in senior age [12], this test demonstrated its validity as a measure of walking performance in neurologically injured subjects [13]. This tool measures the time (in seconds) that patients take to get up from a chair, walk 3 m, and sit back. Walk 3 m is the traditional test TUG, but there are adaptations in which the patient has to walk 10 or 7 m. The score ranges from one (normal) to five points (very abnormal). Times above 20 s are predictors of falls. This test captures the complex interaction between balance and movement, including planning, initiation, and implementation, and completes a series of linked movements that are common in activities of daily living. The validity of the TUG has been studied in different works and found to have a sensitivity and specificity of 87%.

3.4. 10-meter walk test (10MWT)

This test quantifies the walking speed by measuring the time (in seconds) that the patient takes to travel a distance of 10 m [13]. This scale was firstly proposed to assess gait in patients with stroke and Parkinson's disease, and then transferred as an alternative to evaluate patients with

SCI. A study [14] comparing several clinical scales of motion concluded that 10MWT is a more reliable and easier handling tool than the test of 6-minute walk test (see next section). As a drawback, this test requires additional information on technical aids needed during walking.

3.5. 6-minute walk test (6MWT)

This test calculates the distance (in meters) that patients are able to walk in six minutes [15]. Initially, it was used to measure cardiovascular exercise capacity in elderly patients with heart or lung disease, as a submaximal test of the aerobic capacity of the individual. It is one of the most widely used tests to evaluate gait motor recovery in neurologically injured subjects [16].

3.6. Spinal cord (functional) independence measures (FIM and SCIM)

The functional independence measure (FIM) scale was originally developed to assess disability of individuals with stroke [17]. This tool has been then widely applied for the evaluation of the functionality in the SCI. It is a standard and validated scale studying the state of functional recovery of patients from hospital admission to discharge. It is also used globally to monitor the progress of the functionality of patients throughout the rehabilitation treatment. It measures 18 activities, of which 13 items refer to the motor area and five to the cognitive status. These 18 items are grouped into six blocks: self-care, sphincter control, transfers, locomotion, communication, and awareness of the external world. It includes seven levels ranging from total dependence to full independence [18,19].

The SCIM scale was developed specifically to improve some aspects of the FIM scale [13]. This scale consists of 16 items (score range 0–100) and includes three levels of activity: (1) self-care (feeding, grooming, bathing, and dressing), (2) respiration and sphincter management, and (3) mobility (bed and transfers and indoor/outdoor). Scores are obtained by adding up the individual items. The item scores are weighted related to the assumed clinical relevance.

4. Scales to assess clinical conditions of spasticity

The correct measurement of spasticity is of vital importance in SCI for three main reasons: (i) evaluating the effectiveness of anti-spasticity treatments, (ii) optimizing individually the amount of antispastic medication to patients, and (iii) understanding the pathophysiological mechanisms underlying this disorder [20]. However, although spasticity is usually easy to recognize, its quantification is a much more complex process [21]. A unique scale that can provide a general and objective assessment of spasticity is still not available in the literature; therefore, the various tests and clinical measures are usually combined in order to evaluate different aspects of spasticity. The existing clinical measurements include scales that measure muscle hypertonia (modified Ashworth scale (MAS), EAM) [22], the spasms often suffered by patients (frequency spasms scale Penn) [23], and the reflected hyperexcitability after SCI (scale of severity of spasms (SCATS) [24]. In the following sections, these three methods will be briefly described.

4.1. Modified Ashworth scale (MAS)

This scale measures the resistance of muscle to passive stretching [22]. The resistance value is scored between 0 and 4, being "0" the absence of any increase in tone during movement; "1" slight increase in tone and muscle response at the start of movement or increased resistance at the end of the movement; "1+" slight increase in muscle resistance movement followed by minimal resistance throughout the remainder of the range of motion; "2" significant increase in muscle endurance during most arc joint movement, but the joint moves easily; "3" marked increase in muscle strength or passive movement is difficult in flexion or extension; and "4" the affected joints are rigid in flexion or extension. Two physiotherapists should perform this test independently.

4.2. Penn spasm frequency scale (PSFS)

The PENN scale is a tool to quantify spasm frequency suffered by the patient during the 24 h prior to the test [25]. The scores on this scale are between 0 and 4, where "0" is the total absence of spasms, "1" spasms caused only by stimulation, "2" spasms that occur less than once every hour, "3" spasms occur more than once every hour, and "4" spasms that occur more than 10 times an hour. As for the MAS scale, two physiotherapists should perform this test independently.

4.3. Spinal cord assessment tool for spastic reflexes (SCATS)

This scale is a physiologically based measure for spastic reflexes for use in individuals with SCI. It measures the reflected hyperexcitability, which includes clonus, flexor spasms, and cramps in the extensors. This scale is developed to provide a measure of primary spastic reaction, addressing categories of spasms as follows: (1) clonus, (2) flexor spasms, and (3) extensor spasms. The spasm is triggered and rated with a score ranging from 0 to 3. The SCATS does not provide information on patient perspective, which is an important aspect since spasms are sometimes perceived beneficial to the patient. This tool is simple and quick (<5 s) to administer but despite its simplicity it has not been widely accepted yet. The measure could be conducted during a home visit or at a clinic/hospital. A study [24] evaluated the validity of this scale, demonstrating that it correlated significantly with kinematic and electromyographic measures, and with Ashworth scores.

5. Emerging metrics to assess sensorimotor impairments after spinal cord injury

Despite its ability to assess and provide information about underlying mechanisms and changes in motor control, electromyography (EMG) is still rarely employed in the clinical setting to assess SCI patients [26]. Thus, novel approaches using EMG should be explored, as EMG can be very valuable to understand compensatory strategies and for further rehabilitation processes.

This section describes novel techniques based on muscle synergies and frequency-domain analysis of EMG signals (muscle coherence). Such techniques are illustrated as potential tools for assessment of motor function after SCI with experimental data and a case study describing a diagnostic scenario.

5.1. EMG coherence

Neurophysiological studies demonstrate only limited spontaneous recovery of voluntary motor function after incomplete SCI diagnosed with the American Spinal Injury Association (ASIA) Impairment Scale (AIS) [9,27]. Thus, there is a clinical need to identify new comprehensive outcome measures that may be used to assess sensorimotor impairments after incomplete SCI (iSCI). Effective neurophysiological measures should have clinical relevance, reflecting the recovery of volunteer motor force and gait function, as well as the development of maladaptive motor plasticity, such as the spasticity syndrome, which is known to limit the recovery of voluntary motor strength, gait, and daily life activities following SCI [28–34]. These measures may facilitate clinical diagnosis and guidance of individualized neurorehabilitation programs.

5.1.1. Muscle coherence

Lower limb EMG coherence analysis has been used as an indirect measure of voluntary motor control, gait function [35], and spasticity [27] after iSCI. This is a frequency-domain measure of the similarity between two independent EMG signals, having the potential to assess the descending motor drive [36]. The fact that it just needs EMG recording to be calculated makes it suitable for clinical applications. On the other hand, muscle coherence activity estimation can be obtained from the same muscle (intramuscular coherence) [37,38], as well as between two different muscles (intermuscular coherence) [38–40].

Smith et al. [41] have shown that the synchronization of motoneuron discharges (coherence) was reduced after spinal cord injury and also that it could be better recorded during isometric muscle contractions. The analysis of muscle coherence has been used to diagnose lesions in voluntary motor control mechanisms and functionality of SCI patients, for example, gait control [37,38]. Several studies support the use of muscle coherence analysis as an indirect measure of the common descending tracts during the execution of specific motor tasks. For instance, it has been suggested the existence of an association between the force of a maximum isometric contraction and corticospinal activity, based on the evidence of a reduction of intracortical inhibition modulated by training muscle strength [42–45]. Despite the potential of this technique, few studies have investigated which type of movement would be optimal for the use of muscle coherence calculation as a greater diagnostic measure.

Measuring the residual activity of tibialis anterior may represent an interesting diagnostic measure of functionality after SCI, mainly because this muscle receives increased innervation from the corticospinal system [45]. In fact, ankle dorsiflexion movement has been used as an indirect measure of adaptive neuroplasticity during the rehabilitation phase [46], while the recording of tibialis anterior co-activation during plantarflexion may be also used as indicator of maladaptive mechanisms after SCI, such as spasticity or its associated symptoms [47].

5.1.2. An emerging methodology to assess muscle coherence

This section sums up the methodology and main results presented by [27], who analyzed intramuscular TA coherence within specific frequency bands between 10–60 Hz from subjects who suffered an iSCI, while they performed different movement tasks.

Muscle coherence between two TA EMG signals (intramuscular coherence) was calculated during the periods of activation of this muscle during controlled ankle dorsiflexion movements. Specifically, EMG was recorded during the following ankle dorsiflexion tasks: (I) isometric activation at 50, 75, and 100% of maximal voluntary torque (MVT), (II) isokinetic activation at 60 and 120°/s and III) isotonic dorsiflexion at 50% MVT. Periods of activation were visually determined after processing EMG signals. This analysis of EMGs started with demeaning of raw signals, followed by band-pass filtering (3–700 Hz) and rectification.

Muscle coherence was computed using the function "mscohere" of Matlab (Version 7.11). The output of this function is the magnitude-squared coherence estimate of the input signals (both TA signals), using Welch's averaged modified periodogram method [48]. Finally, four bandwidths were analyzed: 10–16, 15–30, 24–40, and 40–60 Hz. For each band, it was computed the mean magnitude squared coherence estimate. A non-significant higher level of coherence activity was identified within the 10–16 Hz band in the iSCI spasticity group, when comparing the isometric activation at 100% of MVT for subjects diagnosed without or with spasticity. For the other bands of frequency, no differences were identified for TA intramuscular coherence [27].

There was also a negative correlation between the TA muscle coherence measured during isometric activation at 100% of MVT and specific symptoms of SCI spasticity muscle hypertonia, passive resistive torque, and involuntary muscle contractions. The modified Ashworth scores correlated negatively with TA coherence within the 24–60 Hz frequency band. The severity spasms measured with the SCATS scale also presented a negative correlation the 40–60 Hz band. On the other hand, a positive correlation was found between the Penn score and the TA coherence for the 15–30 Hz band. A positive correlation was also identified between the degree of clonus activity and TA coherence within the 10–16 Hz bandwidth [27].

TA coherence calculated as the ratio of 120/60°/s isokinetic activation was higher in the iSCI spastic subgroup, when compared with the non-spastic group [27]. In summary, the results presented by Bravo-Esteban et al. [27] suggest that TA muscle coherence activity estimation during the execution of controlled ankle dorsiflexion movements may be used to assess the level of spasticity in iSCI patients.

5.2. Analysis of muscle synergies during cycling

Given the redundancy of the musculoskeletal system, a long-stand idea is that the central nervous system (CNS) controls muscle activation through the use of a synergistic organization constituted by basic control elements called synergies (or motor modules) [49–51]. In 1967, Nikolai Bernstein [52] proposed the existence of muscle synergies as a simplified strategy of motor control. Muscle synergies are functional sets of muscles, co-activated by varying their timing and/or neural drive. This synergistic control is thought to underlie the execution of different biomechanical tasks [53].

Muscle synergies may offer new insight into the underlying motor strategies responsible for impaired locomotion [1]. Thus, muscle synergies have been proposed as a potential technique to measure motor recovery [4]. Nevertheless, it is still difficult to assess or predict motor performance in those patients who lack the required muscle strength to walk during the early stage of the rehabilitation, even with some body weight supports. Given the similarities in kinematics and muscle control with walking [54], cycling may be explored as a novel framework to assess motor performance in iSCI patients.

5.2.1. Comparison of two iSCI patients

Based on the findings presented in our previous research [3], confirming the hypothesis that similar synergistic features are shared between walking and cycling, we further performed a research testing the hypothesis that muscle synergies outcomes extracted during cycling can be used as indicators of gait performance in iSCI patients. Preliminary results of two patients are presented in this section.

5.2.1.1. Subjects

Two iSCI patients gave their written consent to participate in this study and for data publication, after being informed about the procedures and possible discomfort associated with the experiments, in accordance with the Declaration of Helsinki. The local Toledo Paraplegics Hospital (Spain) Clinical Ethical Committee approved this study (07/05/2013 N°47).

Patient ID	Age (years)	Gender	Time post-SCI (months)	Level of lesion	Most affected side	AIS	WISCI II	TUG (s)	10-meter (s)
01	25	M	5	T4	Left	D	15	29.3	27.7
02	77	M	13	C7	Right	D	19	25.1	10.2

M, male; F, female; Level of lesion: C – Cervical, T – Thoracic; AIS, American Spinal Injury Association (ASIA) Impairment Scale. WISCI II, walking index for spinal cord injury; TUG, timed up and go.

Table 1. Individual iSCI patients' description, as well as the amount of physical assistance needed and gait performance.

Detailed information of the patients is presented in **Table 1**. Both patients received the standard rehabilitation program of the hospital. Inclusion criteria were as follows: aged between 18 and 80 years; motor incomplete spinal lesion (AIS C-D) of traumatic and non-traumatic etiology, with a prognosis of recovery of the walking function; evolution of at least 1.5 months. Exclusion criteria were as follows: supraspinal or peripheral neurological involvement; history of epilepsy; musculoskeletal involvement of lower limbs or spasticity higher than 3 (measured with the Modified Ashworth Scale) for each joint, either for extension or flexion.

5.2.1.2. Experimental protocol

Prior to the experiment, a trained physiotherapist performed a set of clinical evaluations in order to inform about the functional status of the patients. The gait performance was evaluated using the timed up and go (TUG) test [55] and the 10-meter test [56]. In order to quantify the amount of assistance required by the subjects (10 m walk), the walking index for spinal cord injury (WISCI II) was applied. This is a 21-point scale that ranges from 0 (patient unable to stand and/or participate in assisted walking) to 20 (patient ambulates 10 m with no devices, no braces and no physical assistance) [10].

On the day of the experiment, patients received their standard rehabilitation therapy in the morning. In the afternoon, each iSCI patient performed four cycling trials (at 30, 42, 50, and 60 rpm, revolutions per minute) of 30 s duration each, with 60 s resting between trials. These trials were performed on an electronically braked cycle ergometer (MOTOmed viva2, Reck, Betzenweiler, Germany) in the passive mode. For each patient, the order of the trials was randomized to avoid biased results. Patients were asked to perform the experiment while sat on a regular chair.

An auditory metronome was used in order to synchronize patients' cycling frequency with the desired cadence. An EMG amplifier (EMG-USB, OT Bioelettronica, Torino, Italy) with recording bandwidth of 10–750 Hz, overall gain of 1000 V/V, and acquisition frequency of 2048 Hz was used to record surface electromyography (sEMG) of 13 muscles of the most affected leg of patients. The recorded muscles were as follows: Gluteus Medius, Adductor Longus, Sartorius, Tibialis Anterior, Rectus Femoris, Tensor Fascia Latae, Vastus Lateralis, Vastus Medialis, Biceps Femoris, Semitendinosus, Soleus, Gastrocnemius Lateralis, and Gastrocnemius Medialis. The most affected side was determined based on the muscle score [57] of quadriceps, hamstrings, TA, and gastrocnemius for both limbs.

Bipolar sEMG electrodes (Ag-AgCl, Ambur Neuroline 720, Ambu, Ballerup, Denmark) were fastened with a 2-cm inter-electrode distance on each recorded muscle, following SENIAM recommendations for sEMG recording procedures [58]. One angular sensor (Vishay, Malvern, PA) was applied to estimate the crank angle at a sampling frequency of 100 Hz. Segmentation of pedaling cycles was then performed based on the bottom dead center (BDC) position of the pedal.

5.2.1.3. Muscle synergies analysis

For each patient and trial, 10 continuous pedaling cycles were selected for analysis. The selected raw EMG signals were pre-processed using high-pass filtering at 20 Hz, demeaning, rectification, and low-pass filtering at 5 Hz, resulting in the EMG envelopes [49,59]. Muscle synergies were extracted using a Non-Negative Matrix Factorization (NNMF) algorithm [60]. A detailed explanation of the procedure to extract muscles synergies is presented in [49] and [3]. For each trial, the NNMF algorithm was run four times, considering as input two to five synergies. In order to avoid local minima, for each run, the NNMF was repeated 40 times and the repetition with the lowest reconstruction error was selected.

To assess whether the recorded EMGs were well described as a combination of the identified synergies, two indicators of the quality of reconstruction of the EMG data were used: the *variability accounted for* (VAF$_{total}$) [49] and the *coefficient of determination* (r^2) [61]. Both VAF$_{total}$ and r^2 have been adopted in most studies on muscle synergies [49,61]. VAF$_{total}$ has been suggested to be more stringent than r^2, since it is sensitive to both shape and amplitude of the signals, whereas r^2 only addresses similarity in shape.

5.2.1.4. Results

Patient 02 presented better motor performance than patient 01. In the case of WISCI II, patient 01 scored 15 points, whereas patient 02 score 19 points. Patient 01 needed 19.3 s to perform TUG test, whereas patient 02 needed 25.1 s to perform the same test. Patient 01 needed 27.7 to perform the 10-meter test, whereas patient 02 just needed 10.2 s to perform the same test.

As a general trend, patient 02 presented higher values of VAF$_{total}$ and r^2 than patient 01, for all speeds and number of synergies. Also, the higher the number of synergies used to reconstruct EMG data, the better the data were reconstructed (higher VAF$_{total}$ and r^2 values). Both patients reached their minimum values of VAF$_{total}$ at 50 rpm, using two synergies to reconstruct EMG data. VAF$_{total}$ values in such condition were 79% (**Figure 1A**) for patient 01 and 76% (**Figure 1B**) for patient 02. Patient 01 reached 92% as maximum VAF$_{total}$ value. This value was observed when using five synergies at 60 rpm. For patient 02, a maximum VAF$_{total}$ of 95% was reached when using five synergies at 42 rpm.

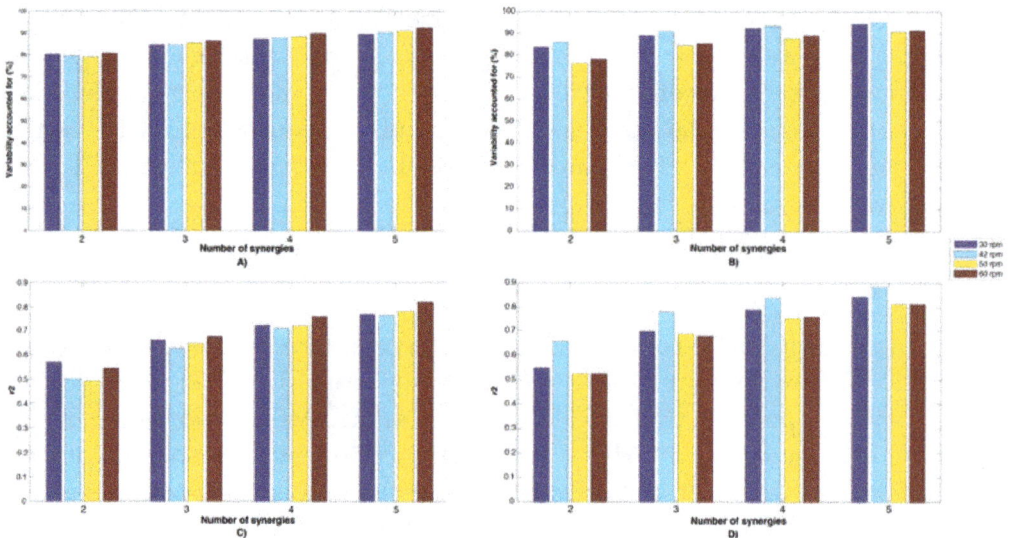

Figure 1. Variability accounted for (VAF_{total}) for patient 01 (A) and patient 02 (B), as well as coefficient of determination (r^2) for patient 01 (C) and patient 02 (D), according to the number of synergies, for each of the four speeds (30, 42, 50, and 60 rpm).

In the case of r^2 values, a minimum of 0.49 (**Figure 1C**) and 0.52 (**Figure 1D**) were obtained for patient 01 (at 50 rpm) and patient 02 (at 60 rpm), respectively. Both values were obtained using two synergies. On the other hand, maximum r^2 values of 0.82 and 0.89 were obtained for patient 01 (at 60 rpm) and patient 02 (at 42 rpm), respectively. Both values were obtained using five synergies. The quality of reconstruction indicators seems to correlate positively with WISCI II scores, that is, patient 02 presented higher values of VAF_{total} and r^2 and also higher values of WISCI II. On the other hand, quality of reconstruction indicators seem to correlate negatively with TUG and 10-meter tests, that is, patient 02 presented higher values of VAF_{total} and r^2 and also needed less time to perform these two gait performance tests.

5.2.1.5. Discussion

Based on the observed common muscle synergies between cycling and walking [3], this preliminary study tested the hypothesis that the analysis of muscle synergies during cycling correlates with gait performance scales in iSCI patients. These preliminary results corroborate this hypothesis.

Results showed positive correlations between WISCI II and EMG reconstruction goodness scores (VAFtotal and r^2) when recording a set of 13 muscles of the most affected leg. In the case of gait speed tests, reconstruction goodness scores correlated negatively with TUG and 10-meter tests. Our results are in agreement with the fact that patients with lower amount of required assistance and good walking performance present higher signal-to-noise ratio in EMG signals than patients with poor walking performance, as severely impaired subjects usually present reduced signal-to-noise ratio in the EMG signals due to reduced signal strength [60]. As a consequence of lower signal-to-noise, lower VAF_{total}, and r^2 values are expected [5].

6. Conclusions

Recovery after SCI is greatly dependent on the severity of the injury as well as the treatment provided in each phase of the lesion, being the subacute phase (up to approximately 6 months) the best phase to promote plastic changes in the CNS. Functional Improvements such as the increase of gait speed increased recovered distance or better WISCI II scores have been observed in acute SCI patients if compared to chronic SCI patients [62].

The application of simple diagnostic measures that might provide comprehensive information regarding the state of adaptive and maladaptive motor control mechanisms after SCI could play a crucial role in guiding rehabilitation strategies in the clinic. Neurophysiological measures should be preferred over qualitative clinical measures, as they are more independent, provide objective data and can be performed in less cooperative patients [63]. However, standardization and clinical validation should be achieved to allow for wide use in the clinical setting.

The analysis of muscle synergies during cycling can be explored as a novel approach for the quantitative assessment of gait performance. This analysis can complement current assessment procedures. On the other hand, the analysis of intramuscular coherence of tibialis anterior can also be explored as a measure of spasticity during the subacute phase of recovery in SCI patients, as it provides information on the mechanisms of maladaptive plasticity (specifically spasticity) [27].

In the future, additional researches are needed in order to validate TA muscle coherence analysis and use it in the clinical setting for the assessment of sensorimotor impairments in SCI patients. Specifically, longitudinal studies have to be performed since the initial stage of recovery, comparing muscle coherence with clinical and functional scales. This will be also useful to provide new information on the neurophysiological mechanisms present during the recovery stage in SCI patients. This work has been partially funded by grant from the European Commission, within the Seventh Framework Programme (IFP7-ICT-2013-10-611695: BioMot - Smart Wearable Robots with Bioinspired Sensory-Motor Skills).

Author details

Filipe Barroso[1,2], Diego Torricelli[2] and Juan C. Moreno[2*]

*Address all correspondence to: jc.moreno@csic.es

1 Department of Physiology, Feinberg School of Medicine – Northwestern University, Chicago, IL, USA

2 Neural Rehabilitation Group, Cajal Institute, Spanish National Research Council (CSIC), Madrid, Spain

References

[1] SAFAVYNIA, S. A.; TORRES-OVIEDO, G.; TING, L. H. Muscle synergies: implications for clinical evaluation and rehabilitation of movement. Top Spinal Cord Inj Rehabil, v. 17, n. 1, p. 16-24, 2011.

[2] NADEAU, S. et al. Guiding task-oriented gait training after stroke or spinal cord injury by means of a biomechanical gait analysis. Progress in Brain Research, v. 192, p. 161-180, 2011.

[3] BARROSO, F. O. et al. Shared muscle synergies in human walking and cycling. Journal of Neurophysiology, v. 112, n. 8, p. 1984-1998, 2014.

[4] ROUTSON, R. L. et al. The influence of locomotor rehabilitation on module quality and post-stroke hemiparetic walking performance. Gait Posture, v. 38, n. 3, p. 511-517, 2013.

[5] STEELE, K. M.; TRESCH, M.; PERREAULT, E. The number and choice of muscles impact the results of muscle synergy analyses. Front Comput Neurosci, v. 7, 2013.

[6] DUFFELL, L. D.; BROWN, G. L.; MIRBAGHERI, M. M. Facilitatory effects of anti-spastic medication on robotic locomotor training in people with chronic incomplete spinal cord injury. J Neuroeng Rehabil, v. 12, n. 29.

[7] REICHENFELSER, W. et al. Monitoring of spasticity and functional ability in individuals with incomplete spinal cord injury with a functional electrical stimulation cycling system. J Rehabil Med, v. 44, n. 5, p. 444-449, 2012.

[8] SAVIC, G. et al. Inter-rater reliability of motor and sensory examinations performed according to American Spinal Injury Association standards. Spinal Cord, v. 45, p. 444-451, 2007.

[9] MAYNARD, F. M. J. et al. International standards for neurological and functional classification of spinal cord injury. American Spinal Injury Association. Spinal Cord, v. 35, n. 5, p. 266-274, 1997.

[10] DITTUNO, P. L.; DITUNNO, J. F. Walking index for spinal cord injury (WISCI II): scale revision. Spinal Cord, v. 39, n. 12, p. 654-656, 2001.

[11] SAENSOOK, W. et al. Discriminative ability of the three functional tests in independent ambulatory patients with spinal cord injury who walked with and without ambulatory assistive devices. J Spinal Cord Med, v. 37, n. 2, p. 212-217, 2014.

[12] PODSIADLO, D.; RICHARDSON, S. The timed "Up & Go": a test of basic functional mobility for frail elderly persons. J Am Geriatr Soc, v. 39, n. 2, p. 142-148, 1991.

[13] FURLAN, J. C. et al. Assessment of disability in patients with acute traumatic spinal cord injury: a systematic review of the literature. J Neurotrauma, v. 28, p. 1413-1430, 2011.

[14] VAN HEDEL, H. J.; WIRZ, M.; DIETZ, V. Assessing walking ability in subjects with spinal cord injury: validity and reliability of 3 walking tests. Arch Phys Med Rehabil., v. 86, n. 2, p. 190-196, 2005.

[15] GUYATT, G. H. et al. The 6-miunte walk: a new measure of exercise capacity in patients with chronic heart failure. Can Med Assoc J, v. 8, n. 919-923, p. 132, 1985.

[16] MAANUM, G. et al. Walking ability and predictors of performance on the 6-minute walk test in adults with spastic cerebral palsy. Dev Med Child Neurol, v. 6, n. e126-e132, p. 52, 2010.

[17] HAMILTON, B. B.; GRANGER, C. V. Disability outcomes following inpatient rehabilitation for stroke. Physical Therapy, v. 74, n. 5, p. 494-503, 1994.

[18] KIRSHBLUM, S. et al. Late neurologic recovery after traumatic spinal cord injury. Arch Phys Med Rehabil, v. 85, p. 1811-1817, 2004.

[19] CATZ, A. et al. A multicenter international study on the spinal cord independence measure, version III: Rasch psychometric validation. Spinal Cord, v. 4, n. 275-291, p. 45, 2007.

[20] BURRIDGE, J. H. et al. Theoretical and methodological considerations in the measurement of spasticity. Disabil Rehabil, v. 27, n. 1-2, p. 69-80, 2005.

[21] BIERING-SORENSEN, F.; NIELSEN, J. B.; KLINGE, K. Spasticity-assessment: a review. Spinal Cord, v. 12, n. 708-722, p. 44, 2006.

[22] BOHANNON, R. W.; SMITH, M. B. Interrater reliability of a modified Ashworth scale of muscle spasticity. Phys Ther, v. 67, n. 2, p. 206-207, 1987.

[23] PENN, R. D. Intrathecal baclofen for severe spasticity. Ann N Y Acad Sci, v. 531, p. 157-166, 1988.

[24] BENZ, E. N.; HORNBY, T. G. A physiologically based clinical measure for spastic reflexes in spinal cord injury. Arch Phys Med Rehabil, v. 86, n. 1, p. 52-59, 2005.

[25] Development and Use of a Knowledge Translation Tool: The Rehabilitation Measures Database Moore, Jennifer L. et al. Archives of Physical Medicine and Rehabilitation, Volume 95, Issue 1, 197–202 January 2014.

[26] WANG, P. et al. Detection of abnormal muscle activations during walking following spinal cord injury (SCI). Res Dev Disabil, v. 34, n. 4, p. 1226-1235, 2013.

[27] BRAVO-ESTEBAN, E. et al. Tibialis anterior muscle coherence during controlled voluntary activation in patients with spinal cord injury: diagnostic potential for muscle strength, gait and spasticity. J Neuroeng Rehabil, v. 11, n. 23, 2014.

[28] BEAUPARLANT, J. et al. Undirected compensatory plasticity contributes to neuronal dysfunction after severe spinal cord injury. Brain, v. 136, n. Pt 11, p. 3347-3361, 2013.

[29] D'Amico, J. M., Condliffe, E. G., Martins, K. J. B., Bennett, D. J., & Gorassini, M. A. (2014). Recovery of neuronal and network excitability after spinal cord injury and implications for spasticity. Frontiers in Integrative Neuroscience, 8, 36. http://doi.org/10.3389/fnint.2014.00036

[30] ZORNER, B. et al. Clinical algorithm for improved prediction of ambulation and patient stratification after incomplete spinal cord injury. J Neurotrauma., v. 27, n. 1, p. 241-252, 2010.

[31] BOAKYE, M. et al. Quantitative testing in spinal cord injury: overview of reliability and predictive validity. J Neurosurg Spine., v. 17, n. 1, p. 141-150, 2012.

[32] PETERSEN, J. A. et al. Spinal cord injury: one-year evolution of motor-evoked potentials and recovery of leg motor function in 255 patients. Neurorehabil Neural Repair, v. 26, n. 8, p. 939-948, 2012.

[33] CURT, A.; KECK, M. E.; DIETZ, V. Functional outcome following spinal cord injury: significance of motor-evoked potentials and ASIA scores. Arch Phys Med Rehabil, v. 79, p. 81-86, 1998.

[34] YANG, J. F. et al. Volitional muscle strength in the legs predicts changes in walking speed following locomotor training in people with chronic Spinal Cord Injury. Phys Ther, v. 91, n. 6, p. 931-943, 2011.

[35] HANSEN, N. L. et al. Reduction of common synaptic drive to ankle dorsiflexormotoneurons during walking in patients with spinal cord lesion. J Neurophysiol, v. 94, p. 934-942, 2005.

[36] Boonstra, T. W. (2013). The potential of corticomuscular and intermuscular coherence for research on human motor control. Frontiers in Human Neuroscience, 7, 855. http://doi.org/10.3389/fnhum.2013.00855

[37] HALLIDAY, D. M. et al. Functional coupling of motor units is modulated during walking in human subjects. J Neurophysiol, v. 89, p. 960–968, 2003.

[38] BARTHELEMY, D. et al. Impaired transmission in the corticospinal tract and gait disability in spinal cord injured persons. J Neurophysiol, v. 104, p. 1167–1176, 2010.

[39] HANSEN, N. L. et al. Synchronization of lower limb motor unit activity during walking in human subjects. J Neurophysiol, v. 86, p. 1266–1276, 2001.

[40] NORTON, J. A.; GORASSINI, M. A. Changes in cortically related intermuscular coherence accompanying improvements in locomotor skills in incomplete spinal cord injury. J Neurophysiol, v. 95, p. 2580–2589, 2006.

[41] SMITH, H. C. et al. Motor unit discharge characteristics during voluntary contraction in patients with incomplete spinal cord injury. Exp Physiol, v. 84, p. 1151–1160, 1999.

[42] CROS, D.; SOTO, O.; CHIAPPA, K. H. Transcranial magnetic stimulation during voluntary action: directional facilitation of outputs and relationships to force generation. Brain Res, v. 1185, p. 103–116, 2007.

[43] ZOGHI, M.; NORDSTROM, M. A. Progressive suppression of intracortical inhibition during graded isometric contraction of a hand muscle is not influenced by hand preference. Exp Brain Res, v. 177, n. 2, p. 266–274, 2007.

[44] WEIER, A. T.; PEARCE, A. J.; KIDGELL, D. J. Strength training reduces intracortical inhibition. Acta Physiol (Oxf), v. 206, n. 2, p. 109–119, 2012.

[45] BROUWER, B.; ASHBY, P. Corticospinal projections to lower limb motoneurons in man. Exp Brain Res, v. 89, p. 649–654, 1992.

[46] WIRTH, B.; VAN HEDEL, H. J.; CURT, A. Changes in corticospinal function and ankle motor control during recovery from incomplete spinal cord injury. J Neurotrauma, v. 25, p. 467–478, 2008.

[47] GOMEZ-SORIANO, J. et al. Voluntary ankle flexor activity and adaptive coactivation gain is decreased by spasticity during subacute spinal cord injury. Exp Neurol, v. 224, p. 507–516, 2010.

[48] WELCH, P. The use of fast Fourier transform for the estimation of power spectra: a method based on time averaging over short, modified periodograms. IEEE Transactions on Audio and Electroacoustics, v. 15, p. 70–73, 1967.

[49] CLARK, D. J. et al. Merging of healthy motor modules predicts reduced locomotor performance and muscle coordination complexity post-stroke. J Neurophysiol, v. 103, n. 2, p. 844-857, 2010.

[50] NEPTUNE, R. R.; MCGOWAN, C. P. Muscle contributions to whole-body sagittal plane angular momentum during walking. J Biomech, v. 44, n. 1, p. 6-12, 2011.

[51] Ilngle, D. (1968). The Co-ordination and Regulation of Movements. Papers translated from Russian and German. N. Bernstein. Pergamon, New York, 1967. xii + 196., illus. $8. Science, 159(3813), 415–416. Retrieved from http://science.sciencemag.org/content/159/3813/415.2.abstract.

[52] Santello M, Bianchi M, Gabiccini M, Ricciardi E, Salvietti G, Prattichizzo D, Ernst M, Moscatelli A, Jörntell H, Kappers AM, Kyriakopoulos K, Albu-Schäffer A, Castellini C, Bicchi A. Hand synergies: Integration of robotics and neuroscience for understanding the control of biological and artificial hands. Phys Life Rev. 2016 Feb 3. pii: S1571-0645(16)00026-9. doi: 10.1016/j.plrev.2016.02.001. [Epub ahead of print] Review. PubMed PMID: 26923030.

[53] ZEHR, E. P. et al. Neural regulation of rhythmic arm and leg movement is conserved across human locomotor tasks. J Physiol, v. 582, p. 209-227, 2007.

[54] WALL, J. C. et al. The timed get-up-and-go test revisited: measurement of the component tasks. J Rehabil Res Dev, v. 37, n. 1, p. 109-113, 2000.

[55] FORREST, G. F. et al. Are the 10 meter and 6 minute walk tests redundant in patients with spinal cord injury? PLoS One, v. 9, n. 5, 2014.

[56] SEDDON, H. W. J. Medical Research Council: Aids to the Exam of the Peripheral Nervous System. [S.l.]: London: Her Majesty's Stationery Office, 1976.

[57] HERMENS, H. J.; FRERIKS, B.; MERLETTI, R. European Recommendations for Surface ElectroMyoGraphy: Results of the SENIAM Project. Enschede, The Netherlands: Roessingh Research and Development, 1999.

[58] HUG, F. et al. Is interindividual variability of EMG patterns in trained cyclists related to different muscle synergies? J Appl Physiol, v. 108, n. 6, p. 1727-1736, 2010.

[59] LEE, D. D.; SEUNG, S. Learning the parts of objects by non-negative matrix factorization. Nature, v. 401, p. 788-791, 1999.

[60] TORRES-OVIEDO, G.; MACPHERSON, J. M.; TING, L. H. Muscle synergy organization is robust across a variety of postural perturbations. J Neurophysiol, v. 96, n. 3, p. 1530-1546, 2006.

[61] DOBKIN, B. et al. Weight-supported treadmill vs over-ground training for walking after acute incomplete SCI. Neurology, v. 66, n. 4, p. 484–493, 2006.

[62] XIE, J.; BOAKYE, M. Electrophysiological outcomes after spinal cord injury. Neurosurg Focus, v. 25, n. 5, p. E11, 2008.

[63] YANG, J. F.; MUSSELMAN, K. E. Training to achieve over ground walking after spinal cord injury: a review of who, what, when, and how. J Spinal Cord Med, v. 35, n. 5, p. 293-304, 2012.

3

Infectious Complications after Spinal Cord Injury

Farhad Abbasi and Soolmaz Korooni

Abstract

Infectious diseases after spinal cord injury (SCI) are important. They can cause mortality and morbidity. The SCI patients usually stay in hospital or rehabilitation units for a long time, and this can cause several complications for them.

Infectious complications: There are several infectious complications in these patients. Pressure ulcers that may be infected, soft tissue infections, osteomyelitis, pneumonia, urinary tract infection, bacteremia, meningitis, epidural abscess, and subdural empyema are important complications. These diseases should be diagnosed and managed promptly, before leading to irreversible complications or death.

Diagnosis: Diagnosis is made by physical examinations; laboratory tests like wound, urine, tracheal secretion, and blood culture with antibiogram; and radiologic evaluation like plain X-ray and magnetic resonance imaging may be used.

Treatment: Appropriate antibiotics are cornerstone of infectious complications. Offloading is important for treatment of pressure ulcers and subsequent complications such as soft tissue infection and osteomyelitis.

Prevention: Intermittent urinary catheterization and prophylactic antibiotic therapy can decrease UTI. Pressure relief, position changes, and regular and frequent observation of skin will prevent pressure ulcers, soft tissue infections, and osteomyelitis. Pulmonary toilet, appropriate positioning, and cough assistance can be useful for clearing retained secretions and preventing pneumonia.

Keywords: infectious, spinal cord, complications

1. Introduction

Infectious complications are supposed to be an important cause of morbidity and mortality in patients with spinal cord injury (SCI). Infectious diseases may lead to death and several complications such as prolonged hospital stay and increased cost of management of patients. Several organs may be affected and problems in these organs can be even more important than the primary event. The types of infections in these patients are different and related to several factors. Inabilities to changing position or ineffective cough, using several necessary devices, prolonged hospitalization, and several other factors, in patients with SCI, predispose them to different types of infections. Inability to walk, sit, or change position may lead to pressure ulcers, skin and soft tissue infection, and osteomyelitis. Reduced tissue perfusion increases the spinal cord-injured patient's susceptibility to pressure ulcers [1] during the acute and rehabilitation phases, most frequently over bony prominences such as the sacrum, tuber ischii, heel, malleolus, and trochanter [2]. Physical and psychosocial elements such as nutrition, past history of pressure ulcers, and social supports can be important in developing ulcers [3]. Ineffective cough and retained pulmonary secretion may lead to pneumonia. Most of the patients need intubation in the course of hospitalization that predisposes them to ventilator-associated pneumonia. Ventilator-associated pneumonia is the most frequent nosocomial infection in patients receiving mechanical ventilation and contributes to a longer intensive care unit stay and high morbidity and mortality [4, 5]. Use of high doses of corticosteroid for management of some patients with SCI can increase the risk of infection. In those patients who need surgical intervention, the operation time is usually prolonged. Sometimes, the use of an external device is mandatory for fixation of unstable vertebral column. The SCI patients may develop bloodstream infection during the hospital admission. During bloodstream infection occurrence in an SCI population, multidrug-resistant organisms are frequent [6]. ICU-acquired bloodstream infection in the intensive care unit is still associated with a high mortality rate. The increase of antimicrobial drug resistance makes its treatment increasingly challenging. ICU bloodstream infection is associated with a 40% increase in the risk of 30-day mortality, particularly if the early antimicrobial therapy is not adequate [7]. Paying attention to antibiotic therapy is important in SCI patients. Antibiotic resistance is of great concern for both infection control and the treatment of infectious diseases. Drug-resistant pathogens, such as methicillin-resistant *Staphylococcus aureus* (MRSA), *Pseudomonas aeruginosa*, *Acinetobacter* and extended-spectrum β-lactamase (ESBL)-producing Enterobacteriaceae, are associated with inappropriate antibiotic treatment that resulted in adverse outcomes. In addition, unnecessary use of broad-spectrum antibiotics for patients with non-drug-resistant pathogens increases mortality [8].

These can be the risk factors for developing infections in SCI patients. In this chapter, the cause of infections, predisposing factors, diagnosis, management, and prevention will be discussed.

2. Infectious diseases after spinal cord injury

2.1. Urinary tract infection

Urinary tract infections (UTI) still cause significant morbidity in patients with spinal cord injury, although mortality due to urinary tract complications has decreased dramatically [9]. Patients with spinal cord injuries (SCIs) and complete or incomplete paraplegia are prone to frequent, recurrent, or chronic UTI. The reason for the increased risk of acquiring UTI is multifactorial, including reduced sensation of classical UTI symptoms, incomplete bladder emptying, frequent catheterizations, or chronic urinary tract catheters [10]. The rate of UTI in an SCI patient is 2.5 episodes in patient per year. UTI is the second leading cause of mortality in SCI patients [11]. Patients with SCI who have urinary catheters have an increased risk of UTI. Urinary tract infection can be important and can cause serious complications including sepsis and septic shock if it is not diagnosed and treated.

Using Foley catheter is usually accompanied with colonization of microorganisms and infection [12]. Bacterial biofilm formation of Foley catheter can cause cystitis [10]. About 80% of UTIs follow urinary catheter insertion. Nitrofurazone-coated and silver alloy-coated catheters can decrease asymptomatic bacteriuria during short-term (<30 days) use in comparison with latex or silicon catheters. The risk of infection is higher with long-term catheterization, and it is safe to remove it early after surgery. Latex and silicone catheters have the same infection rates, but Foley catheters cause more symptomatic bacteriuria and UTI than intermittent catheterizations. Changing the drainage bags and adding antiseptic solution to bags cannot prevent UTI in patients [13]. There are several risk factors for UTI in SCI patients. Reflux of vesicoureteral, postvoiding residuals, outlet obstruction, urinary tract stones, and bladder overdistension [14]. These patients are exposed to antibiotics because of frequent infections that may be an important risk factor for resistant microorganism infection [15]. Today, UTI may be difficult to treat in SCI patients because of antibiotic-resistant organisms. The SCI patients are also colonized by resistant organisms because of recurrent and prolonged hospitalization [16]. The main causative agent of UTI in SCI population is usually derived from the patient's flora. The indwelling catheter has a great role in infection and the duration of catheterization is the most important risk factor. If the patient carries a catheter more than 30 days, the risk of infection with multiple organisms will increase. Although short-term catheterization can be risk factor for bacteriuria, it is usually asymptomatic and often by a single microorganism [17]. It is better to use hydrophilic-coated catheter for intermittent catheterization in SCI patients during acute inpatient rehabilitation. These kinds of catheters can postpone the development of UTI. They also reduce the incidence of bacteriuria and infection. Reduction of complications and treatment costs and preventing the emergence of antibiotic-resistant organisms are other benefits of hydrophilic-coated catheters [18]. Substitution of indwelling catheter with intermittent catheterization during the rehabilitation phase will reduce development of UTI [9]. The unitary catheter should work in a closed system so that no organism can enter the system. It is also important to reduce the duration of catheterization. Sometimes intermittent catheterization, condom sheet catheter, and suprapubic catheters may substitute indwelling catheterization to reduce the risk of infection [17]. Intermittent catheterization is safe and is advised to prevent UTI in SCI patients. Condom sheet catheter can be used in patients who are able to urinate and there is no pathology or injury in urethra. In some patients, where using condom sheet catheter or intermittent catheterization is not suitable or possible, the physician may decide to use suprapubic catheter. The physicians should be aware of these two points that SCI patients may not have the classic symptoms of UTI and urinary infection may cause urologic complications [15].

2.1.1. Diagnosis

Diagnosis of UTI is usually based on the results of urine culture, although in some condition like low titer of organism in urine, slow-growing pathogens and unusual organisms, results of culture may be unreliable [12]. The physician should be aware of how to diagnose UTI and distinguish it from colonization. These patients are at increased risk of acquiring multi-drug-resistant bacteria because they are admitted due to UTI or other infectious diseases and take antibiotics. Several resistant organisms may cause UTI in SCI patients including mul-tidrug-resistant *Pseudomonas aeruginosa*, ESBL (extended-spectrum β-lactamase-producing) *Escherichia coli*, resistant *Klebsiella* spp. and MRSA (methicillin-resistant *Staphylococcus aureus*) [10]. Due to multiple risk factors for acquisition of infection, especially with resistant organisms, complicated UTI may develop with unusual and resistant bacteria. The infection may be polymicrobial. Proteus, Providencia, Serratia, and enterococci may also cause UTI in these groups [9]. For the diagnosis of UTI, culture is needed to find to causative agent, but if the patient is not symptomatic, it is not necessary to get culture, because the patients usually do not need treatment [17]. When UTI is diagnosed in SCI patient, the physician should evaluate the patient for anatomical and functional disorders. It is important to correct any correctable disorder for optimal treatment success [9].

2.1.2. Treatment

Differentiating infection from colonization and asymptomatic bacteriuria from symptomatic infection is an important point in treatment of UTI in SCI patient. A symptomatic patient needs to be treated, and after treatment, long duration of antibiotic suppressive therapy is not necessary [17]. For treatment of UTI, usually, there are many antibiotic options. It is better to postpone the treatment until the result of culture. Sometimes it is necessary to treat the patient empirically. Some variables like probable organism and susceptibility, adminis-tration route (oral vs. intravenous), the patient tolerance, renal function, and the patients' other medications should be considered for choosing appropriate antibiotic [19]. Duration of treatment of chronic UTI in SCI patient may need to be extended. Some studies recommend and some do not. It seems more studies are needed for certain recommendations [10]. The best antibiotics are those that have the most therapeutic effect on causative agent, without any or with less impact on the host normal flora. This antibiotic is best chosen according to result of urine culture and antibiogram. Duration of treatment is usually 5 days but may be extended to 7–14 days when reinfection or relapse occurs [9]. Some studies recommend treating urinary infection between 10 and 14 days in SCI patients, especially when it is not possible to discontinue the urinary catheter. To determine the optimal duration of treatment, multicentral and randomized clinical trial may be necessary [19]. Darouiche's study demon-strates that the 5-day treatment with urinary catheter exchange can be as effective as a 10-day regimen with catheter retention [20]. Antibiotics usually are chosen according to urine cul-ture. Third generation of cephalosporines, carbapenems, and quinolones are often used to treat Gram-negative organisms. For treatment of *Enterococcus* and *Staphylococcus aureus* that usually are resistant in these patients (i.e., methicillin-resistant *S. aureus* or MRSA), vanco-mycin is appropriate.

2.1.3. Prevention and prophylaxis

Prevention of UTI in SCI patients plays an important role in hospital and even in rehabilitation courses of these patients. Paying attention to urinary tract hygiene is necessary. Some patients may encounter relapse or reinfection. In these patients, evaluation of structural and functional disorders should be performed. Duration of previous treatment and probable complications like urine residue and urinary stone should be assessed. Antibiotics may be used as prophylaxis, but it is important to notice that it can be used when recurrent UTI occurs and when all structural and functional abnormalities are corrected. Prophylaxis is not recommended for patients carrying indwelling catheters, and for those who have intermittent catheterization, it is contraventional [9]. Physicians can most effectively prevent UTI by avoiding use of long-term catheters, short duration of catheter use, and substituting intermittent catheterization with indwelling catheter. Daily washing of the catheter or perianal or periurethral areas has no preventive effect. It is recommended to use antibiotic immediately before any invasive procedure on urinary tract system [19]. Probiotics may be useful as prophylactic agents. They may decrease the number of resistant organisms' colonization and may be an attractive substitution for antibiotics for prophylaxis in future [16]. Non-antibiotic prophylaxis may be used for preventing UTI. Some studies may recommend cranberry juice as prophylaxis of UTI, but there is not any reliable clue to prove its effectiveness [9]. In Linsenmeyer's study, cranberry was used for prophylaxis of UTI in patients with neurogenic bladder after spinal cord injury. Cranberry tablets could not effectively decrease the risk of UTI in patients with neurogenic bladders [21].

2.2. Skin and soft tissue infection

One of the most important, serious, and chronic complications of spinal cord injury is pressure ulcer [22]. Pressure ulcers may cause long-term morbidity and even mortality and effectively have severe influence on SCI patients' lives [23]. These patients have more risk of developing pressure ulcer. The ulcers are often chronic wounds that debilitate the patient and increase hospital course [24]. Pressure ulcers are common in SCI patients and usually are complicated. Treatment is often difficult and expensive. It is important to pay special attention to pressure ulcer in SCI population [25]. Several risk factors are associated with pressure ulcer. These risk factors include: decreased activity, complete cord injury that cause paralysis, cervical collar and back board that cause restricted activity, diabetes mellitus, cigarette smoking, hypoalbuminemia, nursing home residence or long duration hospital stay [26], loss of sensation, wet area due to urinary or fecal incontinence, poor nutrition, and muscular atrophy. Pressure ulcers usually occur in about 30–40% of SCI patients. Ulcers usually develop on bony prominences. Sacrum, ischial tuberosity, trochanteric area and malleolus are usual areas for developing ulcers [2]. Patients with pressure ulcers may have good outcomes if rapid diagnosis and proper treatment is performed for them. The ulcer may heal completely without any sequelae. Some ulcers may have slow course of healing and some even may not heal. Some studies emphasize on the role of fibronectin on ulcer healing course. Fibronectin may have a role in opsonizing macro-aggregate debris for phagocytosis, increasing revascularization, and facilitating fibroblast proliferation and migration. Plasma fibronectin increases in ulcers with rapid healing but stay in low level in ulcers with poor healing. So plasma fibronectin level may predict the speed of healing of pressure ulcers [27]. The SCI patients may also suffer from other soft tissue infection rather than pressure ulcers including fungal infections and seborrheic dermatitis [28].

2.2.1. Diagnosis

Diagnosis of pressure ulcers is clinical. The ulcer smear and culture can be useful for recognizing the causative organism and determining the antibiotic sensitivity. *Staphylococcus aureus*, *Pseudomonas aeruginosa*, *Proteus mirabilis*, and *Enterococcus faecalis* are the most common organisms causing pressure ulcers [24].

2.2.2. Treatment

Offloading is the cornerstone of treatment of pressure ulcers. Ultrasound (low-frequency and nonthermal) may have a therapeutic role in intact skin ulcers. If the ulcer is superficial, foam dressing and collagenase may be used. For deep pressure ulcers, usually debridement and surgical intervention is needed. Osteomyelitis beneath the ulcer is so important and should be considered in treatment of deep ulcers [23]. In SCI patients, flap surgery may be needed to cover the place of debridement [25]. In Schryvers's study on large number of SCI patients with pressure ulcers during 20 years, a large number of patients needed surgical intervention. Pelvic area ulcers were the most common (468 of 598 pressure ulcers), of which 431 (92%) were treated surgically. Fasciocutaneous or cutaneous flaps, muscle or musculocutaneous flaps and primary closures were the most common surgical intervention. During the ulcer management, some bone intervention is unavoidable [29]. Medical honey has a substantial efficacy on wound management and control of infection of pressure ulcer, as shown by low bacterial growth, decreased wound size, and improved healing stage [30].

Electric stimulation therapy (EST) accelerates pressure ulcer healing in SCI patients. Pressure ulcer healing is determined by decrease in wound size and improvement in wound appearance after 3 months of treatment with EST [31]. Use of ultraviolet light C (light wavelength 200–290 nm) may be effective in treatment. It can be because of its potency in killing antibiotic-resistant microorganisms. *Staphylococcus aureus*, methicillin-resistant *Staphylococcus aureus* (MRSA) and *Pseudomonas aeruginosa* that may be resident on superficial layer of wound may be killed by ultraviolet light C [32]. Maggot therapy may also be used a subsidiary way to treat wound ulcer. Live blowfly larvae in wound dressings accelerate wound healing by increasing debridement. They can debride necrotic tissue within 1 week that is so rapid in nonsurgical wound management. It is safe, simple, and inexpensive, and it seems that it has no complications, so it can be used for treatment of pressure ulcers in SCI patients [33].

2.2.3. Prevention

Pressure ulcers certainly have a great influence on daily activity and life of SCI patients [34]. The best position and the turning frequency are not clear, but avoiding the 90° lateral position is recommended. This position will bring about high pressure over the trochanters with the risk of pressure ulcer development. The risk of developing pressure ulcer is highly individualized and the SCI patient is at a significant risk. Prevention strategies in seating position and in bed are very important in this group to prevent pressure ulcer, and so, pressure relief maneuvers can be important [35]. Pressure relief, position changes, and regular and frequent observation of skin, especially on the pressure areas, that is, over the bony prominences can prevent pressure ulcer development [2]. Pressure ulcers can also be prevented by improvement of neurologic functions and reducing the time of hospitalization and rehabilitation stay [36]. Pressure ulcer prevention is strongly associated with lifestyle modification [35]. Frequent change of position and use of pressure-relieving devices have important roles in reducing the pressure ulcer development. Some risk factors other than pressure may be important in developing ulcer. In SCI patients who do not have vasomotor control below the level of the lesion, hypoxemia will develop, and it can be an important risk factor. So, pressure ulcers may be prevented not only by reducing external pressure by pressure relief, but also by increasing the patient's resistance to pressure, by increasing tissue oxygenation [37]. One of the important risk factors that may increase skin and soft tissue infections is resistant bacterial colonization. Some activities such as hand hygiene, contact precautions, and cultural changes are associated with significant declines in bacterial infection, especially MRSA colonization and infection [28].

2.3. Osteomyelitis

One of the complications of spinal cord injury is osteomyelitis. Osteomyelitis may develop by extension of infection from pressure ulcers [38]. After spinal fixation surgery, osteomyelitis may be developed, as a complication of surgery. Osteomyelitis increases the treatment cost and may lead to other complications [39].

2.3.1. Diagnosis

There are several diagnostic methods for diagnosis of osteomyelitis in SCI patients.

Bone biopsy is the gold standard, and magnetic resonance imaging (MRI) is usually used as a sensitive and specific modality. Several organisms are known as causative agents. The most common isolated organisms are *Staphylococcus aureus*, Peptostreptococcus, and Bacteroides. Coagulase-negative staphylococci, group B Streptococcus, Proteus, and group milleri Streptococcus may also be isolated as less common agents. The diagnosis of pelvic osteomyelitis is difficult and may need multiple bone biopsies. At least three bone samples may be necessary to detect the pathogen and exclusion of contamination. In one study, sensitivity of MRI for diagnosis of pelvic pressure ulcer osteomyelitis was 94% and specificity was 22% [40].

However, Huang's study demonstrates that MRI is a sensitive method for diagnosis of osteomyelitis in SCI population. MRI can be used to demonstrate the extension of infection and to guide limited surgical resection and preserve viable tissue [41]. Pelvic pressure ulcers that accompany osteomyelitis may show cortical erosion and bone marrow edema in MRI [42]. In SCI patients, abscesses, fluid collections, and sinus tracts can be detected by MRI [43]. For diagnosis of osteomyelitis, gallium scan and plain pelvis X-ray may be used. Negative bone scan can rule out osteomyelitis. However, chronic ulcers usually accompany osteomyelitis. Delayed healing or recurrence of pressure ulcers has no clear association with osteomyelitis [44]. Computerized tomography and Technetium-99 m bone scans are not usually used for diagnosis of osteomyelitis in SCI patients with pressure sores [45].

2.3.2. Treatment

Treatment of osteomyelitis is composed of two parts: surgical management and medical treatment. Surgical approach is in fact debridement and in some patients, muscle flap. Medical therapy is in fact antibiotic therapy and wound care. Hyperbaric oxygen may be used in refractory osteomyelitis [46]. Treatment of osteomyelitis is prolonged and so, expensive. Using surgical debridement can shorten the duration of antibiotic therapy for osteomyelitis in SCI patients. In SCI patients with bony prominence osteomyelitis, surgical debridement and flap coverage of the sore can influence the outcome of antibiotic treatment [47]. Antibiotics for treatment are chosen according to the results of culture.

2.3.3. Prevention

Measures for prevention of osteomyelitis are in fact those that were mentioned in Section 2.3.1 for prevention of pressure ulcer and skin and soft tissue infection. The main preventive measures are pressure relief, regular change of position, and frequent observation of the skin over bony prominences.

2.4. Pneumonia

Pulmonary complications in SCI patients are important, as they may be life threatening. Pneumonia, pulmonary infarction, pulmonary thromboembolism, chest injury, and atelectasis are the most frequent and important complications in these patients. Pneumonia is one of the most important pulmonary complications. It may have developed shortly after spinal cord injury, during hospitalization or even in rehabilitation periods. The risk of pneumonia is greater in post-injury period. In this phase, the patients usually do not have effective cough. If the phrenic and intercostal nerves have been damaged, the respiration cycle may be influenced and the patients may be prone to pneumonia [48]. After intubation and mechanical ventilation, ventilator-associated pneumonia (VAP) may develop. VAP is in fact the occurrence of pneumonia in patients with mechanical ventilation, occurring more than 48 h after endotracheal intubation [49]. VAP is the most frequent nosocomial infection in patients with mechanical ventilation and is associated with longer intensive care unit stay, longer duration of mechanical ventilation, and high morbidity and mortality [4].

2.4.1. Diagnosis

Pneumonia is diagnosed by signs and symptoms of respiratory infection and according to criteria for diagnosis of nosocomial pneumonia and VAP. By endotracheal culture, the causative organism is found and an antibiotic is chosen according to the result of culture. The most common organisms are *Pseudomonas aeruginosa*, *Klebsiella pneumonia*, *Acinetobacter baumannii* [50],

Serratia marcescens [51] and methicillin-resistant *Staphylococcus aureus* [52]. Chest radiograph accompanied by clinical and laboratory findings are required for diagnosis of patients with suspected VAP [53].

2.4.2. Treatment

Antibiotics are chosen according to endotracheal secretion culture. For empirical treatment, combination antibiotic therapy is necessary. In this combination, an anti-pseudomonas agent (that is usually effective on other gram negative organisms) such as imipenem, meropenem, piperacillin-tazobactam or cefepime in addition to an aminoglycoside or a quinolone is used. For coverage of Methicillin-resistant *Staphylococcus aureus* (MRSA), vancomycin is usually added to this combination. For a special situation such as multidrug-resistant Acinetobacter or Pseudomona, the appropriate antibiotic (like colistin) is elected according to culture. The rising rates of antimicrobial resistance have led to the routine empiric administration of broad-spectrum antibiotics even when bacterial infection is not documented [52].

2.4.3. Prevention

One important risk factor for developing pneumonia is retained secretion. So, pulmonary toilet is important in these patients. Appropriate positioning and cough assistance can be useful for clearing retained secretions. Sometimes early intubation may be necessary to prevent secretion retaining by frequent suctioning [48]. Using effective oral care with antiseptics is associated with the reduction of the incidence of ventilator-associated pneumonia. Oral care solutions have been widely used to prevent ventilator-associated pneumonia [49]. Routine cleaning and disinfection of ventilators can play an important role in VAP prevention and management approach [53].

2.5. Other infections

Blood stream infection secondary to urinary tract infections, pneumonia, pressure ulcers [48], catheter-related bloodstream infections [54], and infections at other sites may occur in SCI patients. Meningitis may occur after penetrating injuries or as a result of CSF leakage at the time of injury or subsequent to surgery [48]. Epidural abscess and subdural empyema can be developed with the same mechanisms. Ventilator-associated tracheobronchitis (VAT) is an infective complication of mechanical ventilation and is a part of the spectrum of ventilator-associated respiratory infections [55].

3. Conclusion

Infectious diseases after spinal cord injury are important and should be considered in patients with fever and other signs and symptoms of infections. Appropriate approach, diagnosis, and treatment and surgical interventions, if needed, can be lifesaving and can decrease mortality and morbidity.

Acknowledgements

With special thanks to Dr. Hadi Niknam, my dear neurosurgeon colleague, and Mrs. Shadi Nasrizadeh Moghaddam.

Author details

Farhad Abbasi* and Soolmaz Korooni

*Address all correspondence to: f_abbasi55@yahoo.com

Bushehr University of Medical Sciences, Bushehr, Iran

References

[1] Mawson AR, Biundo JJ Jr, Neville P, Linares HA, Winchester Y, Lopez A. Risk factors for early occurring pressure ulcers following spinal cord injury. American Journal of Physical Medicine & Rehabilitation. 1988;**67**(3):123-127

[2] Hoff JM, Bjerke LW, Gravem PE, Hagen EM, Rekand T. Pressure ulcers after spinal cord injury. Tidsskrift for den Norske Lægeforening. 2012;**132**(7):838-839

[3] Lehman CA. Risk factors for pressure ulcers in the spinal cord injured in the community. SCI Nursing. 1995;**12**(4):110-114

[4] Sachdeva D, Singh D, Loomba P, Kaur A, Tandon M, Bishnoi I. Assessment of surgical risk factors in the development of ventilator-associated pneumonia in neurosurgical intensive care unit patients: Alarming observations. Neurology India. 2017;**65**(4):779-784

[5] Chacko R, Rajan A, Lionel P, Thilagavathi M, Yadav B, Premkumar J. Oral decontamination techniques and ventilator-associated pneumonia. The British Journal of Nursing. 2017;**26**(11):594-599

[6] Dinh A, Saliba M, Saadeh D, Bouchand F, Descatha A, Roux AL, Davido B, Clair B, Denys P, Annane D, Perronne C, Bernard L. Blood stream infections due to multidrug-resistant organisms among spinal cord-injured patients, epidemiology over 16 years and associated risks: A comparative study. Spinal Cord. 2016;**54**(9):720-725

[7] Adrie C, Garrouste-Orgeas M, Ibn Essaied W, Schwebel C, Darmon M, Mourvillier B, Ruckly S, Dumenil AS, Kallel H, Argaud L, Marcotte G, Barbier F, Laurent V, Goldgran-Toledano D, Clec'h C, Azoulay E, Souweine B, Timsit JF. Attributable mortality of ICU-acquired bloodstream infections: Impact of the source, causative micro-organism, resistance profile and antimicrobial therapy. The Journal of Infection. 2017;**74**(2):131-141

[8] Shindo Y, Hasegawa Y. Regional differences in antibiotic-resistant pathogens in patients with pneumonia: Implications for clinicians. Respirology. 2017;**22**(8):1536-1546

[9] Biering-Sorensen F, Bagi P, Hoiby N. Urinary tract infections in patients with spinal cord lesions: Treatment and prevention. Drugs. 2001;**61**(9):1275-1287

[10] Tofte N, Nielsen AC, Trøstrup H, Andersen CB, Von Linstow M, Hansen B, Biering-Sorensen F, Hoiby N, Moser C. Chronic urinary tract infections in patients with spinal cord lesions—Biofilm infection with need for long-term antibiotic treatment. APMIS. 2017;**125**(4):385-391

[11] Siroky MB. Pathogenesis of bacteriuria and infection in the spinal cord injured patient. The American Journal of Medicine. 2002;**113**(Suppl 1A):67S-79S

[12] Bossa L, Kline K, McDougald D, Lee BB, Rice SA. Urinary catheter-associated microbiota change in accordance with treatment and infection status. PLoS One. 2017;**12**(6):e0177633. DOI: 10.1371/journal.pone.0177633. eCollection 2017

[13] Moola S, Konno R. A systematic review of the management of short-term indwelling urethral catheters to prevent urinary tract infections. JBI Library of Systematic Reviews. 2010;**8**(17):695-729

[14] National Institute On Disability And Rehabilitation Research. Prevention and management of urinary tract infections among people with SCI: Consensus statement. NeuroRehabilitation. 1994;**4**(4):222-236

[15] García Leoni ME, Esclarín De Ruz A. Management of urinary tract infection in patients with spinal cord injuries. Clinical Microbiology and Infection. 2003;**9**(8):780-785

[16] Lee BB, Toh SL, Ryan S, Simpson JM, Clezy K, Bossa L, Rice SA, Marial O, Weber G, Kaur J, Boswell-Ruys C, Goodall S, Middleton J, Tudehope M, Kotsiou G. Probiotics versus placebo as prophylaxis for urinary tract infection in persons with spinal cord injury: A study protocol for a randomised controlled trial. BMC Urology. 2016;**16**:18

[17] Tenke P, Kovacs B, Bjerklund Johansen TE, Matsumoto T, Tambyah PA, Naber KG. European and Asian guidelines on management and prevention of catheter-associated urinary tract infections. International Journal of Antimicrobial Agents. 2008;**31**(Suppl 1): S68-S78

[18] Cardenas DD, Moore KN, Dannels-McClure A, Scelza WM, Graves DE, Brooks M, Busch AK. Intermittent catheterization with a hydrophilic-coated catheter delays urinary tract infections in acute spinal cord injury: A prospective, randomized, multicenter trial. PM & R. 2011;**3**(5):408-417

[19] Nicolle LE. Catheter-related urinary tract infection. Drugs & Aging. 2005;**22**(8):627-639

[20] Darouiche RO, Al Mohajer M, Siddiq DM, Minard CG. Short versus long course of antibiotics for catheter-associated urinary tract infections in patients with spinal cord injury: A randomized controlled noninferiority trial. Archives of Physical Medicine and Rehabilitation. 2014;**95**(2):290-296

[21] Linsenmeyer TA, Harrison B, Oakley A, Kirshblum S, Stock JA, Millis SR. Evaluation of cranberry supplement for reduction of urinary tract infections in individuals

with neurogenic bladders secondary to spinal cord injury. A prospective, double-blinded, placebo-controlled, crossover study. The Journal of Spinal Cord Medicine. 2004;**27**(1):29-34

[22] Guihan M, Bombardier CH. Potentially modifiable risk factors among veterans with spinal cord injury hospitalized for severe pressure ulcers: A descriptive study. The Journal of Spinal Cord Medicine. 2012;**35**(4):240-250

[23] Sunn G. Spinal cord injury pressure ulcer treatment: An experience-based approach. Physical Medicine and Rehabilitation Clinics of North America. 2014;**25**(3):671-680

[24] Dana AN, Bauman WA. Bacteriology of pressure ulcers in individuals with spinal cord injury: What we know and what we should know. The Journal of Spinal Cord Medicine. 2015;**38**(2):147-160

[25] Biglari B, Büchler A, Reitzel T, Swing T, Gerner HJ, Ferbert T, Moghaddam A. A retrospective study on flap complications after pressure ulcer surgery in spinal cord-injured patients. Spinal Cord. 2014;**52**(1):80-83

[26] Salzberg CA, Byrne DW, Cayten CG, van Niewerburgh P, Murphy JG, Viehbeck M. A new pressure ulcer risk assessment scale for individuals with spinal cord injury. American Journal of Physical Medicine & Rehabilitation. 1996;**75**(2):96-104

[27] Vaziri ND, Eltorai I, Gonzales E, Winer RL, Pham H, Bui TD, Said S. Pressure ulcer, fibronectin, and related proteins in spinal cord injured patients. Archives of Physical Medicine and Rehabilitation. 1992;**73**(9):803-806

[28] Han ZA, Choi JY, Ko YJ. Dermatological problems following spinal cord injury in Korean patients. The Journal of Spinal Cord Medicine. 2015;**38**(1):63-67

[29] Schryvers OI, Stranc MF, Nance PW. Surgical treatment of pressure ulcers: 20-year experience. Archives of Physical Medicine and Rehabilitation. 2000;**81**(12):1556-1562

[30] Biglari B, Linden PH, Simon A, Aytac S, Gerner HJ, Moghaddam A. Use of Medihoney as a non-surgical therapy for chronic pressure ulcers in patients with spinal cord injury. Spinal Cord. 2012;**50**(2):165-169

[31] Houghton PE, Campbell KE, Fraser CH, Harris C, Keast DH, Potter PJ, Hayes KC, Woodbury MG. Electrical stimulation therapy increases rate of healing of pressure ulcers in community-dwelling people with spinal cord injury. Archives of Physical Medicine and Rehabilitation. 2010;**91**(5):669-678

[32] Thai TP, Keast DH, Campbell KE, Woodbury MG, Houghton PE. Effect of ultraviolet light C on bacterial colonization in chronic wounds. Ostomy/Wound Management. 2005;**51**(10):32-45

[33] Sherman RA, Wyle F, Vulpe M. Maggot therapy for treating pressure ulcers in spinal cord injury patients. The Journal of Spinal Cord Medicine. 1995;**18**(2):71-74

[34] Lala D, Dumont FS, Leblond J, Houghton PE, Noreau L. Impact of pressure ulcers on individuals living with a spinal cord injury. Archives of Physical Medicine and Rehabilitation. 2014;**95**(12):2312-2319

[35] Groah SL, Schladen M, Pineda CG, Hsieh CH. Prevention of pressure ulcers among people with spinal cord injury: A systematic review. PM &R. 2015;**7**(6):613-636

[36] Celani MG, Spizzichino L, Ricci S, Zampolini M, Franceschini M. Spinal cord injury in Italy: A multicenter retrospective study. Archives of Physical Medicine and Rehabilitation. 2001;**82**(5):589-596

[37] Mawson AR, Siddiqui FH, Biundo JJ Jr. Enhancing host resistance to pressure ulcers: A new approach to prevention. Preventive Medicine. 1993;**22**(3):433-450

[38] Eltorai I, Hart GB, Strauss MB. Osteomyelitis in the spinal cord injured: A review and a preliminary report on the use of hyperbaric oxygen therapy. Paraplegia. 1984;**22**(1):17-24

[39] Rennert R, Golinko M, Yan A, Flattau A, Tomic-Canic M, Brem H. Developing and evaluating outcomes of an evidence-based protocol for the treatment of osteomyelitis in Stage IV pressure ulcers: A literature and wound electronic medical record database review. Ostomy/Wound Management. 2009;**55**(3):42-53

[40] Brunel AS, Lamy B, Cyteval C, Perrochia H, Téot L, Masson R, Bertet H, Bourdon A, Morquin D, Reynes J, Le Moing V. Diagnosing pelvic osteomyelitis beneath pressure ulcers in spinal cord injured patients: A prospective study. Clinical Microbiology Infection. 2016;**22**(3):267

[41] Huang AB, Schweitzer ME, Hume E, Batte WG. Osteomyelitis of the pelvis/hips in paralyzed patients: Accuracy and clinical utility of MRI. Journal of Computer Assisted Tomography. 1998;**22**(3):437-443

[42] Hauptfleisch J, Meagher TM, Hughes RJ, Singh JP, Graham A, López de Heredia L. Interobserver agreement of magnetic resonance imaging signs of osteomyelitis in pelvic pressure ulcers in patients with spinal cord injury. Archives of Physical Medicine and Rehabilitation. 2013;**94**(6):1107-1111

[43] Ruan CM, Escobedo E, Harrison S, Goldstein B. Magnetic resonance imaging of non-healing pressure ulcers and myocutaneous flaps. Archives of Physical Medicine and Rehabilitation. 1998;**79**(9):1080-1088

[44] Thornhill-Joynes M, Gonzales F, Stewart CA, Kanel GC, Lee GC, Capen DA, Sapico FL, Canawati HN, Montgomerie JZ. Osteomyelitis associated with pressure ulcers. Archives of Physical Medicine and Rehabilitation. 1986;**67**(5):314-318

[45] Lewis VL, Bailey MH, Pulawski G, Kind G, Bashioum RW, Hendrix RW. The diagnosis of osteomyelitis in patients with pressure sores. Plastic and Reconstructive Surgery. 1988;**81**(2):229-232

[46] Deloach ED, DiBenedetto RJ, Womble L, Gilley JD. The treatment of osteomyelitis underlying pressure ulcers. Decubitus. 1992;**5**(6):32-41

[47] Marriott R, Rubayi S. Successful truncated osteomyelitis treatment for chronic osteomyelitis secondary to pressure ulcers in spinal cord injury patients. Annals of Plastic Surgery. 2008;**61**(4):425-429

[48] John Z. Montgomerie. Infections in patients with spinal cord injuries. Clinical Infectious Diseases. 1997;**25**:1285-1292

[49] Zhang Z, Hou Y, Zhang J, Wang B, Zhang J, Yang A, Li G, Tian J. Comparison of the effect of oral care with four different antiseptics to prevent ventilator-associated pneumonia in adults: Protocol for a network meta-analysis. Systmatic Review. 2017;**6**(1):103

[50] Ergul AB, Cetin S, Altintop YA, Bozdemir SE, Ozcan A, Altug U, Samsa H, Torun YA. Evaluation of microorganisms causing ventilator-associated pneumonia in a pediatric intensive care unit. The Eurasian Journal of Medicine. 2017;**49**(2):87-91

[51] Souza LCD, Mota VBRD, Carvalho AVDSZ, Corrêa RDGCF, Libério SA, Lopes FF. Association between pathogens from tracheal aspirate and oral biofilm of patients on mechanical ventilation. Brazilian Oral Research. 2017;**31**:e3

[52] Kollef MH, Burnham CD. Ventilator-associated pneumonia: The role of emerging diagnostic technologies. Seminars in Respiratory and Critical Care Medicine. 2017;**38**(3):253-263

[53] Guo L, Li G, Wang J, Zhao X, Wang S, Zhai L, Jia H, Cao B. Suspicious outbreak of ventilator-associated pneumonia caused by Burkholderia cepacia in a surgical intensive care unit. American Journal of Infection Control. 2017;**45**(6):660-666

[54] Saliba M, Saadeh D, Bouchand F, Davido B, Duran C, Clair B, Lawrence C, Annane D, Denys P, Salomon J, Bernard L, Dinh A. Outcome of bloodstream infections among spinal cord injury patients and impact of multidrug-resistant organisms. Spinal Cord. 2017;**55**(2):148-154

[55] Ray U, Ramasubban S, Chakravarty C, Goswami L, Dutta S. A prospective study of ventilator-associated tracheobronchitis: Incidence and etiology in intensive care unit of a tertiary care hospital. Lung India. 2017;**34**(3):236-240

4

Normal Distribution and Plasticity of Serotonin Receptors after Spinal Cord Injury and Their Impacts on Motor Outputs

Mengliang Zhang

Abstract

Following spinal cord injury (SCI) a series of anatomical and functional plastic changes occur in the spinal cord, including reorganization of the spinal neuronal network, alteration of properties of interneurons and motoneurons as well as up- or down-regulation of different neurotransmitter receptors. In mammalian spinal cord, one of the important neurotransmitters, serotonin (5-HT), plays an essential role in modulating sensory, motor and autonomic functions. Following SCI, especially complete spinal cord lesion, the descending supply of 5-HT is lost. As a consequence different 5-HT receptors undergo variant degrees of plastic changes.

In this chapter I have systematically reviewed the distribution of different 5-HT receptors in the spinal cord and their plastic changes following SCI where applicable. In addition, the plastic changes of 5-HT supplying system in reaction to SCI have also been reviewed. These results indicate that 5-HT receptors are important factors not only for modulation of normal motor function, their plastic changes are also critical for motor functional recovery and, quite often, for the development of certain pathological states after SCI. Pharmacological and/or genetic intervention of selected 5-HT receptors and/or intrinsic 5-HT producing system in the spinal cord may pave new ways for the restoration of motor functions after SCI.

Keywords: monoamine, monoamine receptor, spinal cord, motor control, intraspinal 5-HT cell

1. Introduction

Spinal cord injury (SCI) is a devastating condition with an incidence of 10–83 per million people per year worldwide according to statistical data from different countries [1]. It leads to an extensive and usually irreversible loss of sensory functions, voluntary motor control, and autonomic functions below injury level. A variety of primary and secondary complications occur depending on the severity of the injury and time course of its development. These symptoms may involve different systems, manifesting as, e.g., paralysis, spasticity, neuropathic pain, pulmonary and cardiovascular problems, osteoporosis, anemia, pressure ulcers, bladder and bowel problems, and sexual dysfunction [2–8]. Currently, there is no cure for SCI and thus improving quality of life, such as restoration of partial motor and sensory functions, has become a priority for setting up the treatment strategy. The primary cause of these problems is the loss of both descending and ascending projecting pathways in the spinal cord. The descending pathways include direct motor-initiating pathways, such as cortical spinal tracts, and modulatory pathways, such as serotonergic, dopaminergic, and noradrenergic pathways. These monoaminergic systems are so important that in either acute or chronic SCI direct stimulation of the receptors of these monoamines with drugs could regain locomotor activity in animals [9–17]. Thus, restoring the function of monoaminergic systems has become a key strategy to restore motor function and ameliorate secondary symptoms [18–23].

So far a great number of studies have been focusing on the serotonergic system in SCI. In the mammalian spinal cord, serotonin (5-HT) originates mainly in the raphe nuclei of the brainstem and plays an important role in modulating sensory, motor, and autonomic function [24–27]. Following SCI, especially complete spinal cord lesion, the descending supply of 5-HT is lost and as a consequence different 5-HT receptors undergo variant degrees of plastic changes [22, 28–36]. In addition, a potential intraspinal 5-HT-producing system in the spinal cord, i.e., aromatic L-amino acid decarboxylase (AADC) cells, also undergoes plastic changes to increase their potency to produce 5-HT from its precursor [37–40]. Although these plastic changes may induce pathological symptoms such as spasticity and chronic central pain [34, 41, 42], they are essential for spinal function recovery (for review see [43–45]). In this chapter, I will make a systematic review according to up-to-date literature related to the distribution and plastic changes of 5-HT receptors in the spinal cord in normal or SCI states with a note on the intraspinal 5-HT-producing cells.

2. 5-HT in the spinal cord in health

In mammals, including humans, 5-HT axons in the spinal cord almost exclusively originate from the brainstem raphe nuclei [46–49]. Their terminals are distributed in all parts of the gray matter at all levels of the spinal cord [50, 51]. The cell bodies with descending 5-HT projections are located in the caudal part of the raphe nuclei, which include the raphe magnus, raphe obscurus, raphe pallidus, ventral lateral medulla, and the area postrema [52]. In the spinal cord, 5-HT projecting fibers descend in the white matter through two different routes: one with fibers from the raphe magnus in the dorsal part of the lateral funiculus which terminates mainly in the dorsal horn, and the other with fibers from raphe obscurus and raphe pallidus in the ventral funiculus which terminates mainly in the ventral horn and the intermediate zone.

In addition to the descending projecting system, there are indeed 5-HT neurons in the spinal cord although in normal states their contribution of 5-HT can be ignored. So far a small number of intraspinal 5-HT neurons have been reported in macaque monkey (ca. 150 cells per monkey [53]), rat (3–9 cells per rat [54, 55]), and mouse [51]. In the rat spinal cord, 5-HT cells were distributed in different parts of the spinal cord with the exception of cervical segments; in the monkey spinal cord most of the cells were observed in the cervical segments with a small number in other segments; whereas in the mouse spinal cord they were exclusively located in the sacral segments. In the rat spinal cord, the 5-HT cells were found to be located in laminae VII and X in the gray matter, whereas in monkey and mouse spinal cord they were exclusively found in lamina X.

Serotonin in the spinal cord plays an important role in sensory information processing, motor control, and autonomic function. Traditionally, it is hypothesized that 5-HT in the spinal cord exerts its effects by inhibiting sensory systems and facilitating motor systems [56]. However, now it is known that the effects of 5-HT are very complicated both in sensory and motor aspects. In sensory aspect, 5-HT not only has antinociceptive but also pronociceptive effects (e.g., [57, 58]). In motor aspect, except for facilitating motor output, 5-HT also inhibits motor behavior (e.g., [59, 60]). The different functions that 5-HT exert at different circumstances depend on many factors, such as the brainstem origins of the descending projections, the termination localizations of these fibers in the spinal cord, and the activation states of its different receptors.

3. 5-HT receptors in the spinal cord in health

The diverse functions of 5-HT in the spinal cord are achieved through the activation of different 5-HT receptors. As seen in **Table 1**, seven families (or types) and at least 14 subfamilies (or subtypes) of 5-HT receptors have been identified so far [61]. In these seven families, with exception of 5-HT3 receptors that are ligand-gated ion channels, all other families are G protein-coupled receptors [62]. To better understand the diversity of 5-HT functions, it is fundamentally important to have the knowledge of the anatomical localizations of different 5-HT receptors in the spinal cord. A majority, though not all, of 5-HT receptor subfamilies have been found to be expressed in the spinal cord (for reviews see [63, 64]). Here, I will make a systematic review of these receptors in terms of their cellular as well as subcellular localizations in the spinal cord based on available data. One should keep in mind that due to the existence of a great number of splices and editing variants for several 5-HT receptors, a greater degree of operational diversity could be expected, though this issue is not the focus of the present review.

Receptor family (year of molecular gene clone)*	Receptor subfamily (year of molecular gene clone)*	Expression in the spinal cord	Functions at normal states	Expression changes following SCI	Functions at SCI states
5-HT1	1A (1987)	Primary afferent fibers in dorsal horn [66]; neuronal somata in different laminae of gray matter [31,69]; axon initial segments [31,71];	Antinociception [73,76]; pronociception [77]; increases motoneuron excitability [60]; induces central fatigue [81]	Upregulation at least to 30 days after SCI [28,31]	Promotes motor functional recovery [13,14,172]
	1B (1992)	Primary afferent fibers in dorsal horn [83]; neuronal somata at least in intermediate zone [38]	Antinociception [72]; autoreceptor [89]; inhibits activity of AADC cells [38]	--	Inhibits mono- and polysynaptic reflexes [99,174]
	1D (1991)	Primary afferent fibers in dorsal horn [92]; gamma motoneurons in ventral horn [94]	Antinociception, [93]; modulates proprioceptive circuits [94]	--	Inhibits polysynaptic reflex [95]??
	1E (1992)	--	--	--	--
	1F (1993)	Substantia gelatinosa of spinal dorsal horn [98]	Antinociception [101,102]??	--	Inhibits polysynaptic reflex [99]??
5-HT2	2A (1988)	Different laminae of the spinal gray matter but largely in the superficial dorsal horn and lamina IX	Pronociceptive [57,112]; antinociceptive [115]; excites motoneuron [117]; facilitates micturition reflex [119]; facilitates sexual behavior	Upregulation [32,33,35]	Locomotor functional recovery [12,14,43]; 5-HT supersensitivity and muscle spasm [42]

Receptor family (year of molecular gene clone)*	Receptor subfamily (year of molecular gene clone)*	Expression in the spinal cord	Functions at normal states	Expression changes following SCI	Functions at SCI states
		[104,107,108]	[120,121]		
	2B (1992)	Dorsal horn (probably primary afferent fibers) [109]	Pronociception [109,124,126]	Constitutive activation [182]	Motoneuron hyperexcitability and muscle spasm [182]
	2C (1988) (Named 1C before 1993)	Different laminae of the spinal gray matter [36,104,107]	Pronociception [57,112]; antinociception [96,115,133]; induces long-lasting amplification of spinal reflexes [73,134]; inhibits micturition reflex [127,138]	Constitutive activation [34,182]; upregulation [22,36,177]	Motor functional recovery [34,182]; 5-HT supersensitivity, motoneuron hyperexcitability, and muscle spasm [34,42,182]
5-HT3	3A (1991) 3B (1999) 3C (2003) 3D (2003) 3E (2003) [62,139]	Different laminae of the spinal gray matter [107,142]	Antinociception [145,146]; pronociception [149]; mediates tail-flick reflexes [117]; inhibits bladder function [152]	--	Promotes motor function recovery [151]
5-HT4 (1995)		Ventral horn, some sympathetic neurons [153]	Pronociception [154]	--	--
5-HT5	5A (1994)	Dorsal horn, intermediate lateral nucleus, and Onuf's nucleus [110,156]	Antinociception [58,157]; autonomic and micturition control [156]	--	--
	5B (1993)	--	--	--	--
5-HT6 (1993)		Different laminae of the spinal gray matter [159]	Pronociception [160]	--	--
5-HT7 (1993)		Dorsal horn, intermediate zone, and ventral horn	Pronociception [164–166]; promotes locomotion		Promotes locomotor functional

Receptor family (year of molecular gene clone)*	Receptor subfamily (year of molecular gene clone)*	Expression in the spinal cord	Functions at normal states	Expression changes following SCI	Functions at SCI states
		with a dorsoventral density gradient [16,162]	[16,167,169]		recovery [43,172]

* Year of molecular gene clone is based on Wikipedia (https://en.wikipedia.org/wiki/5HT_receptor) except 5-HT3 receptors; --: no data available; ??: data not conclusive.

Table 1. 5-HT receptors in the spinal cord and plastic changes following SCI.

3.1. 5-HT1 receptors

As listed in **Table 1**, 5-HT1 receptors include five subfamilies: 1A, 1B, 1D, 1E, and 1F. Although all of these receptors have been detected in the brain by different techniques [65], there is no report to my knowledge demonstrating the expression of 5-HT1E receptors in the spinal cord. In addition, the evidence of the existence of 5-HT1F in the spinal cord is mainly from physiological experiments. Nonetheless, I will describe 5-HT1A, 1B, 1D, and 1F in the spinal cord according to the available data.

5-HT1A receptors: Data from both autoradiographic (radioligand binding) and immunohistochemical experiments have demonstrated the presence of 5-HT1A receptors in different regions of the spinal gray matter across different spinal segments in rats [31, 66–69]. 5-HT1A receptor binding sites were predominantly seen in the dorsal horn especially laminae I and II [67], where they were partly located in the primary afferent fibers [66]. In autoradiographic images, it is difficult to identify the components located in cell bodies; however, with immunohistochemistry with a 5-HT1A antibody generated from an intracellular epitope, it was clear that 5-HT1A receptors were expressed in cell bodies in the spinal cord [31]. The immunolabeled cell bodies were located in different spinal regions in the gray matter including the dorsal horn, intermediate zone, and ventral horn [31, 69, 70]. In addition, using a different 5-HT1A antibody generated from an extracellular epitope, the receptors were also shown to be present in the axon hillock [31, 71]. There are no studies to investigate 5-HT1A receptor localization at an ultrastructural level and therefore no data available for their subcellular distribution.

It is commonly believed that 5-HT1A receptors exert an inhibitory effect in sensory information transmission including nociception in the spinal dorsal horn (e.g., [72–76]). For example, in mice intrathecal injection of 5-HT1A receptor agonist 8-hydroxy-2-(di-*n*-propylamino) tetralin (8-OH-DPAT) could inhibit the tail-flicks induced by noxious radiant heat [72]. In neonatal rat spinal cord in vitro experiments, Hochman et al. [73] showed that 8-OH-DPAT depressed evoked excitatory postsynaptic potentials (EPSPs) in the deep dorsal horn neurons, whereas 5-HT1A receptor antagonist WAY-100635 (*N*-[2-[4-(2-methoxyphenyl)-1-

piperazinyl]ethyl]-N-(2-pyridyl)cyclohexanecarboxamide) facilitated evoked EPSPs. Data from the same group also indicated that the activation of 5-HT1A receptors facilitated long-term depression in the dorsal horn neurons. However, the effects of 5-HT1A receptors in the dorsal horn are not always inhibitory. For example, the activation of 5-HT1A receptors has been reported to facilitate nociceptive [77, 78] and itch transmission [79], and to induce spontaneous tail-flicks [80].

As 5-HT1A receptors have been found to be present both at the neuronal somata and the axon initial segments in spinal ventral horn neurons, including motoneurons [31], it is speculated that 5-HT1A receptors may have heterogeneous functions on motor outputs, i.e., both excitatory and inhibitory [59, 60]. Indeed, using a turtle spinal cord, slice preparation, and intracellular recording technique, Perrier and Cotel [60] demonstrated that the activation of 5-HT1A receptors by 8-OH-DPAT induced an increased excitability in a large fraction (9/11) of sampled motoneurons; whereas in a small fraction of motoneurons (2/11) 8-OH-DPAT gave a hyperpolarizing effect. Subsequent data from the same research group have demonstrated that the inhibitory effect was due to the activation of extrasynaptic 5-HT1A receptors located at the axon initial segments, a mechanism supposed to underlie central fatigue [81, 82].

5-HT1B receptors: To the best of my knowledge, there are no systematic immunohistochemical studies on the distribution of 5-HT1B receptors in the spinal cord. Previous studies using autoradiography have demonstrated that 5-HT1B receptors did not have any dominant expression region in the spinal gray matter although the intermediate zone seemed to dwell slightly higher labeled profiles [67, 68]. Although it is difficult to differentiate labeled cell bodies from nerve fibers with autoradiography, results from studies using other methods including lesion, pharmacology, and reverse transcription polymerase chain reaction (RT-PCT) indicated the existence of this receptor subfamily both at presynaptic (primary afferent fibers) [83] and postsynaptic locations (motoneurons) [84, 85]. Recently by using immunohistochemistry, Wienecke et al. [38] have found that 5-HT1B receptors were indeed expressed in the cell bodies at least in the intermediate zone in the rat spinal cord.

Similar to 5-HT1A receptors, a major role of 5-HT1B receptors is inhibition in sensory transmission, especially nociception [72, 86, 87]. For example, Eide et al. [72] showed that in mice intrathecal injection of 5-HT1B receptor antagonist RU-24969 (5-methoxy-3(1,2,3,6-tetrahydropyridin-4-yl)-1H-indole) induced a significant increase of tail-flick latencies. Another role of 5-HT1B receptors is to inhibit the release of 5-HT from its fibers via autoreceptor mechanism. Although both 5-HT1A and 1B receptors have been demonstrated to be autoreceptors in the brain, in the spinal cord it is most likely that 5-HT1B receptors play a more important role than 5-HT1A receptors in controlling the release of 5-HT from 5-HT fiber terminals [88–90]. Thus, Brown et al. [89] using rat spinal cord synaptosomes preparation showed that the 5-HT1B receptor agonists 1-(m-trifluoromethylphenyl)piperazine and 1-(m-chlorophenyl) piperazine concentration-dependently decreased [3H]5-HT release. In addition, 5-HT1B receptors could also inhibit the production of 5-HT from AADC cells in the spinal cord through feed-forward mechanism so that the AADC cells do not produce 5-HT in normal physiological states [38]. Another function of 5-HT1B receptors, as noted in mice, is to delay the maturation of γ-aminobutyric acid (GABA) phenotype in spinal cord during its development [91].

5-HT1D receptors: Data concerning the anatomical localization of 5-HT1D receptors in the spinal cord are relatively poor. The available data indicate that 5-HT1D receptors exist both in the dorsal and the ventral horn. Using immunohistochemistry, 5-HT1D receptors were found to be expressed in the primary afferent fibers in the superficial dorsal horn of the rat spinal cord [92, 93]. At the ultrastructural level, 5-HT1D receptors in the spinal cord dorsal horn were found to be localized exclusively within dense core vesicles of synaptic terminals and not the plasma membrane [92]. Using in situ hybridization and transgenic mouse model, Enjin et al. [94] found that 5-HT1D receptors were specifically expressed in γ motoneurons in the ventral horn as well as in some proprioceptive sensory neurons in different spinal regions which were coexpressed with parvalbumin (used as a proprioceptive neuronal marker in the study).

The available data indicate an effect of 5-HT1D receptors in the suppression of sensory, especially nociceptive, information transmission [58, 93, 95]. However, different results were also present. For example, in a formalin-induced hindpaw pain model, Jeong et al. [96] showed that the 5-HT1D receptor agonist GR-46611 (3-[3-(2-dimethylaminoethyl)-1*H*-indol-5-yl]-*N*-(4-methoxybenzyl)acrylamide) did not suppress the formalin-induced flinching responses and the 5-HT1D receptor antagonist BRL-15572 (3-(4-(4-chlorophenyl)piperazin-1-yl)-1,1-diphenyl-2-propanol) failed to reverse the antinociceptive effects of 5-HT. Other functions of 5-HT1D receptors include, e.g., depressing the spinal monosynaptic reflex induced by endogenously released 5-HT [97], and shaping proprioceptive circuits to receive and relay accurate sensory information in the spinal cord motor network [94]. In addition, since 5-HT1D receptors were expressed in γ, but not α, motoneurons, they could be used as a marker to identify γ motoneurons in the spinal cord [94].

5-HT1F receptors: To my knowledge, there is no systematic investigation concerning the expression of 5-HT1F receptors in the spinal cord of any species. However, there are indeed some pieces of evidence from studies using radioligand or physiological technique indicating that this receptor subfamily is present in the spinal cord dorsal horn. Castro et al. [98] used [3*H*]sumatriptan as a radioligand in the presence of suitable concentrations of 5-carboxamidotryptamine (5-CT) to define 5-HT1F receptors in the human spinal cord, and they found significant levels of binding sites in substantia gelatinosa in the cervical spinal cord. However, because 5-CT is not a specific 5-HT1F agonist, the data cannot be taken as granted. Using an in vitro sacrocaudal spinal cord preparation from spinal transected rats, Murray et al. [99] showed that the EPSPs and associated long polysynaptic reflexes were consistently inhibited by 5-HT1F-specific agonist LY-344864 (*N*-[(3*R*)-3-(dimethylamino)-2,3,4,9-tetrahydro-1*H*-carbazol-6-yl]-4-fluorobenzamide), indicating the existence of 5-HT1F in the spinal cord. However, the exact locations of these receptors are yet to be determined.

Due to the lack of related anatomical data, it is difficult to unveil the functions of 5-HT1F in the spinal cord. Considering that 5-HT1F receptors are expressed in the trigeminal and spinal dorsal root ganglia [100] and their agonists have been used to treat migraine [101, 102], it is most likely that this receptor subfamily exerts an antinociceptive effect in spinal cord.

3.2. 5-HT2 receptors

As listed in **Table 1**, 5-HT2 receptors include three subfamilies, i.e., 5-HT2A, 2B, and 2C. Before 1993, 5-HT2C receptors were named 5-HT1C receptors. [103]. By using different experimental techniques including autoradiography, in situ hybridization, Western blot and immunohistochemistry all these three receptor subfamilies have been detected in the spinal cord in different species [104–109] although 5-HT2C subfamily is probably not expressed in cat spinal cord [105]. 5-HT2A and 2C receptors are likely among the most thoroughly investigated 5-HT receptors in the spinal cord due to their important functions in both sensory information processing and motor control.

5-HT2A receptors: Using various techniques, the existence of 5-HT2A receptors has been confirmed at both mRNA and protein level in the spinal cord of different species [104–108, 110]. By using polymerase chain reaction (PCR) together with Southern hybridization technique, Helton et al. [105] showed that spinal cord tissues from rat, cat, monkey, and human contained 5-HT2A receptor mRNAs. By using in situ hybridization, Pompeiano et al. [104] showed that 5-HT2A receptor mRNAs were present at intermediate density in the ventral horn. This distribution pattern has been confirmed with immunohistochemistry [106, 108]. Doly et al. [108] systematically investigated the distribution of 5-HT2A receptor immunoreactivity in rat spinal cord and the results indicated that 5-HT2A receptors were distributed in all the spinal segments with a similar immunolabeling pattern. The most prominent labeling was found in lamina IX, where many, but not all, motoneurons were labeled. At lumbar five to six level, 5-HT2A receptors were densely expressed in Onuf's nucleus that contains the motoneurons innervating pelvic striated muscles controlling sexual behavior and micturition [110]. Another region with dense immunolabeling was lamina II. The remaining laminae of the gray matter displayed a weak to moderate labeling. Doly et al. [108] also examined the subcellular localization of 5-HT2A receptors in laminae II and IX and they demonstrated that most immunolabeled profiles were postsynaptic, i.e., dendrites and cell somata, although a small number of axons and axon terminals were also labeled. The immunoreactive product was localized mainly on the plasma membrane where synaptic specifications were lacking.

The localization of 5-HT2A receptors in the neurons in both the spinal dorsal and ventral horn endows their functions in both sensory information transmission and motor control. For the sensory information modulation, evidence to date largely favors in their pronociceptive role [57, 111–114]. For example, Kjørsvik et al. [112] showed that in formalin-induced pain model, intrathecal injection of DOI ((±)-2,5-dimethoxy-4-iodoamphetamine hydrochloride), a 5-HT2A/2C receptor agonist, augmented nociceptive response in rats. This effect could be completely abolished when ketanserin (a 5-HT-2A receptor antagonist) was coadministrated. Rahman et al. [57] investigated the effects of DOI, ketanserin, and ritanserin (another 5-HT2A/2C antagonist) on the evoked responses of dorsal horn neurons to electrical, mechanical, and thermal stimulation, and found that the activation of 5-HT2A receptors facilitated the spinal nociceptive transmission under normal physiological states. However, there is also evidence indicating that 5-HT2A receptors exert an antinociceptive effect [115, 116]. For example, using a rat spinal cord slice preparation Xie et al. [115] found that bath application of 5-HT increased the frequency of spontaneous inhibitory postsynaptic currents in GABAergic and glycinergic neurons in substantia gelatinosa. TCB-2 (4-bromo-3,6-dimethoxybenzocyclobut-en-1-yl)methylamine hydrobromide), a 5-HT2A receptor agonist, could mimic the 5-HT effect, and ketanserin could partially inhibit the effect of 5-HT and completely inhibit the effect of TCB-2.

It is not surprising that 5-HT2A receptors play a significant role in motor control considering their intensive expression in ventral horn motoneurons. Indeed, direct stimulation of 5-HT2 receptors in motoneurons in vivo with selective 5-HT2 receptor agonist DOI or DOM (2,5-dimethoxy-alpha,4-dimethylbenzene ethamine hydrochloride) produced dose-related back muscle contractions and wet dog shakes which could be markedly attenuated by ritanserin, ketanserin, or mianserin, suggesting an effect from 5-HT2A receptors [117]. Their direct facilitating effect on spinal motoneurons was also evidenced by application of DOI in rat spinal cord in vitro experiments [118]. In addition, pharmacological experiments showed that 5-HT2A receptor activation facilitated micturition reflex and activated the external urethral sphincter in female rats [119], whereas in both male and female rats 5-HT2A receptors seemed to involve sexual behavior [120, 121].

5-HT2B receptors: In comparison with 5-HT2A and 5-HT2C, 5-HT2B receptors in the spinal cord have been less investigated and the available data are inconsistent. Using in situ hybridization expression of 5-HT2B receptors was not found in rat spinal cord and even brain [104]. However, using several other techniques, the receptors have been detected in the spinal cord. Thus, using reverse transcription polymerase chain reaction (RT-PCR) 5-HT2B receptor mRNAs have been detected in spinal cord tissue in many different species including rat, cat, monkey, and human [105]. Using microarray global gene expression technique [122] and immunohistochemistry [123], 5-HT2B receptors have been detected in the rat spinal cord motoneurons. In addition, using Western blot it was shown that the receptor proteins were also present in the dorsal part of the spinal cord [109]. Considering that with Western blot and immunohistochemistry 5-HT2B receptors have been demonstrated to be expressed in the dorsal root ganglia [109, 124], their expression in the spinal dorsal horn is likely originating from the primary afferent fibers from the dorsal root ganglia, although it cannot be excluded that they might be also expressed in neuronal somata (e.g., [125]).

It is presumable that 5-HT2B receptors are largely related with sensory information transmission considering their localization in dorsal root ganglia and dorsal horn. Thus, evidence from a few studies related to 5-HT2B receptor functions in the spinal cord favors that the receptors are responsible for facilitating mechanical hyperalgesia, tactile allodynia, and nociception [109, 124, 126]. Studies concerning the receptors' motor function are rare. One study showed that 5-HT2B receptors likely increased urethral smooth muscle tone since the 5-HT2B receptor antagonist RS-127445 (3-(4-(4-chlorophenyl)piperazin-1-yl)-1,1-diphenyl-2-propanol) blocked increase in urethral pressure in female rats [127]. In frog, the activation of 5-HT2B receptors by α-methey-5-HT (a 5-HT2B receptor agonist) facilitates N-methyl-D-aspartate (NMDA)-induced depolarization of motoneurons [128]. In addition, 5-HT2B receptors seemed to modulate respiratory activity in rats [123].

5-HT2C receptors: 5-HT2C receptor mRNAs and proteins were widely distributed in different laminae of the spinal gray matter including motoneurons as demonstrated by different experimental methods, such as PCR [105], autoradiography [68, 129], in situ hybridization [104, 107], and immunohistochemistry [36, 130–132]. Using PCR combined with Southern hybridization 5-HT2C receptor mRNAs were detected in spinal cord tissue from rat, monkey, and human, but not in cat spinal cord [105]. By using in situ hybridization, Fonseca et al. [107] showed that 5-HT2C receptor mRNAs were present at high levels in most parts of the spinal gray matter, except lamina II. Using immunohistochemistry, Ren et al. [36] have investigated 5-HT2C receptor expression in both normal and spinalized rats and the results showed that 5-HT2C receptors were widely distributed in different regions of the spinal gray matter (except lamina II) and were predominantly located in the neuronal somata and their dendrites although they also seemed to be present in axonal fibers in the superficial dorsal horn. Thus, the data from in situ hybridization and immunohistochemistry fit very well for this receptor subfamily.

The wide distribution of 5-HT2C receptors in different laminae of the spinal cord endows the receptors' role both in sensory information transmission and motor control. For the sensory information transmission available data point to that 5-HT2C receptors play roles both in pronociception [57, 112] and antinociception [96, 115, 133]. For their role on pronociception, refer to the part concerning 5-HT2A receptors since most studies used DOI (a common agonist for 5-HT2A and 2C receptors) to stimulate and ketanserin to inhibit the receptors in response to different nociceptive stimulations. However, because ketanserin is mainly a 5-HT2A receptor antagonist some researchers argued that the pronociception effect should preferably attribute to 2-HT2A than 2C receptors. Their effects on antinociception seem to be adequately evidenced. For instance, in one study Jeong et al. [96] showed that in formalin-induced pain model 5-HT2C receptor specific antagonist D-MC (N-ormethylclozapine/8-chloro-11-(1-piperazinyl)-5H-dibenzo[b,e][1,4]diazepine) could block the suppression effect of 5-HT, whereas 5-HT2C receptor specific agonist MK-212 (6-chloro-2-(1-piperazinyl)pyrazine hydrochloride) could suppress the formalin response. In another study, Xie et al. [115] showed that a 5-HT2C receptor agonist WAY-161503 (8,9-dichloro-2,3,4,4a-tetrahydro-1H-pyrazino[1,2-a]quinoxalin-5(6H)) mimicked the 5-HT antinociceptive effect in dorsal horn neurons and this effect could be blocked by a 5-HT2C receptor antagonist, N-desmethylclozapine.

In motor control, one of the functions of 5-HT2C receptors is the induction of a long-lasting amplification of spinal reflex [73, 134–136]. Machacek et al. [134] showed that, in an in vitro neonatal rat spinal cord preparation, superfusion of 5-HT depressed reflex responses recorded in the ventral roots which was induced by electrical stimulation of primary afferents. However, following 5-HT washout, a long-lasting reflex facilitation was observed. Further pharmacological analysis indicated that it was the activation of 5-HT2C but not 5-HT2A receptors that was required for this long-lasting reflex. Although 5-HT2C receptors play a major role in long-term motor reflexes, they also play an inhibitory role in some physiological states. For example, in mice, when activated by DOI, 5-HT2C receptors inhibited the locomotor activity which opposed the effects of 5-HT2A receptors [137]. In addition, 5-HT2C receptors were also demonstrated to inhibit the micturition reflex [119, 127, 138]. Thus, Conlon et al. [138] showed that, in guinea pigs, Ro-600175 ((αS)-6-chloro-5-fluoro-α-methyl-1Hindole-1-ethanamine fumarate), a 5-HT2C receptor agonist, increased peak urethral pressure in a dose-dependent manner. This effect was reversed by a selective 5-HT2C receptor antagonist SB-242084 (6-chloro-2,3-dihydro-5-methyl-N-[6-[(2-methyl-3-pyridinyl)oxy]-3-pyridinyl]-1H-indole-1-carboxyamide) but not a 5-HT2A or 2B receptor antagonist. Similar results were also observed in rats [119, 127]. Clinically, duloxetine, a serotonin-norepinephrine reuptake inhibitor, has been used to treat stress urinary incontinence. One possible mechanism for this effect may be the activation of 5-HT2C receptors in motoneurons in Onuf's nucleus, which leads to an increased activity of pudendal motor neurons and a subsequent increase in the strength of urethral sphincter contractions.

3.3. 5-HT3 receptors

Although genes encoding the molecular structures of five different 5-HT3 receptor subfamilies (A–E) have been cloned, it is demonstrated so far that only the 5-HT3A subfamily is functional in homomeric form, and all other subfamilies require coassembling with 5-HT3A as functional heteromers [62, 139]. Therefore, here 5-HT3 receptors will be described together as one receptor unity. In the spinal cord, 5-HT3 receptors in the beginning were detected mainly in the dorsal horn with autoradiography and immunohistochemistry in rats and humans [140, 141]. Later by using in situ hybridization and immunohistochemistry, they were found to be expressed in different laminae across the spinal gray matter [107, 142]. By using immunohistochemistry, Morales et al. [142] observed labeled cell bodies in the dorsal horn among the densely labeled fiber terminals. In the ventral horn, large neurons, likely motoneurons, were densely labeled. By using in situ hybridization, Fonseca et al. [107] found that 5-HT3 receptor mRNAs were expressed in different laminae in the rat spinal cord with very low levels in the dorsal horn, slightly higher levels in laminae VI through X and the highest level in lamina IX. Maxwell et al. [143] have studied the ultrastructure of 5-HT3 immunolabeled profiles in the dorsal horn of the rat spinal cord. They found that 5-HT3-immunopositive terminals invariably formed asymmetric synaptic junctions with dendritic profiles and often contained a mixture of granular and agranular vesicles. Immunoreactive cells were found to contain intense patches of reaction product within their cytoplasm. Although there are no data available regarding the subcellular morphology of 5-HT3 receptors in the ventral horn neurons, from the light microscopic data, it can be concluded that the receptor immunoreactive product was located at least in the cytoplasm [142].

It has long been known that 5-HT3 receptors modulate spinal nociceptive reflexes [144]. A large part of literature demonstrated a role of 5-HT3 receptors in antinociception in the spinal cord (e.g., [145, 146]). This is likely due to, for instance, that the receptors interact with inhibitory interneurons such as GABA interneurons in the dorsal horn [147]. However, there are also data indicated that 5-HT3 receptors have a pronociceptive effect. For example, Guo et al. [148] showed that when the spinal 5-HT3 receptors were activated by intrathecal injection of a selective 5-HT3 receptor agonist SR-57227 (1-(6-chloropyridin-2-yl)piperidin-4-amine) spinal glial hyperactivity, neuronal hyperexcitability, and pain hypersensitivity were induced in rats. These diverse effects could be explained by, e.g., the expression of 5-HT3 receptors in different neuronal components and/or the different effects of assemblies formed from different receptor subfamilies [149, 150].

Although 5-HT3 receptors are expressed in the ventral horn neurons data concerning their motor functions are scarce. A study by Guertin and Steuer [151] showed that in hindlimb paralyzed mice 5-HT3 receptor agonist SR-57227 could produce hindlimb movements although with a low score. This result indicates that 5-HT3 receptors might also modulate spinal motoneuron activity in normal states. In addition, the activation of 5-HT3 receptors by 2-methyl-5-HT, another 5-HT3 receptor agonist, could induce sideward tail-flick reflex in rats [117], which might likely involve both sensory and motor components in the spinal cord. Further, 5-HT3 receptors have been reported to inhibit micturition in cats in both normal and spinalized situation [152].

3.4. 5-HT4 receptors

Data concerning 5-HT4 receptors in the spinal cord are scarce. As far as I know, so far only one article reported the expression of 5-HT4 receptors in the spinal cord [153]. Using immunohistochemistry, Suwa et al. [153] investigated 5-HT4 receptor cell distribution in the brain and spinal cord in juvenile rats and found a high density of immunostained neurons in the ventral horn of the spinal cord. In addition, several sympathetic neurons were also seen to be immunopositive.

Similarly, studies about the functions of 5-HT4 receptors in the spinal cord are also rare. Using pharmacological method, Godínez-Chaparro et al. [154] showed that 5-HT in the spinal cord promotes the development and maintenance of secondary allodynia and hyperalgesia caused by formalin stimulation via the activation of 5-HT4/6/7 receptors. Considering the anatomical distribution of 5-HT4 receptors in the spinal cord, they should also play a role in some motor functions. Whether this is the case needs to be investigated further.

3.5. 5-HT5 receptors

The 5-HT5 receptor family comprises two members: 5-HT5A and 5-HT5B. Although 5-HT5B receptors have been found in some structures in rat and mouse brain, they are not expressed in humans [155]. Therefore, I will only describe the 5-HT5A receptors in this chapter.

5-HT5A receptors were first identified in the rat spinal cord by Doly et al. [156]. They showed that in the rat spinal cord, 5-HT5A receptors were expressed with high density in the superficial dorsal horn (laminae I and II) especially in lamina II. In addition, they were also expressed in other regions including the intermediolateral nucleus in the thoracolumbar region and Onuf's nucleus in lumbosacral region. Ventral horn motoneurons in different regions were weakly labeled. Subcellularly, the receptors were found both in the cytoplasm and on the cell membrane of neuronal somata and dendrites. In the cytoplasm, they were associated with Golgi apparatus, rough endoplasmic reticulum, and vesicles. On the membrane, they were exclusively located on the postsynaptic density that was in clear contrast with the subcellular localization of 5-HT2A receptors [108, 110].

According to their locations in the spinal cord, it is speculated that 5-HT5A receptors are related to spinal modulation of pain, autonomic function, and control of micturition. Indeed, data from recent pharmacological studies have demonstrated that 5-HT-induced antinociceptive effect was mediated by spinal 5-HT5A receptors in several pain models, such as that induced by formalin, capsaicin, or acetic acid [58, 157]. For example, injection of 5-HT or 5-CT (an agonist of 5-HT5A receptors) could dose-dependently prevent nociception induced by formalin [157]. However, the speculated effects of the receptors on autonomic function and control of micturition yet need to be demonstrated.

3.6. 5-HT6 receptors

Using RT-PCR, Gérard et al. [158] discovered the existence of 5-HT6 receptor mRNAs at a moderate level in the rat spinal cord. Later, using immunoautoradiogram, data from the same group showed that 5-HT6 receptor immunoreactive product seemed to be present across all laminae of the spinal gray matter with a denser labeling in the superficial dorsal horn and lamina IX [159]. No data are available about the subcellular distribution of 5-HT6 receptors in the spinal cord. However, according to the electron microscopic data from other brain regions such as the striatum and the hippocampus, 5-HT6 receptors were mainly associated with postsynaptic dendrites and no immunopositive axon terminals were found [159].

The exclusive roles of 5-HT6 receptors in the spinal cord yet remain to be elaborated. Using a formalin pain model in rats, Castañeda-Corral et al. [160] suggested that 5-HT6 receptors play a pronociceptive role in the spinal cord since intrathecal injection of EMD-386088 (5-chloro-2-methyl-3-(1,2,3,6-tetrahydro-4-pyridinyl)-1H-indole), a selective 5-HT6 receptor agonist, enhanced formalin-induced nociception. It is unknown whether 5-HT6 receptors play any role in motor control.

3.7. 5-HT7 receptors

As there were no specific radioligands for 5-HT7 receptors available, data concerning their distribution in the spinal cord acquired using autoradiography had been inconclusive [161] until 2005 when Doly et al. [162] used immunohistochemistry to study their distribution in the rat spinal cord. Doly et al. [162] showed that in the rat lumbar spinal cord 5-HT7 receptors were mainly located in two superficial laminae of the dorsal horn. Except in the Onuf's nucleus where the labeling was relatively denser, immunolabeling in the ventral horn motoneuron region was generally weak. At subcellular level, the receptors were found in the postsynaptic locations in neuronal cell bodies and dendrites as well as presynaptic locations in unmyelinated and thin myelinated axonal fibers. In addition, immunolabeling was also found in astrocytes. In cats, Noga et al. [16] found that in thoracolumbar spinal cord 5-HT7-immunolabeled cells spread across different laminae in the gray matter with a dorsoventral density gradient.

Available data showed that 5-HT7 receptors exert multiple roles in modulating both sensory and motor behavior. In sensory aspect 5-HT7 receptors have been demonstrated to exert dual but diverse actions in nociception depending on the different situations. In healthy rats, 5-HT7 receptor agonists exerted a pronociceptive action but in neuropathic animals they exerted an antinociceptive action [163]. Yesilyurt et al. [164] showed that intrathecal application of SB-269970 ((2R)-1-[(3-hydroxyphenyl)sulfonyl]-2 -(2-(4-methyl-1-piperidinyl)ethyl)pyrrolidine), a 5-HT7 receptor antagonist, blocked both opioid and nonopioid type stress-induced analgesia, and this effect was mediated by descending serotonergic pathways and the spinal 5-HT7 receptors. Several pieces of evidence have indicated that the nonopioid analgesic drug Nefopam also took its effects via activation of 5-HT7 receptors [165, 166].

5-HT7 receptors have been demonstrated to be critical for 5-HT-induced locomotor-like activity [16, 167–169]. Liu and Jordan [167] showed that in rats 5-HT7 receptor antagonists blocked locomotor-like activity induced by stimulating mid-medulla region and also decreased step cycle duration. These results have been verified in 5-HT7 knockout mice [169]. Considering that 5-HT7 receptor antagonists blocked locomotor-like activity when applied only above the L3 segments [167], it is possible that they activated the central pattern generator neurons above this level that expressed 5-HT7 receptors and responded to 5-HT stimulation. Indeed, in decerebrated cats in which locomotion was induced by electrical stimulation of the mesencephalic locomotor region abundant c-Fos immunoreactive cells were observed in laminae VII and VIII throughout the thoracolumbar segments [16].

4. Expression changes of different 5-HT receptors and their significance in motor outputs following SCI

Following SCI the descending 5-HT projections are interrupted and as a consequence, a number of 5-HT receptors undergo different degrees of plastic changes below the lesion depending on the severity of injury, which on one hand will facilitate the re-establishment of neuronal circuits in the spinal cord below the lesion and thus promote functional recovery, and on the other hand will result in pathological symptoms. These changes can occur at both anatomical and functional levels. However, due to the fact that more functional than anatomical data are available, for some receptors only functional changes have been reported. So far 5-HT receptors that have been confirmed to undergo anatomical changes include, but are not limited to, 5-HT1 and 5-HT2 receptor families. In some other receptors, functional (activity) changes are indeed detected although there are no data revealing their anatomical changes. This group of receptors includes 5-HT3 and 5-HT7 receptors. So far there are no reports as to the anatomical or functional changes for 5-HT4, 5-HT5, and 5-HT6 receptors following SCI. Below I will mainly describe the 5-HT receptors that have been clearly demonstrated to undergo anatomical and/or functional changes in relation to their impact on motor outputs.

4.1. 5-HT1 receptors

Among the different 5-HT1 subfamilies, 5-HT1A receptors were mostly investigated in terms of their anatomical and functional changes probably due to their direct involvement in functional recovery following SCI. For other subfamilies, such as 5-HT1B, 1D, and 1F, related studies were less abundant and results relating to their roles in motor functional outputs were also less conclusive.

5-HT1A receptors: Using autoradiography, the expression of 5-HT1A receptors have been shown to increase in the rat spinal cord 3 weeks following destruction of descending serotonergic fibers with 5,7-dihydroxytryptamine [83]. In cats, using the same technique, it was found that after spinal cord transection at T13 level binding density was significantly increased in laminae II, III, and X of lumbar segments at 15 and 30 days, but at 60 days the binding density recovered to the control level [28]. It should be addressed that using binding technique it is difficult to differentiate whether the labeled profiles were from neuronal cell bodies, their dendrites or axon fiber terminals. Using immunohistochemistry with two different 5-HT1A antibodies, one labeling neuronal somata and the other labeling the axon initial segments, Otoshi et al. [31] reported that 8 weeks following complete spinal transection at T7-T8 level the expression of 5-HT1A receptors in axon hillock was increased in laminae III, IV, VII, and IX, whereas the expression in neuronal somata and dendrites were increased in laminae VII and IX. This upregulation, both in the axon hillock and neuronal somata and dendrites, was dependent on the sensory input since the receptors were not upregulated when the spinal cord was isolated. Using in situ hybridization, Cornide-Petronio et al. [170] saw a similar upregulation time course for 5-HT1A receptors in lampreys as in cats. They reported an acute upregulation of 5-HT1A receptors in the spinal cord after SCI both in the rostral and caudal part of the lesion site, and the upregulation recovered to normal levels at 3 weeks. This quick recovery of 5-HT1A receptor expression may be due to that in lamprey serotonergic descending projecting neurons in the rhombencephalon could regenerate their axons across the lesion site after complete spinal cord transection [171]. Thus, the variation of results from these studies may partly reflect the different receptor responses to SCI in different species.

There is ample evidence that the activation of 5-HT1A receptors could induce motor functional recovery after SCI [13, 84, 172]. Antri et al. [13] found that, in thoracic spinal cord transected rats, after daily systemic application of 5-HT1A receptor agonist 8-OH-DPAT, locomotor function was significantly improved when compared with control spinalized animals. The agonist had both short- and long-term effects for motor functional improvement. A similar result was also demonstrated by Jackson and White [84] that in acute C1 spinal cord transected rats, after intravenous administration of 8-OH-DPAT, the excitability of spinal motoneurons was markedly enhanced. However, local application of 8-OH-DPAT directly into the ventral horn by microiontophoresis inhibited the glutamate-evoked firing of motoneurons. These results indicate that when 8-OH-DPAT was directly applied into the vicinity of the motoneurons it may activate 5-HT1A receptors in the axon hillock which inhibits the motoneuron firing [81]. However, the marked increase in firing of motoneurons induced by systemic administration of 8-OH-DPAT suggests that 5-HT1A receptors in other locations, likely at sites presynaptic to the motoneurons, have also been activated. In addition to the functions described above, 5-HT1A receptors have been reported to increase bladder capacity under saline or acid infused conditions in SCI cats [173].

5-HT1B receptors: In comparison with 5-HT1A receptors, studies concerning plastic changes of 5-HT1B receptors following SCI are sparse. Using autoradiography, Laporte et al. [83]

reported that when descending serotonergic projections were destroyed by 5,7-dihydroxy-tryptamine the labeling of 5-HT1B receptors was decreased (−12%) in the dorsal horn at the cervical but not at the lumbar level in rats. Interestingly, when noradrenergic systems had been lesioned by DSP-4 (N-(2-chloroethyl)-N-ethyl-2-bromobenzylamine) there was an increase of labeling of 5-HT1B receptors both at the cervical level (+31%) and the lumbar level (+17%). In a C2 hemisection rat model, using quantitative RT-PCR, Mantilla et al. [86] did not detect expression changes of 5-HT1B receptors in phrenic motoneurons 2 or 3 weeks following the injury.

Similar to their functions in normal physiological states, in SCI states 5-HT1B receptors also play an inhibitory role for motor outputs possibly through inhibitions on both mono- and polysynaptic reflexes. In acute C1 spinalized rats, Honda et al. [174] showed that serotoner-gic depression of monosynaptic reflex transmission induced by application of 5-HTP was mediated by 5-HT1B receptors. In S2 spinal cord transection model (also called tail spasticity model), Murray et al. [99] showed that polysynaptic EPSPs that trigger muscle spasms after SCI were inhibited by 5-HT1B receptors.

5-HT1D and 1F receptors: To my knowledge, no studies have investigated the expression changes of these two receptors following SCI. Functionally, the activation of 5-HT1D recep-tors seemed to reduce sensory transmission in both monosynaptic and polysynaptic reflexes in humans [95], and to inhibit bladder activity in cats after SCI [175]. The activation of 5-HT1F seemed to inhibit long polysynaptic reflexes in rats after SCI [99]. However because the agonists used in these studies were not specific enough for selected receptors the results were not conclusive.

4.2. 5-HT2 receptors

5-HT2, especially 5-HT2A and 2C, receptors are the most intensely studied receptors among all 5-HT receptor families mostly due to their considerable effects on the motor functional recovery and perhaps also on the pathological symptoms developed following SCI such as spasticity. Due to the close relationship and similar functions of these three receptor subfami-lies, their influences on the motor outputs after SCI will be described together.

5-HT2A receptors: Using different SCI animal models such as contusion, hemisection, and complete spinal transection, it is confirmed that 5-HT2A receptors underwent different degrees of plastic changes following SCI. In thoracic contusive rats using immunohistochem-istry, Lee et al. [30] found a moderate yet significantly increased 5-HT2A receptor expres-sion (~1.2-fold of control) in the motoneurons at L5-L6 level after 4 weeks of injury. With the same method in a C2 hemisection rat model Fuller et al. [29] demonstrated a significant upregulation (~1.7-fold of control) of 5-HT2A receptors in the ipsilateral phrenic motoneur-ons after 2 weeks of injury. In a S2 spinal transection model, Kong et al. [32, 33] reported a dramatic increase of 5-HT2A receptor immunoreactivity (~5.6-fold of control) in the moto-neurons below the lesion. The upregulation began as early as 1 day after injury, reached a maximal level by 28 days and lasted at least until 60 days, the longest time interval investi-gated. Similarly an upregulation of 5-HT2A receptors were also observed in chronic (6 weeks) thoracic spinal transected rats. Navarrett et al. [35] reported a ~1.3-fold increase of 5-HT2A receptor mRNAs in the spinal tissue (including both white and gray matter) below the lesion with RT-PCR. Upregulation of 5-HT2A receptor mRNAs was also reported in mice subjected to an acute thoracic spinal transection. Thus, Ung et al. [176] found that 3 h after the lesion 5-HT2A receptor mRNA expression levels were increased 2.5-fold in the lateral intermediate zone in L1-L2 segments and they remained to be elevated for at least 2 weeks. However, no significant change was found in the ventral horn motoneuron regions, which was strikingly different from that in the rat.

5-HT2B receptors: No expression changes have been reported for this receptor subfamily in the spinal cord following SCI. With microarray global gene analysis technique, Wienecke et al. [122] did not detect significant changes of 5-HT2B receptor mRNAs in S2 spinal transected rats.

5-HT2C receptors: Similar to 5-HT2A receptors, 5-HT2C receptor expression changes have been investigated in different SCI animal models with different techniques. However, discrepancies exist as to whether 5-HT2C receptors are upregulated or not following SCI. In chronic SCI rats (~15 weeks) severe contusion or transection at thoracic level (T9) could induce a significant increase of 5-HT2C receptor immunoreactivity in lumbar spinal cord [22]. The increase could reach 4–7-fold in the ventral horn and ~17-fold in the dorsal horn over control level. In thoracic (T8-T9) spinal transected neonatal rats, following 4 weeks injury 5-HT2C receptor immunoreactivity was seen to increase 4–5-fold both in the spinal dorsal and ventral horn [177]. In a S2 spinal transection rat model, data from our group [36] indicated that 5-HT2C receptor immunoreactivity increased in all parts of the spinal gray matter below the lesion from 2 weeks but did not reach a significant level until 3 weeks (~1.4-fold over control animals). The increase sustained thereafter and a maximal level was reached at 45 days (~1.7-fold) and maintained at 60 days, the longest investigated interval. It is somehow perplexing that although upregulation was observed at protein level no significant increase at mRNA level was detected in different SCI animal models [34, 35, 122, 178]. However, although no significant changes of the total amount of 5-HT2C receptor mRNAs were detected, Murray et al. [34] did detect certain constitutive isoforms, such as INI isoform, that were significantly increased in the motoneurons 6 weeks after S2 spinal transection.

Functional significance for motor outputs of 5-HT2 receptors: The activation of 5-HT2 receptors has different effects on motor outputs after SCI, which include promoting motor functional recovery and causing maladaptive pathological motor symptoms such as spasticity. Due to uncertainty of the expression of 5-HT2B receptors in the spinal cord most studies have been focused on 5-HT2A and 2C receptors. There is ample evidence for the roles of 5-HT2A and 2C receptors in motor functional recovery following SCI from different studies (e.g., [9, 12, 14, 34, 43, 84, 134, 176, 179, 180], for reviews see [44, 45]). For example, in thoracic spinalized cats, when a 5-HT2A/C receptor agonist (e.g., quipazine or DOI) was administrated α-motoneuron excitability was increased and hindlimb motor activity was enhanced [9]. Similar results were also demonstrated in SCI rats [12, 14] and mice [176]. Although 5-HT2A and 2C receptors both play a common role for motor functional recovery each subfamily may also exert different functions in different aspects of the motor outputs. Using different agonists and antagonists specific for each of these two receptor subfamilies it is found that 5-HT2A receptors might contribute to locomotor network activation and locomotor-like movement generation

[15, 43, 176]. Direct stimulation of 5-HT2C receptors with its agonist meta-chlorophenylpiper-azine improved weight-supported locomotion in adult rats spinalized as neonates [177, 181]. 5-HT2C, probably also 2B, but not 2A, receptors could become constitutively active which could contribute to motor functional recovery following SCI [34, 182].

One maladaptive consequence for 5-HT2 receptor plastic changes is the induction of muscle spasm due to increased motoneuron excitability. The rapid and robust upregulation of 5-HT2A receptors in spinal motoneurons might be responsible for 5-HT supersensitivity after SCI [32, 33]. Activation of 5-HT2C receptors could induce long-lasting reflexes of motoneurons in the in vitro spinal cord preparations [134, 135]. These long-lasting reflexes could be enhanced when 5-HT2C receptors became constitutively active following SCI [34, 182]. One of the cellular mechanisms for the increased motoneuron excitability is that the activation of 5-HT2 recep-tors could enhance calcium and/or sodium persistent inward currents [42, 183].

In addition to promoting locomotion, 5-HT2 (especially 2A) receptors also play a significant role for respiratory functional recovery after cervical spinal hemisection [179] and in enhanc-ing bladder function in thoracic spinal transected rats [184].

It should be addressed that the upregulation of 5-HT2 receptors does not by all means lead the motoneurons toward a hyperexcitatory state. Recently one interesting finding is present-ed by Bos et al. [185] who showed that the activation of 5-HT2A receptors could increase K(+)-Cl(−) cotransporter (KCC2) expression on cell membrane in the spinal cord motoneurons after SCI. The upregulation of KCC2 receptors in turn increased the activity of GABA A and glycine receptors which would restore endogenous inhibition and reduce spasticity after SCI in rats [186]. These results indicate that the upregulation of 5-HT2A receptors would not simply produce an excitatory effect. Rather, their activation will trigger an inhibitory factor which attempts to balance the excitatory effect. This effect seems to be paradoxical to the 5-HT2A receptors' direct excitatory effect on motoneurons. However, this might be one of the com-mon functional mechanisms of a spinal network—different factors interact and compensate each other, and the final motor output is determined by a summed vector of these push-pull forces acted on the motoneurons. In fact, any motor action cannot be arisen solely from the activation of a single factor; instead it needs a concert activity of multiple factors including both excitatory and inhibitory. For instance, Hayashi et al. [22] have showed that in contu-sive SCI rats, application of 5-HT1A or 5-HT2C receptor agonists alone or in combination could not improve hindlimb motor function; rather, motor functional improvement could be achieved only when the 5-HT precursor 5-HTP was administrated, indicating that simultane-ously multiple 5-HT receptor activations are needed for motor functional recovery. This concept is reinforced by the results from Noga et al. [16] who showed that in paralyzed, decerebrated cats, when locomotion was induced by electrical stimulation of the mesence-phalic locomotor region, most locomotor-activated cells, labeled with c-Fos, colocalized with 5-HT1A, 5-HT2A, and 5-HT7 receptors in laminae VII and VIII in the thoracolumbar spinal region.

4.3. 5-HT3 receptors

There are no data demonstrating the expression changes of 5-HT3 following SCI. Laporte et al. [83] did not detect 5-HT3 receptor expression changes with binding technique in rat spinal cords whose descending serotonergic projections had been destroyed by 5,7-dihydroxytrypt-amine. However, lesions in peripheral nerves could reduce 5-HT3 receptor expression in the spinal motoneurons in rats [187].

Most studies concerning 5-HT3 receptor functions have been focused on sensory aspects, especially nociception. Studies relating to their functions in motor outputs after SCI are scarce. So far there is only one study having investigated the influence of the activation of 5-HT3 receptors on motor outputs in SCI mice. In this study, Guertin and Steuer [152] showed that in hindlimb paralyzed mice 5-HT3 receptor agonist SR-57227 could produce hindlimb movements although with a low score. This result, anyhow, provided the first evidence that 5-HT3 receptors could modulate spinal motoneuron activity after SCI.

4.4. 5-HT7 receptors

So far there are no data available with respect to the expression changes of 5-HT7 receptors following SCI. However, the activation of 5-HT7 receptor has been shown to be related to locomotor functional recovery in SCI states [23, 43, 172]. Landry et al. [172] showed that in thoracic spinal transected mice systemic application of 8-OH-DPAT, an agonist for both 5-HT1A and 5-HT7 receptors, acutely induced hindlimb movements with characteristics similar to normal locomotion. When the animals were pretreated with SB-269970, a selective 5-HT7 receptor antagonist, 8-OH-DPAT-induced movements were reduced. Sławińska et al. [23] showed that, in thoracic spinal transected rats, grafting of neurons from the B1, B2, and B3 descending 5-HT system from the brainstem into the spinal cord below the lesion effectively restored coordinated plantar stepping, and the application of SB-269970 disrupted the inter- and intralimb coordination. Further evidence from the same group indicated that 8-OH-DPAT facilitated plantar stepping in chronic spinalized rats [43]. Since 5-HT7 receptor agonists mainly improved coordination movement the authors assumed that 5-HT7 receptors mainly facilitated the activity of the central pattern generator interneurons. This assumption is supported by anatomical data that 5-HT7 receptors were mainly expressed in the neurons in the dorsal horn and the intermediate zone of the spinal gray matter [16]. In addition to the effects on locomotion, it has been reported that the activation of 5-HT7 receptors by their agonist LP44 (4-[2-(methylthio)phenyl]-N-(1,2,3,4-tetrahydronaphthalen-1-yl)-1-piperazine-hexanamide) increased bladder voiding efficiency in chronic thoracic spinal transected rats [188].

5. Plasticity of 5-HT innervations after SCI

It is evidenced that a small number of 5-HT receptors, or more precisely receptor isoforms, could become active following SCI without ligand activation—so-called constitutive activation. However, for most of the 5-HT receptors that do not have constitutive isoforms the presence of their ligand—5HT is a necessity for their activation. Then, where could 5-HT originate following SCI? After contusion spinal cord injury or partial spinal cord transections there are still spared supraspinal serotonergic projections and these serotonergic fibers could undergo plastic changes to eventually supplement lost 5-HT supply in the injured spinal cord. For example, in contusion injury the density of spared 5-HT fibers below the lesion varies depending on the locations along the dorsoventral axis and the severity of the injury [22, 189, 190], and 5-HT innervation could be partially restored with time which is responsible at least partly for motor functional recovery [190]. In thoracic hemisection injury, the density of 5-HT fibers in the ipsilateral ventral horn varied from 8% to 30% of the control value according to studies with a postinjury interval 4–7 days [39, 191–194]. The data are inconsistent as to whether 5-HT fibers increase with time following hemisection. Some researchers reported a gradual increase of 5-HT fibers on the ipsilateral side below the lesion (e.g., [193, 195]), whereas some others did not see apparent changes (e.g., [39, 194]). For example, Saruhashi et al. [193] observed that 5-HT-immunoreactive fibers recovered from 20% to about 75% of the normal value in the ventral horn during first 4 weeks. Camand et al. [195] also reported a similar finding in the intermediate zone. However, Filli et al. [194] reported a decrease to about 10% by 4 weeks from about 30% at day 4 in ventral horn motoneuron region. Azam et al. [39] reported that by 60 days the density of 5-HT-immunoreacitve fibers in the intermediate zone was reduced to 11% from 23% at 5 days, whereas in the ventral horn it was not reduced (23% vs. 22%). Following complete spinal transection, some 2–15% of the normal content of 5-HT remained in the spinal cord below the lesion ([196]; for review see [25]).

The next question would be then where the residual 5-HT originates following complete spinal transection. One origin might be the intraspinal serotonergic neurons. However, intraspinal serotonergic neurons are very few in number and sparsely distributed (see Section 1). Then, what are the other possible sources? Recent findings from our [38] and Bennett's group [37] indicated that AADC cells in the spinal cord might be another origin. AADC is an essential enzyme for the synthesis of 5-HT, dopamine, and certain trace amines from their respective precursors. AADC cells are widely distributed in different regions of the spinal cord [38], not limiting to the area around the central canal as reported previously [197]. Following SCI the ability of AADC cells in the spinal cord to synthesize 5-HT/dopamine from 5-HTP/L-dopa was dramatically increased and 5-HT/dopamine produced in the AADC was responsible for the increased motoneuron ability recorded both in vivo and in vitro [37, 38, 40, 198]. Nonetheless, we have to admit that without 5-HTP application 5-HT could not be detected in the spinal AADC cells. This might be due to that the detecting techniques used in related studies were not sensitive enough to disclose a small amount of 5-HT, or the turnover rate of 5-HT produced in the AADC cells was so high that once produced it was immediately metabolized. One piece of evidence to support the speculation that monoamine transmitters could be produced from AADC cells in the spinal cord after SCI comes from Hou et al. [199], who showed that the number of dopamine-producing cells, which contained both AADC and tyrosine hydroxylase, was increased in lumbosacral spinal cord in thoracic spinal transected rats; and with enzyme-linked immunosorbent assay (ELISA) dopamine with a content of about 10% of its normal value could be detected in this part of the spinal cord even without L-dopa application. At the same time they also showed that dopamine produced from the spinal cord below the lesion was implicated for micturition functional recovery following SCI.

6. Conclusions

The serotonin system in the spinal cord is an important modulator for sensory, motor as well as autonomic function. This system normally exercises its function via the interaction between ligand 5-HT and a number of 5-HT receptors expressed in different structures in the spinal cord. Among the 14 5-HT receptor subfamilies at least 12 have been detected in the spinal cord, in which 5-HT1A, 2A, 2C, and 7 receptors have been demonstrated to be more important for motor control. In normal physiological states, these receptors coordinate with each other and also with other monoamine systems to enable smooth and controllable motor outputs for our physical activity [200]. Following SCI extensive plastic changes occur for a number of 5-HT receptor subfamilies, mostly with increased receptor numbers and/or constitutive activity. In addition, plasticity also occurs for descending serotonergic fibers (in the case of incomplete SCI) and intraspinal serotonin-producing cells. The coeffects of these plastic changes, together with the plastic changes of other monoamine systems, ultimately lead to increased motoneuron excitability in the chronic phase [17, 21, 108]. These plastic changes have both beneficial and detrimental effects for spinal motor outputs after SCI. Although the plastic changes can result in an adaptive compensation of the lost transmitters and thus assist in motor functional recovery, they can also result in a plethora of maladaptive problems, such as spasticity. In clinical practice, a strategy needs to be set so as to maximally take advantage of the positive side of the plasticity to promote motor functional recovery and meanwhile to reduce negative effects to a minimal extent. To reach this endpoint, pharmacological and/or genetic interferences need to be utilized so that the activity of different 5-HT receptors and 5-HT supply in the spinal cord reach a new balance and consequently an appropriate motor behavior is generated. Such a strategy would certainly have great implications for future treatment of SCI patients.

Acknowledgements

This work was supported by the Lundbeck Foundation and the Danish Medical Research Council.

Abbreviations

5-CT: 5-carboxamidotryptamine

5-HT: 5-hydroxytryptomine, serotonin

8-OH-DPAT: 8-hydroxy-2-(di-*n*-propylamino) tetralin

AADC: aromatic L-amino acid decarboxylase

BRL-15572: 3-(4-(4-chlorophenyl)piperazin-1-yl)-1,1-diphenyl-2-propanol

C, T, L, and S: cervical, thoracic, lumbar, and sacral spinal cord, respectively

D-MC: N-ormethylclozapine/8-chloro-11-(1-piperazinyl)-5H-dibenzo[b,e][1,4]diazepine

DOI: (±)-2,5-dimethoxy-4-iodoamphetamine hydrochloride

DOM: 2,5-dimethoxy-alpha,4-dimethyl-benzene ethamine hydrochloride

DSP-4: N-(2-chloroethyl)-N-ethyl-2-bromobenzylamine

ELISA: enzyme-linked immunosorbent assay

EMD-386088: 5-chloro-2-methyl-3-(1,2,3,6-tetrahydro-4-pyridinyl)-1H-indole

EPSP: excitatory postsynaptic potential

GABA: γ-aminobutyric acid

GR-46611: 3-[3-(2-dimethylaminoethyl)-1H-indol-5-yl]-N-(4-methoxybenzyl)acrylamide

KCC2: K(+)-Cl(−) cotransporter

L-dopa: L-3,4-dihydroxyphenylalanine

LP44:   4-[2-(methylthio)phenyl]-N-(1,2,3,4-tetrahydronaphthalen-1-yl)-1-piperazinehexanamide

LY-344864:   N-[(3R)-3-(dimethylamino)-2,3,4,9-tetrahydro-1H-carbazol-6-yl]-4-fluorobenzamide

MK-212: 6-chloro-2-(1-piperazinyl)pyrazine hydrochloride

mRNA: messenger ribonucleic acid

NMDA: N-methyl-D-aspartate

PCR: polymerase chain reaction

Ro-600175: (αS)-6-chloro-5-fluoro-α-methyl-1H-indole-1-ethanamine fumarate

RS-127445: (3-(4-(4-chlorophenyl)piperazin-1-yl)-1,1-diphenyl-2-propanol)

RT-PCT: reverse transcription polymerase chain reaction

RU-24969: 5-methoxy-3(1,2,3,6-tetrahydropyridin-4-yl)-1H-indole

SB-242084: 6-chloro-2,3-dihydro-5-methyl-N-[6-[(2-methyl-3-pyridinyl)oxy]-3-pyridinyl]-1H-indole-1-carboxyamide

SB-269970:   (2R)-1-[(3-hydroxyphenyl)sulfonyl]-2 -(2-(4-methyl-1-piperidinyl)ethyl)pyrrolidine

SCI: spinal cord injury

SR-57227: 1-(6-chloropyridin-2-yl)piperidin-4-amine

TCB-2: 4-bromo-3,6-dimethoxybenzocyclobuten-1-yl)methylamine hydrobromide

WAY-100635: *N*-[2-[4-(2-methoxyphenyl)-1-piperazinyl]ethyl]-*N*-(2-pyridyl)cyclohexanecar-boxamide

WAY-161503: 8,9-dichloro-2,3,4,4a-tetrahydro-1*H*-pyrazino[1,2-*a*]quinoxalin-5(6*H*)

Author details

Mengliang Zhang[1,2]

Address all correspondence to: mzhang@sund.ku.dk

1 Department of Neuroscience and Pharmacology, University of Copenhagen, Copenhagen, Denmark

2 Neuronano Research Center, Department of Experimental Medical Science, Lund University, Lund, Sweden

References

[1] Witiw CD, Fehlings MG. Acute spinal cord injury. J Spinal Disord Tech. 2015;28:202–210. DOI: 10.1097/BSD.0000000000000287.

[2] Jensen MP, Kuehn CM, Amtmann D, Cardenas DD. Symptom burden in persons with spinal cord injury. Arch Phys Med Rehabil. 2007;88:638–645. DOI: 10.1016/j.apmr.2007.02.002.

[3] Nielsen JB, Crone C, Hultborn H. The spinal pathophysiology of spasticity-from a basic science point of view. Acta Physiol (Oxf). 2007;189:171–180. DOI: 10.1111/j.1748-1716.2006.01652.x.

[4] Sheean G, McGuire JR. Spastic hypertonia and movement disorders: pathophysiology, clinical presentation, and quantification. PM R. 2009;1:827–833. DOI: 10.1016/j.pmrj.2009.08.002.

[5] Gunduz H, Binak DF. Autonomic dysreflexia: an important cardiovascular complication in spinal cord injury patients. Cardiol J. 2012;19:215–219. DOI: 10.5603/CJ.2012.0040.

[6] Felix ER. Chronic neuropathic pain in SCI: evaluation and treatment. Phys Med Rehabil Clin N Am. 2014;25:545–571. DOI: 10.1016/0006-8993(88)91548-X.

[7] Nas K, Yazmalar L, Şah V, Aydın A, Öneş K. Rehabilitation of spinal cord injuries. World J Orthop. 2015;6:8–16. DOI: 10.5312/wjo.v6.i1.8.

[8]   Guertin PA. New pharmacological approaches against chronic bowel and bladder problems in paralytics. World J Crit Care Med. 2016;5:1–6. DOI: 10.5492/wjccm.v5.i1.1.

[9]   Barbeau H, Rossignol S. The effects of serotonergic drugs on the locomotor pattern and on cutaneous reflexes of the adult chronic spinal cat. Brain Res. 1990;514:55–67. DOI: 10.1016/0006-8993(90)90435-E.

[10] Kiehn O, Kjaerulff O. Spatiotemporal characteristics of 5-HT and dopamine-induced rhythmic hindlimb activity in the in vitro neonatal rat. J Neurophysiol. 1996;75:1472–1482.

[11] McEwen ML, Van Hartesveldt C, Stehouwer DJ. L-DOPA and quipazine elicit air-stepping in neonatal rats with spinal cord transections. Behav Neurosci. 1997;111:825–833. DOI: 10.1037/0735-7044.111.4.825.

[12] Antri M, Orsal D, Barthe JY. Locomotor recovery in the chronic spinal rat: effects of long-term treatment with a 5-HT2 agonist. Eur J Neurosci. 2002;16:467–476. DOI: 10.1046/j.1460-9568.2002.02088.x.

[13] Antri M, Mouffle C, Orsal D, Barthe JY. 5-HT1A receptors are involved in short- and long-term processes responsible for 5-HT-induced locomotor function recovery in chronic spinal rat. Eur J Neurosci. 2003;18:1963–1972. DOI: 10.1046/j.1460-9568.2003.02916.x.

[14] Antri M, Barthe JY, Mouffle C, Orsal D. Long-lasting recovery of locomotor function in chronic spinal rat following chronic combined pharmacological stimulation of serotonergic receptors with 8-OHDPAT and quipazine. Neurosci Lett. 2005;384:162–267. DOI: 10.1016/j.neulet.2005.04.062.

[15] Landry ES, Guertin PA. Differential effects of 5-HT1 and 5-HT2 receptor agonists on hindlimb movements in paraplegic mice. Prog Neuropsychopharmacol Biol Psychiatry. 2004;28:1053–1060. DOI: 10.1016/j.pnpbp.2004.05.001.

[16] Noga BR, Johnson DM, Riesgo MI, Pinzon A. Locomotor-activated neurons of the cat. I. Serotonergic innervation and co-localization of 5-HT7, 5-HT2A, and 5-HT1A receptors in the thoraco-lumbar spinal cord. J Neurophysiol. 2009;102:1560–1576. DOI: 10.1152/jn.91179.2008.

[17] Musienko P, van den Brand R, Märzendorfer O, Roy RR, Gerasimenko Y, Edgerton VR, Courtine G. Controlling specific locomotor behaviors through multidimensional monoaminergic modulation of spinal circuitries. J Neurosci. 2011;31:9264–9278. DOI: 10.1523/JNEUROSCI.5796-10.2011.

[18] Feraboli-Lohnherr D, Orsal D, Yakovleff A, Giménez y Ribotta M, Privat A. Recovery of locomotor activity in the adult chronic spinal rat after sublesional transplantation of embryonic nervous cells: specific role of serotonergic neurons. Exp Brain Res. 1997;113:443–454. DOI: 10.1007/PL00005597.

[19] Orsal D, Barthe JY, Antri M, Feraboli-Lohnherr D, Yakovleff A, Giménez y Ribotta M, Privat A, Provencher J, Rossignol S. Locomotor recovery in chronic spinal rat: long-

term pharmacological treatment or transplantation of embryonic neurons? Prog Brain Res. 2002;137:213–230.

[20] Kubasak MD, Jindrich DL, Zhong H, Takeoka A, McFarland KC, Muñoz-Quiles C, Roy RR, Edgerton VR, Ramón-Cueto A, Phelps PE. OEG implantation and step training enhance hindlimb-stepping ability in adult spinal transected rats. Brain. 2008;131:264–276. DOI: 10.1093/brain/awm267.

[21] Courtine G, Gerasimenko Y, van den Brand R, Yew A, Musienko P, Zhong H, Song B, Ao Y, Ichiyama RM, Lavrov I, Roy RR, Sofroniew MV, Edgerton VR. Transformation of nonfunctional spinal circuits into functional states after the loss of brain input. Nat Neurosci. 2009;12:1333–1342. DOI: 10.1038/nn.2401.

[22] Hayashi Y, Jacob-Vadakot S, Dugan EA, McBride S, Olexa R, Simansky K, Murray M, Shumsky JS. 5-HT precursor loading, but not 5-HT receptor agonists, increases motor function after spinal cord contusion in adult rats. Exp Neurol. 2010;221:68–78. DOI: 10.1016/j.expneurol.2009.10.003.

[23] Sławińska U, Miazga K, Cabaj AM, Leszczyńska AN, Majczyński H, Nagy JI, Jordan LM. Grafting of fetal brainstem 5-HT neurons into the sublesional spinal cord of paraplegic rats restores coordinated hindlimb locomotion. Exp Neurol. 2013;247:572–581. DOI: 10.1016/j.expneurol.2013.02.008.

[24] Jacobs BL, Fornal CA. Serotonin and motor activity. Curr Opin Neurobiol. 1997;7:820–825. DOI: 10.1016/S0959-4388(97)80141-9.

[25] Schmidt BJ, Jordan LM. The role of serotonin in reflex modulation and locomotor rhythm production in the mammalian spinal cord. Brain Res Bull. 2000;53:689–710. DOI: 10.1016/S0361-9230(00)00402-0.

[26] Millan MJ. Descending control of pain. Prog Neurobiol. 2002;66:355–474. DOI: 10.1016/S0301-0082(02)00009-6.

[27] Pearlstein E, Ben Mabrouk F, Pflieger JF, Vinay L. Serotonin refines the locomotor-related alternations in the in vitro neonatal rat spinal cord. Eur J Neurosci. 2005;21:1338–1346. DOI: 10.1111/j.1460-9568.2005.03971.x.

[28] Giroux N, Rossignol S, Reader TA. Autoradiographic study of alpha1- and alpha2-noradrenergic and serotonin1A receptors in the spinal cord of normal and chronically transected cats. J Comp Neurol. 1999;406:402–414. DOI: 10.1002/(SICI)1096-9861(19990412)406:3<402::AID-CNE8>3.0.CO;2-F.

[29] Fuller DD, Baker-Herman TL, Golder FJ, Doperalski NJ, Watters JJ, Mitchell GS. Cervical spinal cord injury upregulates ventral spinal 5-HT2A receptors. J Neurotrauma. 2005;22:203–213. DOI: 10.1089/neu.2005.22.203.

[30] Lee JK, Johnson CS, Wrathall JR. Up-regulation of 5-HT2 receptors is involved in the increased H-reflex amplitude after contusive spinal cord injury. Exp Neurol. 2007;203:502–511. DOI: 10.1016/j.expneurol.2006.09.003.

[31] Otoshi CK, Walwyn WM, Tillakaratne NJ, Zhong H, Roy RR, Edgerton VR. Distribution and localization of 5-HT(1A) receptors in the rat lumbar spinal cord after transection and deafferentation. J Neurotrauma. 2009;26:575–584. DOI: 10.1089/neu.2008.0640.

[32] Kong X-Y, Wienecke J, Hultborn H, Zhang M. Robust upregulation of serotonin 2A receptors after chronic spinal transection of rats: an immunohistochemical study. Brain Res. 2010;1320:60–68. DOI: 10.1016/j.brainres.2010.01.030.

[33] Kong XY, Wienecke J, Chen M, Hultborn H, Zhang M. The time course of serotonin 2A receptor expression after spinal transection of rats: an immunohistochemical study. Neuroscience. 2011;177:114–126. DOI: 10.1016/j.neuroscience.2010.12.062.

[34] Murray KC, Nakae A, Stephens MJ, Rank M, D'Amico J, Harvey PJ, Li X, Harris RL, Ballou EW, Anelli R, Heckman CJ, Mashimo T, Vavrek R, Sanelli L, Gorassini MA, Bennett DJ, Fouad K. Recovery of motoneuron and locomotor function after spinal cord injury depends on constitutive activity in 5-HT2C receptors. Nat Med. 2010;16:694–700. DOI: 10.1038/nm.2160.

[35] Navarrett S, Collier L, Cardozo C, Dracheva S. Alterations of serotonin 2C and 2A receptors in response to T10 spinal cord transection in rats. Neurosci Lett. 2012;506:74–78. DOI: 10.1016/j.neulet.2011.10.052.

[36] Ren LQ, Wienecke J, Chen M, Møller M, Hultborn H, Zhang M. The time course of serotonin 2C receptor expression after spinal transection of rats: an immunohistochemical study. Neuroscience. 2013;236:31–46. DOI: 10.1016/j.neuroscience.2012.12.063.

[37] Li Y, Li L, Stephens MJ, Zenner D, Murray KC, Winship IR, Vavrek R, Baker GB, Fouad K, Bennett DJ. Synthesis, transport, and metabolism of serotonin formed from exogenously applied 5-HTP after spinal cord injury in rats. J Neurophysiol. 2014;111:145–163. DOI: 10.1152/jn.00508.2013.

[38] Wienecke J, Ren LQ, Hultborn H, Chen M, Møller M, Zhang Y, Zhang M. Spinal cord injury enables aromatic L-amino acid decarboxylase cells to synthesize monoamines. J Neurosci. 2014;34:11984–12000. DOI: 10.1523/JNEUROSCI.3838-13.2014.

[39] Azam B, Wienecke J, Jensen DB, Azam A, Zhang M. Spinal cord hemisection facilitates aromatic L-amino acid decarboxylase cells to produce serotonin in the subchronic but not the chronic phase. Neural Plast. 2015;2015:549671. DOI: 10.1155/2015/549671.

[40] Zhang M. Aromatic L-amino acid decarboxylase cells in the spinal cord: a potential origin of monoamines. Neural Regen Res. 2015;10:715–717. DOI: 10.4103/1673-5374.156960.

[41] Hains BC, Everhart AW, Fullwood SD, and Hulsebosch CE. Changes in serotonin, serotonin transporter expression and serotonin denervation supersensitivity: involvement in chronic central pain after spinal hemisection in the rat. Exp Neurol. 2002;175:347–362. DOI: 10.1006/exnr.2002.7892.

[42] Harvey PJ, Li X, Li Y, Bennett DJ. 5-HT2 receptor activation facilitates a persistent sodium current and repetitive firing in spinal motoneurons of rats with and without

chronic spinal cord injury. J Neurophysiol. 2006;96:1158–1170. DOI: 10.1152/jn. 01088.2005.

[43] Sławińska U, Miazga K, Jordan LM. 5-HT2 and 5-HT7 receptor agonists facilitate plantar stepping in chronic spinal rats through actions on different populations of spinal neurons. Front Neural Circuits. 2014;8:95. DOI: 10.3389/fncir.2014.00095.

[44] Ghosh M, Pearse DD. The role of the serotonergic system in locomotor recovery after spinal cord injury. Front Neural Circuits. 2015;8:151. DOI: 10.3389/fncir.2014.00151.

[45] Nardone R, Höller Y, Thomschewski A, Höller P, Lochner P, Golaszewski S, Brigo F, Trinka E. Serotonergic transmission after spinal cord injury. J Neural Transm (Vienna). 2015;122:279–295. DOI: 10.1007/s00702-014-1241-z.

[46] Dahlstroem A, Fuxe K. Evidence for the existence of monoamine containing neurons in the central nervous system. I. Demonstration of monamines in the cell bodies of brain stem neurons. Acta Physiol Scand Suppl. 1964;62:1–55.

[47] Takeuchi Y, Kimura H, Sano Y. Immunohistochemical demonstration of serotonin neurons in the brainstem of the rat and cat. Cell Tissue Res. 1982;224:247–267. DOI: 10.1007/BF00216872.

[48] Skagerberg G, Björklund A. Topographic principles in the spinal projections of serotonergic and non-serotonergic brainstem neurons in the rat. Neuroscience. 1985;15:445–480. DOI: 10.1016/0306-4522(85)90225-8.

[49] Hornung JP. The human raphe nuclei and the serotonergic system. J Chem Neuroanat. 2003;26:331–343. DOI: 10.1016/j.jchemneu.2003.10.002.

[50] Azmitia EC, Gannon PJ. The primate serotonergic system: a review of human and animal studies and a report on macaca fasicularis. Adv Neurol. 1986;43:407–468.

[51] Ballion B, Branchereau P, Chapron J, Viala D. Ontogeny of descending serotonergic innervation and evidence for intraspinal 5-HT neurons in the mouse spinal cord. Brain Res Dev Brain Res. 2002;137:81–88. DOI: 10.1016/S0165-3806(02)00414-5.

[52] Jacobs BL, Azmitia EC. Structure and function of the brain serotonin system. Physiol Rev. 1992;72:165–229.

[53] Lamotte CC, Johns DR, de Lanerolle NC. Immunohistochemical evidence of indolamine neurons in monkey spinal cord. J Comp Neurol.1982; 206:359–570. DOI: 10.1002/cne.902060404.

[54] Newton BW, Maley BE, Hamill RW. Immunohistochemical demonstration of serotonin neurons in autonomic regions of the rat spinal cord. Brain Res. 1986;376:155–163. DOI: 10.1016/0006-8993(86)90910-8.

[55] Newton BW, Hamill RW. The morphology and distribution of rat serotoninergic intraspinal neurons: an immunohistochemical study. Brain Res Bull. 1988;20:349–360. DOI: 10.1016/0361-9230(88)90064-0.

[56] Jacobs BL, Fornal CA. 5-HT and motor control: a hypothesis. Trends Neurosci. 1993;16:346–352. DOI: 10.1016/0166-2236(93)90090-9.

[57] Rahman W, Bannister K, Bee LA, Dickenson AH. A pronociceptive role for the 5-HT2 receptor on spinal nociceptive transmission: an in vivo electrophysiological study in the rat. Brain Res. 2011;1382:29–36. DOI: 10.1016/j.brainres.2011.01.057.

[58] Cervantes-Durán C, Rocha-González HI, Granados-Soto V. Peripheral and spinal 5-HT receptors participate in the pronociceptive and antinociceptive effects of fluoxetine in rats. Neuroscience. 2013;252:396–409. DOI: 10.1016/j.neuroscience.2013.08.022.

[59] Beato M, Nistri A. Serotonin-induced inhibition of locomotor rhythm of the rat isolated spinal cord is mediated by the 5-HT1 receptor class. Proc Biol Sci. 1998;265:2073–2080. DOI: 10.1098/rspb.1998.0542.

[60] Perrier JF, Cotel F. Serotonin differentially modulates the intrinsic properties of spinal motoneurons from the adult turtle. J Physiol. 2008;586:1233–1238. DOI: 10.1113/jphysiol.2007.145706.

[61] Nichols DE, Nichols CD. Serotonin receptors. Chem Rev. 2008;108:1614–1641. DOI: 10.1021/cr078224o.

[62] Hannon J, Hoyer D. Molecular biology of 5-HT receptors. Behav Brain Res. 2008;195:198–213. DOI: 10.1016/j.bbr.2008.03.020.

[63] Werry TD, Loiacono R, Sexton PM, Christopoulos A. RNA editing of the serotonin 5HT2C receptor and its effects on cell signalling, pharmacology and brain function. Pharmacol Ther. 2008;119:7–23. DOI: 10.1016/j.pharmthera.2008.03.012.

[64] Perrier JF, Rasmussen HB, Christensen RK, Petersen AV. Modulation of the intrinsic properties of motoneurons by serotonin. Curr Pharm Des. 2013;19:4371–4384. DOI: 10.2174/13816128113199990341.

[65] Lanfumey L, Hamon M. 5-HT1 receptors. Curr Drug Targets CNS Neurol Disord. 2004;3:1–10. DOI: 10.2174/1568007043482570.

[66] Daval G, Vergé D, Basbaum AI, Bourgoin S, Hamon M. Autoradiographic evidence of serotonin1 binding sites on primary afferent fibres in the dorsal horn of the rat spinal cord. Neurosci Lett. 1987;83:71–76. DOI: 10.1016/0304-3940(87)90218-7.

[67] Marlier L, Teilhac JR, Cerruti C, Privat A. Autoradiographic mapping of 5-HT1, 5-HT1A, 5-HT1B and 5-HT2 receptors in the rat spinal cord. Brain Res. 1991;550:15–23. DOI: 10.1016/0006-8993(91)90400-P.

[68] Thor KB, Nickolaus S, Helke CJ. Autoradiographic localization of 5-hydroxytrypta-mine1A, 5-hydroxytryptamine1B and 5-hydroxytryptamine1C/2 binding sites in the rat spinal cord. Neuroscience. 1993;55:235–252. DOI: 10.1016/0306-4522(93)90469-V.

[69] Kia HK, Miquel MC, Brisorgueil MJ, Daval G, Riad M, El Mestikawy S, Hamon M, Vergé D. Immunocytochemical localization of serotonin1A receptors in the rat central

nervous system. J Comp Neurol. 1996;365:289–305. DOI: 10.1002/(SI-CI)1096-9861(19960205)365:2<289::AID-CNE7>3.0.CO;2-1.

[70] Talley EM, Bayliss DA. Postnatal development of 5-HT(1A) receptor expression in rat somatic motoneurons. Brain Res Dev Brain Res. 2000;122:1–10. DOI: 10.1016/S0165-3806(00)00036-5.

[71] Kheck NM, Gannon PJ, Azmitia EC. 5-HT1A receptor localization on the axon hillock of cervical spinal motoneurons in primates. J Comp Neurol. 1995;355:211–220. DOI: 10.1002/cne.903550205.

[72] Eide PK, Joly NM, Hole K. The role of spinal cord 5-HT1A and 5-HT1B receptors in the modulation of a spinal nociceptive reflex. Brain Res. 1990;536:195–200. DOI: 10.1016/0006-8993(90)90025-7.

[73] Hochman S, Garraway SM, Machacek DW, Shay BL. 5-HT receptors and the neuro-modulatory control of spinal cord function. In: Cope TC, editor. Motor Neurobiology of the Spinal Cord. CRC Press: Boca Raton; 2001. p. 47–87.

[74] Nadeson R, Goodchild CS. Antinociceptive role of 5-HT1A receptors in rat spinal cord. Br J Anaesth. 2002;88:679–684. DOI: 10.1093/bja/88.5.679.

[75] Buritova J, Larrue S, Aliaga M, Besson JM, Colpaert F. Effects of the high-efficacy 5-HT1A receptor agonist, F 13640 in the formalin pain model: a c-Fos study. Eur J Pharmacol. 2005;514:121–130. DOI:10.1016/j.ejphar.2005.03.016.

[76] Kim JM, Jeong SW, Yang J, Lee SH, Kim WM, Jeong S, Bae HB, Yoon MH, Choi JI. Spinal 5-HT1A, not the 5-HT1B or 5-HT3 receptors, mediates descending serotoner-gic inhibition for late-phase mechanical allodynia of carrageenan-induced peripheral inflammation. Neurosci Lett. 2015;600:91–97. DOI: 10.1016/j.neulet.2015.05.058.

[77] Alhaider AA, Wilcox GL. Differential roles of 5-hydroxytryptamine1A and 5-hydrox-ytryptamine1B receptor subtypes in modulating spinal nociceptive transmission in mice. J Pharmacol Exp Ther. 1993;265:378–385.

[78] Ali Z, Wu G, Kozlov A, Barasi S. The actions of 5-HT1 agonists and antagonists on nociceptive processing in the rat spinal cord: results from behavioural and electrophy-siological studies. Brain Res. 1994;661:83–90. DOI:10.1016/0006-8993(94)91184-3.

[79] Zhao ZQ, Liu XY, Jeffry J, Karunarathne WK, Li JL, Munanairi A, Zhou XY, Li H, Sun YG, Wan L, Wu ZY, Kim S, Huo FQ, Mo P, Barry DM, Zhang CK, Kim JY, Gautam N, Renner KJ, Li YQ, Chen ZF. Descending control of itch transmission by the serotoner-gic system via 5-HT1A-facilitated GRP–GRPR signaling. Neuron. 2014;84:821–834. DOI: 10.1016/j.neuron.2014.10.003.

[80] Bervoets K, Rivet JM, Millan MJ. 5-HT1A receptors and the tail-flick response. IV. Spinally localized 5-HT1A receptors postsynaptic to serotoninergic neurones mediate spontaneous tail-flicks in the rat. J Pharmacol Exp Ther. 1993;264:95–104.

[81] Cotel F, Exley R, Cragg SJ, Perrier JF. Serotonin spillover onto the axon initial segment of motoneurons induces central fatigue by inhibiting action potential initiation. Proc Natl Acad Sci USA. 2013;110:4774–4779. DOI: 10.1073/pnas.1216150110.

[82] Perrier JF, Cotel F. Serotonergic modulation of spinal motor control. Curr Opin Neurobiol. 2015;33:1–7. DOI: 10.1016/j.conb.2014.12.008.

[83] Laporte AM, Fattaccini CM, Lombard MC, Chauveau J, Hamon M. Effects of dorsal rhizotomy and selective lesion of serotonergic and noradrenergic systems on 5-HT1A, 5-HT1B, and 5-HT3 receptors in the rat spinal cord. J Neural Transm Gen Sect. 1995;100:207–223. DOI: 10.1007/BF01276459.

[84] Jackson DA, White SR. Receptor subtypes mediating facilitation by serotonin of excitability of spinal motoneurons. Neuropharmacology.1990; 29:787–797. DOI: 10.1016/0028-3908(90)90151-G.

[85] Mantilla CB, Bailey JP, Zhan WZ, Sieck G. Phrenic motoneuron expression of serotonergic and glutamatergic receptors following upper cervical spinal cord injury. Exp Neurol. 2012;234:191–199. DOI: 10.1016/j.expneurol.2011.12.036.

[86] el-Yassir N, Fleetwood-Walker SM, Mitchell R. Heterogeneous effects of serotonin in the dorsal horn of rat: the involvement of 5-HT1 receptor subtypes. Brain Res. 1988;456:147–158. DOI: 10.1016/0006-8993(88)90356-3.

[87] Zhang Y, Yang Z, Gao X, Wu G. The role of 5-hydroxytryptamine1A and 5-hydroxytryptamine1B receptors in modulating spinalnociceptive transmission in normal and carrageenan-injected rats. Pain. 2001;92:201–211. DOI: 10.1016/S0304-3959(01)00259-7.

[88] Monroe PJ, Smith DJ. Demonstration of an autoreceptor modulating the release of [3H]5-hydroxytryptamine from a synaptosomal-rich spinal cord tissue preparation. J Neurochem. 1985;45:1886–1894. DOI: 10.1111/j.1471-4159.1985.tb10548.x.

[89] Brown L, Amedro J, Williams G, Smith D. A pharmacological analysis of the rat spinal cord serotonin (5-HT) autoreceptor. Eur J Pharm. 1988;145: 163–171. DOI: 10.1016/0014-2999(88)90227-0.

[90] Murphy RM, Zemlan FP. Selective 5-HT1B agonists identify the 5-HT autoreceptor in lumbar spinal cord of rat. Neuropharmacology. 1988;27:37–42. DOI: 10.1016/0028-3908(88)90198-0.

[91] Allain AE, Ségu L, Meyrand P, Branchereau P. Serotonin controls the maturation of the GABA phenotype in the ventral spinal cord via 5-HT1b receptors. Ann N Y Acad Sci. 2010;1198:208–219. DOI: 10.1111/j.1749-6632.2010.05433.x.

[92] Potrebic S, Ahn AH, Skinner K, Fields HL, Basbaum AI. Peptidergic nociceptors of both trigeminal and dorsal root ganglia express serotonin 1D receptors: implications for the selective antimigraine action of triptans. J Neurosci. 2003;23:10988–10997.

[93] Ahn AH, Basbaum AI. Tissue injury regulates serotonin 1D receptor expression: implications for the control of migraine and inflammatory pain. J Neurosci. 2006;26:8332–8338. DOI: 10.1523/JNEUROSCI.1989-06.2006.

[94] Enjin A, Leão KE, Mikulovic S, Le Merre P, Tourtellotte WG, Kullander K. Sensorimotor function is modulated by the serotonin receptor 1d, a novel marker for gamma motor neurons. Mol Cell Neurosci. 2012;49:322–332. DOI: 10.1016/j.mcn.2012.01.003.

[95] D'Amico JM, Li Y, Bennett DJ, Gorassini MA. Reduction of spinal sensory transmission by facilitation of 5-HT1B/D receptors in noninjured andspinal cord-injured humans. J Neurophysiol. 2013;109:1485–1493. DOI: 10.1152/jn.00822.2012.

[96] Jeong CY, Choi JI, Yoon MH. Roles of serotonin receptor subtypes for the antinociception of 5-HT in the spinal cord of rats. Eur J Pharmacol. 2004;502:205–211. DOI: 10.1016/j.ejphar.2004.08.048.

[97] Honda M, Imaida K, Tanabe M, Ono H. Endogenously released 5-hydroxytryptamine depresses the spinal monosynaptic reflex via 5-HT1D receptors. Eur J Pharmacol. 2004;503:55–61. DOI: 10.1016/j.ejphar.2004.09.045.

[98] Castro ME, Pascual J, Romón T, del Arco C, del Olmo E, Pazos A. Differential distribution of [³H]sumatriptan binding sites (5-HT1B, 5-HT1D and 5-HT1F receptors) in human brain: focus on brainstem and spinal cord. Neuropharmacology. 1997;36:535–542. DOI: 10.1016/S0028-3908(97)00061-0.

[99] Murray KC, Stephens MJ, Rank M, D'Amico J, Gorassini MA, Bennett DJ. Polysynaptic excitatory postsynaptic potentials that trigger spasms after spinal cord injury in rats are inhibited by 5-HT1B and 5-HT1F receptors. J Neurophysiol. 2011;106:925–943. DOI: 10.1152/jn.01011.2010.

[100] Classey JD, Bartsch T, Goadsby PJ. Distribution of 5-HT(1B), 5-HT(1D) and 5-HT(1F) receptor expression in rat trigeminal and dorsal root ganglia neurons: relevance to the selective anti-migraine effect of triptans. Brain Res. 2010;1361:76–85. DOI: 10.1016/j.brainres.2010.09.004.

[101] Agosti RM. 5HT1F- and 5HT7-receptor agonists for the treatment of migraines. CNS Neurol Disord Drug Targets. 2007;6:235–237. DOI: 10.2174/187152707781387242.

[102] Ferrari MD, Färkkilä M, Reuter U, Pilgrim A, Davis C, Krauss M, Diener HC; European COL-144 Investigators. Acute treatment of migraine with the selective 5-HT1F receptor agonist lasmiditan—a randomised proof-of-concept trial. Cephalalgia. 2010;30:1170–1178. DOI: 10.1177/0333102410375512.

[103] Humphrey PP, Hartig P, Hoyer D. A proposed new nomenclature for 5-HT receptors. Trends Pharmacol Sci. 1993;14:233–236. DOI: 10.1016/0165-6147(93)90016-D.

[104] Pompeiano M, Palacios JM, Mengod G. Distribution of the serotonin 5-HT2 receptor family mRNAs: comparison between 5-HT2A and 5-HT2C receptors. Brain Res Mol Brain Res. 1994;23:163–178. DOI: 10.1016/0169-328X(94)90223-2.

[105] Helton LA, Thor KB, Baez M. 5-Hydroxytryptamine2A, 5-hydroxytryptamine2B, and 5-hydroxytryptamine2C receptor mRNA expression in the spinal cord of rat, cat, monkey and human. Neuroreport. 1994;5:2617–2620.

[106] Cornea-Hébert V, Riad M, Wu C, Singh SK, Descarries L. Cellular and subcellular distribution of the serotonin 5-HT2A receptor in the central nervous system of adult rat.   J   Comp   Neurol.   1999;409:187–209.   DOI: 10.1002/(SI-CI)1096-9861(19990628)409:2<187::AID-CNE2>3.0.CO;2-P.

[107] Fonseca MI, Ni YG, Dunning DD, Miledi R. Distribution of serotonin 2A, 2C and 3 receptor mRNA in spinal cord and medulla oblongata. Brain Res Mol Brain Res. 2001;89:11–19. DOI: 10.1016/S0169-328X(01)00049-3.

[108] Doly S, Madeira A, Fischer J, Brisorgueil MJ, Daval G, Bernard R, Verge D, Conrath M. The 5-HT2A receptor is widely distributed in the rat spinal cord and mainly localized at the plasma membrane of postsynaptic neurons. J Comp Neurol. 2004;472:496–511. DOI: 10.1002/cne.20082.

[109] Pineda-Farias JB, Velázquez-Lagunas I, Barragán-Iglesias P, Cervantes-Durán C, Granados-Soto V. 5-HT$_{2B}$ receptor antagonists reduce nerve injury-induced tactile allodynia and expression of 5-HT$_{2B}$ receptors. Drug Dev Res. 2015;76:31–39. DOI: 10.1002/ddr.21238.

[110] Xu C, Giuliano F, Sun XQ, Brisorgueil MJ, Leclerc P, Vergé D, Conrath M. Serotonin 5-HT2A and 5-HT5A receptors are expressed by different motoneuron populations in rat Onuf's nucleus. J Comp Neurol. 2007;502:620–634. DOI: 10.1002/cne.21344.

[111] Eide PK, Hole K. Different role of 5-HT1A and 5-HT2 receptors in spinal cord in the control of nociceptive responsiveness. Neuropharmacology. 1991;30:727–731. DOI: 10.1016/0028-3908(91)90180-J.

[112] Kjørsvik A, Tjølsen A, Hole K. Activation of spinal serotonin(2A/2C) receptors augments nociceptive responses in the rat. Brain Res. 2001;910:179–181. DOI: 10.1016/S0006-8993(01)02652-X.

[113] Nishiyama T. Effects of a 5-HT2A receptor antagonist, sarpogrelate on thermal or inflammatory pain. Eur J Pharmacol. 2005;516:18–22. DOI: 10.1016/j.ejphar.2005.04.026.

[114] Thibault K, Van Steenwinckel J, Brisorgueil MJ, Fischer J, Hamon M, Calvino B, Conrath M. Serotonin 5-HT2A receptor involvement and Fos expression at the spinal level in vincristine-induced neuropathy in the rat. Pain. 2008;140:305–322. DOI: 10.1016/j.pain.2008.09.006.

[115] Xie DJ, Uta D, Feng PY, Wakita M, Shin MC, Furue H, Yoshimura M. Identification of 5-HT receptor subtypes enhancing inhibitory transmission in the rat spinal dorsal horn in vitro. Mol Pain. 2012;8:58. DOI: 10.1186/1744-8069-8-58.

[116] Iwasaki T, Otsuguro K, Kobayashi T, Ohta T, Ito S. Endogenously released 5-HT inhibits A and C fiber-evoked synaptic transmission in the rat spinal cord by the facilitation of

GABA/glycine and 5-HT release via 5-HT(2A) and 5-HT(3) receptors. Eur J Pharmacol. 2013;702:149–157. DOI: 10.1016/j.ejphar.2013.01.058.

[117] Fone KC, Robinson AJ, Marsden CA. Characterization of the 5-HT receptor subtypes involved in the motor behaviours produced by intrathecal administration of 5-HT agonists in rats. Br J Pharmacol. 1991;103:1547–1555. DOI: 10.1111/j. 1476-5381.1991.tb09825.x.

[118] Yamazaki J, Fukuda H, Nagao T, Ono H. 5-HT2/5-HT1C receptor-mediated facilitatory action on unit activity of ventral horn cells in rat spinal cord slices. Eur J Pharmacol. 1992;220:237–242. DOI: 10.1016/0014-2999(92)90753-Q.

[119] Mbaki Y, Gardiner J, McMurray G, Ramage AG. 5-HT 2A receptor activation of the external urethral sphincter and 5-HT 2C receptor inhibition of micturition: a study based on pharmacokinetics in the anaesthetized female rat. Eur J Pharmacol. 2012;682:142–152. DOI: 10.1016/j.ejphar.2012.02.010.

[120] Watson NV, Gorzalka BB. DOI-induced inhibition of copulatory behavior in male rats: reversal by 5-HT2 antagonists. Pharmacol Biochem Behav. 1991;39:605–612. DOI: 10.1016/0091-3057(91)90135-O.

[121] Rössler AS, Bernabé J, Denys P, Alexandre L, Giuliano F. Effect of the 5-HT receptor agonist DOI on female rat sexual behavior. J Sex Med. 2006;3:432–441. DOI: 10.1111/j. 1743-6109.2006.00240.x.

[122] Wienecke J, Westerdahl AC, Hultborn H, Kiehn O, Ryge J. Global gene expression analysis of rodent motor neurons following spinal cord injury associates molecular mechanisms with development of postinjury spasticity. J Neurophysiol. 2010;103:761–778. DOI: 10.1152/jn.00609.2009.

[123] MacFarlane PM, Vinit S, Mitchell GS. Serotonin 2A and 2B receptor-induced phrenic motor facilitation: differential requirement for spinal NADPH oxidase activity. Neuroscience. 2011;178:45–55. DOI: 10.1016/j.neuroscience.2011.01.011.

[124] Lin SY, Chang WJ, Lin CS, Huang CY, Wang HF, Sun WH. Serotonin receptor 5-HT2B mediates serotonin-induced mechanical hyperalgesia. J Neurosci. 2011;31:1410–1418. DOI: 10.1523/JNEUROSCI.4682-10.2011.

[125] Aira Z, Buesa I, García del Caño G, Salgueiro M, Mendiable N, Mingo J, Aguilera L, Bilbao J, Azkue JJ. Selective impairment of spinal mu-opioid receptor mechanism by plasticity of serotonergic facilitation mediated by 5-HT2A and 5-HT2B receptors. Pain. 2012;153:1418–1425. DOI: 10.1016/j.pain.2012.03.017.

[126] Cervantes-Durán C, Vidal-Cantú GC, Barragán-Iglesias P, Pineda-Farias JB, Bravo-Hernández M, Murbartián J, Granados-Soto V. Role of peripheral and spinal 5-HT2B receptors in formalin-induced nociception. Pharmacol Biochem Behav. 2012;102:30–35. DOI: 10.1016/j.pbb.2012.03.015.

[127] Mbaki Y, Ramage AG. Investigation of the role of 5-HT2 receptor subtypes in the control of the bladder and the urethra in the anaesthetized female rat. Br J Pharmacol. 2008;155:343–356. DOI: 10.1038/bjp.2008.273.

[128] Holohean AM, Hackman JC. Mechanisms intrinsic to 5-HT2B receptor-induced potentiation of NMDA receptor responses in frog motoneurones. Br J Pharmacol. 2004;143:351–360. DOI: 10.1038/sj.bjp.0705935.

[129] Pranzatelli MR, Murthy JN, Pluchino RS. Identification of spinal 5-HT1C binding sites in the rat: characterization of [³H]mesulergine binding. J Pharmacol Exp Ther. 1992;261:161–165.

[130] Bancila M, Vergé D, Rampin O, Backstrom JR, Sanders-Bush E, McKenna KE, Marson L, Calas A, Giuliano F. 5-Hydroxytryptamine 2C receptors on spinal neurons controlling penile erection in the rat. Neuroscience. 1999;92:1523–1537. DOI: 10.1016/S0306-4522(99)00082-2.

[131] Clemett DA, Punhani T, Duxon MS, Blackburn TP, Fone KC. Immunohistochemical localisation of the 5-HT2C receptor protein in the rat CNS. Neuropharmacology. 2000;39:123–132. DOI: 10.1016/S0028-3908(99)00086-6.

[132] Holmes GM. 5-Hydroxytryptamine2C receptors on pudendal motoneurons innervating the external anal sphincter. Brain Res. 2005;1057:65–71. DOI: 10.1016/j.brainres.2005.07.047.

[133] Obata H, Saito S, Sakurazawa S, Sasaki M, Usui T, Goto F. Antiallodynic effects of intrathecally administered 5-HT(2C) receptor agonists in rats with nerve injury. Pain. 2004;108:163–169. DOI: 10.1016/j.pain.2003.12.019.

[134] Machacek DW, Garraway SM, Shay BL, Hochman S. Serotonin 5-HT(2) receptor activation induces a long-lasting amplification of spinal reflex actions in the rat. J Physiol. 2001;537:201–207. DOI: 10.1111/j.1469-7793.2001.0201k.x.

[135] Shay BL, Sawchuk M, Machacek DW, Hochman S. Serotonin 5-HT2 receptors induce a long-lasting facilitation of spinal reflexes independent of ionotropic receptor activity. J Neurophysiol. 2005;94:2867–2877. DOI: 10.1152/jn.00465.2005.

[136] Gajendiran M. In vivo evidence for serotonin 5-HT2C receptor-mediated long-lasting excitability of lumbar spinal reflex and its functional interaction with 5-HT1A receptor in the mammalian spinal cord. Brain Res Bull. 2008;75:674–680. DOI: 10.1016/j.brainresbull.2007.11.003.

[137] Halberstadt AL, van der Heijden I, Ruderman MA, Risbrough VB, Gingrich JA, Geyer MA, Powell SB. 5-HT(2A) and 5-HT(2C) receptors exert opposing effects on locomotor activity in mice. Neuropsychopharmacology. 2009;34:1958–1967. DOI: 10.1038/npp.2009.29.

[138] Conlon K, Miner W, McCleary S, McMurray G. Identification of 5-HT(2C) mediated mechanisms involved in urethral sphincter reflexes in a guinea-pig model of urethral function. BJU Int. 2012;110:E113–117. DOI: 10.1111/j.1464-410X.2011.10756.x.

[139] Thompson AJ, Lummis SC. Discriminating between 5-HT₃A and 5-HT₃AB receptors. Br J Pharmacol. 2013;169:736–747. DOI: 10.1111/bph.12166.

[140] Kia HK, Miquel MC, McKernan RM, Laporte AM, Lombard MC, Bourgoin S, Hamon M, Vergé D. Localization of 5-HT3 receptors in the rat spinal cord: immunohistochemistry and in situ hybridization. Neuroreport. 1995;6:257–261.

[141] Laporte AM, Doyen C, Nevo IT, Chauveau J, Hauw JJ, Hamon M. Autoradiographic mapping of serotonin 5-HT1A, 5-HT1D, 5-HT2A and 5-HT3 receptors in the aged human spinal cord. J Chem Neuroanat. 1996;11:67–75. DOI: 10.1016/0891-0618(96)00130-5.

[142] Morales M, Battenberg E, Bloom FE. Distribution of neurons expressing immunoreactivity for the 5HT3 receptor subtype in the rat brain and spinal cord. J Comp Neurol. 1998;402:385–401. DOI: 10.1002/(SICI)1096-9861(19981221)402:3<385::AID-CNE7>3.0.CO;2-Q.

[143] Maxwell DJ, Kerr R, Rashid S, Anderson E. Characterisation of axon terminals in the rat dorsal horn that are immunoreactive for serotonin 5-HT3A receptor subunits. Exp Brain Res. 2003;149:114–124. DOI: 10.1007/s00221-002-1339-7.

[144] Glaum SR, Proudfit HK, Anderson EG. 5-HT3 receptors modulate spinal nociceptive reflexes. Brain Res. 1990;510:12–16. DOI: 10.1016/0006-8993(90)90721-M.

[145] Alhaider AA, Lei SZ, Wilcox GL. Spinal 5-HT3 receptor-mediated antinociception: possible release of GABA. J Neurosci. 1991;11:1881–1888.

[146] Khasabov SG, Lopez-Garcia JA, Asghar AU, King AE. Modulation of afferent-evoked neurotransmission by 5-HT3 receptors in young rat dorsal horn neurones in vitro: a putative mechanism of 5-HT3 induced anti-nociception. Br J Pharmacol. 1999;127:843–852. DOI: 10.1038/sj.bjp.0702592.

[147] Fukushima T, Ohtsubo T, Tsuda M, Yanagawa Y, Hori Y. Facilitatory actions of serotonin type 3 receptors on GABAergic inhibitory synaptic transmission in the spinal superficial dorsal horn. J Neurophysiol. 2009;102:1459–1471. DOI: 10.1152/jn.91160.2008.

[148] Guo W, Miyoshi K, Dubner R, Gu M, Li M, Liu J, Yang J, Zou S, Ren K, Noguchi K, Wei F. Spinal 5-HT3 receptors mediate descending facilitation and contribute to behavioral hypersensitivity via a reciprocal neuron–glial signaling cascade. Mol Pain. 2014;10:35. DOI: 10.1186/1744-8069-10-35.

[149] Conte D, Legg ED, McCourt AC, Silajdzic E, Nagy GG, Maxwell DJ. Transmitter content, origins and connections of axons in the spinal cord that possess theserotonin

(5-hydroxytryptamine) 3 receptor. Neuroscience. 2005;134:165–173. DOI: 10.1016/
j.neuroscience.2005.02.013.

[150] Huang J, Wang YY, Wang W, Li YQ, Tamamaki N, Wu SX. 5-HT(3A) receptor subunit
is expressed in a subpopulation of GABAergic and enkephalinergic neurons in the
mouse dorsal spinal cord. Neurosci Lett. 2008;441:1–6. DOI: 10.1016/j.neulet.
2008.04.105.

[151] Guertin PA, Steuer I. Ionotropic 5-HT3 receptor agonist-induced motor responses in
the hindlimbs of paraplegic mice. J Neurophysiol. 2005;94:3397–3405. DOI: 10.1152/jn.
00587.2005.

[152] Espey MJ, Downie JW. Serotonergic modulation of cat bladder function before and after
spinal   transection.   Eur   J   Pharmacol.   1995;287:173–177.   DOI:
10.1016/0014-2999(95)00614-1.

[153] Suwa B, Bock N, Preusse S, Rothenberger A, Manzke T. Distribution of serotonin4(a)
receptors in the juvenile rat brain and spinal cord. J Chem Neuroanat. 2014;55:67–77.
DOI: 10.1016/j.jchemneu.2013.12.004.

[154] Godínez-Chaparro B, López-Santillán FJ, Orduña P, Granados-Soto V. Secondary
mechanical allodynia and hyperalgesia depend on descending facilitation mediated
byspinal 5-HT4, 5-HT6 and 5-HT7 receptors. Neuroscience. 2012;222:379–391. DOI:
10.1016/j.neuroscience.2012.07.008.

[155] Grailhe R, Grabtree GW, Hen R. Human 5-HT(5) receptors: the 5-HT(5A) receptor is
functional but the 5-HT(5B) receptor was lost during mammalian evolution. Eur J
Pharmacol. 2001;418:157–167. DOI: 10.1016/S0014-2999(01)00933-5.

[156] Doly S, Fischer J, Brisorgueil MJ, Vergé D, Conrath M. 5-HT5A receptor localization in
the rat spinal cord suggests a role in nociception and control of pelvic floor muscula-
ture. J Comp Neurol. 2004;476:316–329. DOI: 10.1002/cne.20214.

[157] Muñoz-Islas E, Vidal-Cantú GC, Bravo-Hernández M, Cervantes-Durán C, Quiñonez-
Bastidas GN, Pineda-Farias JB, Barragán-Iglesias P, Granados-Soto V. Spinal 5-HT5A
receptors mediate 5-HT-induced antinociception in several pain models in rats.
Pharmacol Biochem Behav. 2014;120:25–32. DOI: 10.1016/j.pbb.2014.02.001.

[158] Gérard C, el Mestikawy S, Lebrand C, Adrien J, Ruat M, Traiffort E, Hamon M, Martres
MP. Quantitative RT-PCR distribution of serotonin 5-HT6 receptor mRNA in the
central nervous system of control or 5,7-dihydroxytryptamine-treated rats. Synapse.
1996;23:164–173. DOI: 10.1002/(SICI)1098-2396(199607)23:3<164::AID-SYN5>3.0.CO;
2-6.

[159] Gérard C, Martres MP, Lefèvre K, Miquel MC, Vergé D, Lanfumey L, Doucet E, Hamon
M, el Mestikawy S. Immuno-localization of serotonin 5-HT6 receptor-like material in
the rat central nervous system. Brain Res. 1997;746:207–219. DOI: 10.1016/
S0006-8993(96)01224-3.

[160] Castañeda-Corral G, Rocha-González HI, Araiza-Saldaña CI, Ambriz-Tututi M, Vidal-Cantú GC, Granados-Soto V. Role of peripheral and spinal 5-HT6 receptors according to the rat formalin test. Neuroscience. 2009;162:444–452. DOI: 10.1016/j.neuroscience.2009.04.072.

[161] To ZP, Bonhaus DW, Eglen RM, Jakeman LB. Characterization and distribution of putative 5-ht7 receptors in guinea-pig brain. Br J Pharmacol. 1995;115:107–116. DOI: 10.1111/j.1476-5381.1995.tb16327.x.

[162] Doly S, Fischer J, Brisorgueil MJ, Vergé D, Conrath M. Pre- and postsynaptic localization of the 5-HT7 receptor in rat dorsal spinal cord: immunocytochemical evidence. J Comp Neurol. 2005;490:256–269. DOI: 10.1002/cne.20667.

[163] Viguier F, Michot B, Hamon M, Bourgoin S. Multiple roles of serotonin in pain control mechanisms—implications of 5-HT7 and other 5-HT receptor types. Eur J Pharmacol. 2013;716:8–16. DOI: 10.1016/j.ejphar.2013.01.074.

[164] Yesilyurt O, Seyrek M, Tasdemir S, Kahraman S, Deveci MS, Karakus E, Halici Z, Dogrul A. The critical role of spinal 5-HT7 receptors in opioid and non-opioid type stress-induced analgesia. Eur J Pharmacol. 2015;762:402–410. DOI: 10.1016/j.ejphar.2015.04.020.

[165] Dam LJ, Hai L, Ha YM. Role of the 5-HT(7) receptor in the effects of intrathecal nefopam in neuropathic pain in rats. Neurosci Lett. 2014;566:50–54. DOI: 10.1016/j.neulet.2014.02.021.

[166] Lee HG, Kim WM, Kim JM, Bae HB, Choi JI. Intrathecal nefopam-induced antinociception through activation of descending serotonergic projections involving spinal 5-HT7 but not 5-HT3 receptors. Neurosci Lett. 2015;587:120–125. DOI: 10.1016/j.neulet.2014.12.040.

[167] Liu J, Jordan LM. Stimulation of the parapyramidal region of the neonatal rat brain stem produces locomotor-like activity involving spinal 5-HT7 and 5-HT2A receptors. J Neurophysiol. 2005;94:1392–1404. DOI: 10.1152/jn.00136.2005.

[168] Jordan LM, Liu J, Hedlund PB, Akay T, Pearson KG. Descending command systems for the initiation of locomotion in mammals. Brain Res Rev. 2008;57:183–191. DOI: 10.1016/j.brainresrev.2007.07.019.

[169] Liu J, Akay T, Hedlund PB, Pearson KG, Jordan LM. Spinal 5-HT7 receptors are critical for alternating activity during locomotion: in vitro neonatal and in vivo adult studies using 5-HT7 receptor knockout mice. J Neurophysiol. 2009;102:337–348. DOI: 10.1152/jn.91239.2008.

[170] Cornide-Petronio ME, Fernández-López B, Barreiro-Iglesias A, Rodicio MC. Traumatic injury induces changes in the expression of the serotonin 1A receptor in the spinal cord of lampreys. Neuropharmacology. 2014;77:369–378. DOI: 10.1016/j.neuropharm.2013.10.017.

[171] Cornide-Petronio ME, Ruiz MS, Barreiro-Iglesias A, Rodicio MC. Spontaneous regeneration of the serotonergic descending innervation in the sea lamprey after spinal cord injury. J Neurotrauma. 2011;28:2535–2540. DOI: 10.1089/neu.2011.1766.

[172] Landry ES, Lapointe NP, Rouillard C, Levesque D, Hedlund PB, Guertin PA. Contribution of spinal 5-HT1A and 5-HT7 receptors to locomotor-like movement induced by 8-OH-DPAT in spinal cord-transected mice. Eur J Neurosci. 2006;24:535–546. DOI: 10.1111/j.1460-9568.2006.04917.x.

[173] Gu B, Thor KB, Reiter JP, Dolber PC. Effect of 5-hydroxytryptamine1 serotonin receptor agonists on noxiously stimulated micturition in cats with chronic spinal cord injury. J Urol. 2007;177:2381–2385. DOI: 10.1016/j.juro.2007.01.110.

[174] Honda M, Tanabe M, Ono H. Serotonergic depression of spinal monosynaptic transmission is mediated by 5-HT1B receptors. Eur J Pharmacol. 2003;482:155–161. DOI: 10.1016/j.ejphar.2003.09.070.

[175] Gu B, Olejar KJ, Reiter JP, Thor KB, Dolber PC. Inhibition of bladder activity by 5-hydroxytryptamine1 serotonin receptor agonists in cats with chronicspinal cord injury. J Pharmacol Exp Ther. 2004;310:1266–1272. DOI: 10.1124/jpet.103.063842.

[176] Ung RV, Landry ES, Rouleau P, Lapointe NP, Rouillard C, Guertin PA. Role of spinal 5-HT2 receptor subtypes in quipazine-induced hindlimb movements after a low-thoracic spinal cord transection. Eur J Neurosci. 2008;28:2231–2242. DOI: 10.1111/j. 1460-9568.2008.06508.x.

[177] Kao T, Shumsky JS, Jacob-Vadakot S, Himes BT, Murray M, Moxon K. Role of the 5-HT2C receptor in improving weight-supported stepping in adult rats spinalized as neonates. Brain Res. 2006;1112:159–168. DOI: 10.1016/j.brainres.2006.07.020.

[178] Basura GJ, Zhou SY, Walker PD, Goshgarian HG. Distribution of serotonin 2A and 2C receptor mRNA expression in the cervical ventral horn and phrenic motoneurons following spinal cord hemisection. Exp Neurol. 2001;169:255–263. DOI: 10.1006/exnr. 2001.7682.

[179] Zhou SY, Basura GJ, Goshgarian HG. Serotonin (2) receptors mediate respiratory recovery after cervical spinal cord hemisection in adult rats. J Appl Physiol. 2001;91:2665–2673.

[180] Majczyński H, Maleszak K, Cabaj A, Sławińska U. Serotonin-related enhancement of recovery of hind limb motor functions in spinal rats after grafting of embryonic raphe nuclei. J Neurotrauma. 2005;22:590–604. DOI: 10.1089/neu.2005.22.590.

[181] Kim D, Murray M, Simansky KJ. The serotonergic 5-HT(2C) agonist m-chlorophenyl-piperazine increases weight-supported locomotion without development of toler-ance in rats with spinal transections. Exp Neurol. 2001;169:496–500. DOI: 10.1006/ exnr.2001.7660.

[182] Murray KC, Stephens MJ, Ballou EW, Heckman CJ, Bennett DJ. Motoneuron excitability and muscle spasms are regulated by 5-HT2B and 5-HT2C receptor activity. J Neurophysiol. 2011;105:731–748. DOI: 10.1152/jn.00774.2010.

[183] Perrier JF, Hounsgaard J. 5-HT2 receptors promote plateau potentials in turtle spinal motoneurons by facilitating an L-type calcium current. J Neurophysiol. 2003;89:954–959. DOI: 10.1152/jn.00753.2002.

[184] Chen J, Gu B, Wu G, Tu H, Si J, Xu Y, Andersson KE. The effect of the 5-HT2A/2C receptor agonist DOI on micturition in rats with chronic spinal cord injury. J Urol. 2013;189:1982–1988. DOI: 10.1016/j.juro.2012.11.049.

[185] Bos R, Sadlaoud K, Boulenguez P, Buttigieg D, Liabeuf S, Brocard C, Haase G, Bras H, Vinay L. Activation of 5-HT2A receptors upregulates the function of the neuronal K-Cl cotransporter KCC2. Proc Natl Acad Sci USA. 2013;110:348–353. DOI: 10.1073/pnas.1213680110.

[186] Gackière F, Vinay L. Serotonergic modulation of post-synaptic inhibition and locomotor alternating pattern in the spinal cord. Front Neural Circuits. 2014;8:102. DOI: 10.3389/fncir.2014.00102.

[187] Rende M, Morales M, Brizi E, Bruno R, Bloom F, Sanna PP. Modulation of serotonin 5-HT3 receptor expression in injured adult rat spinal cord motoneurons. Brain Res. 1999;823:234–240. DOI: 10.1016/S0006-8993(99)01180-4.

[188] Gang W, Hongjian T, Jasheng C, Jiemin S, Zhong C, Yuemin X, Baojun G, Andersson KE. The effect of the 5-HT7 serotonin receptor agonist, LP44, on micturition in rats with chronic spinal cord injury. Neurourol Urodyn. 2014;33:1165–1170. DOI: 10.1002/nau.22463.

[189] Faden AI, Gannon A, Basbaum AI. Use of serotonin immunocytochemistry as a marker of injury severity after experimental spinal trauma in rats. Brain Res. 1988;450:94–100. DOI: 10.1016/0006-8993(88)91548-X.

[190] Holmes GM, Van Meter MJ, Beattie MS, Bresnahan JC. Serotonergic fiber sprouting to external anal sphincter motoneurons after spinal cord contusion. Exp Neurol. 2005;193:29–42. DOI: 10.1016/j.expneurol.2005.01.002.

[191] Hadjiconstantinou M, Panula P, Lackovic Z, Neff NH. Spinal cord serotonin: a biochemical and immunohistochemical study following transection. Brain Res. 1984;322:245–254. DOI: 10.1016/0006-8993(84)90114-8.

[192] Bregman BS. Development of serotonin immunoreactivity in the rat spinal cord and its plasticity after neonatal spinal cord lesions. Brain Res. 1987;431:245–263. DOI: 10.1016/0165-3806(87)90213-6.

[193] Saruhashi Y, Young W, Perkins R. The recovery of 5-HT immunoreactivity in lumbosacral spinal cord and locomotor function after thoracic hemisection. Exp Neurol. 1996;39:203–213. DOI: 10.1006/exnr.1996.0094.

[194] Filli L, Zörner B, Weinmann O, Schwab ME. Motor deficits and recovery in rats with unilateral spinal cord hemisection mimic the Brown-Sequard syndrome. Brain. 2011;134:2261–2273. DOI: 10.1093/brain/awr167.

[195] Camand E, Morel MP, Faissner A, Sotelo C, Dusart I. Long-term changes in the molecular composition of the glial scar and progressive increase of serotoninergic fibre sprouting after hemisection of the mouse spinal cord. Eur J Neurosci. 2004;20:1161–1176. DOI: 10.1111/j.1460-9568.2004.03558.x.

[196] Magnusson T. Effect of chronic transection on dopamine, noradrenaline and 5-hydroxytryptamine in the rat spinal cord. Naunyn Schmiedebergs Arch Pharmacol. 1973;278:13–22. DOI: 10.1007/BF00501859.

[197] Jaeger CB, Teitelman G, Joh TH, Albert VR, Park DH, Reis DJ. Some neurons of the rat central nervous system contain aromatic-L-amino-acid decarboxylase but not monoamines. Science. 1983;219:1233–1235. DOI: 10.1126/science.6131537.

[198] Ren LQ, Wienecke J, Hultborn H, Zhang M. Production of dopamine by aromatic L-amino acid decarboxylase cells after spinal cord injury. J Neurotrauma. 2016;33:1–11. DOI: 10.1089/neu.2015.4037.

[199] Hou S, Carson DM, Wu D, Klaw MC, Houlé JD, Tom VJ. Dopamine is produced in the rat spinal cord and regulates micturition reflex after spinal cord injury. Exp Neurol. DOI: 10.1016/j.expneurol.2015.12.001.

[200] Bhattacharyya S, Raote I, Bhattacharya A, Miledi R, Panicker MM. Activation, internalization, and recycling of the serotonin 2A receptor by dopamine. Proc Natl Acad Sci USA. 2006;103:15248–15253. DOI: 10.1073/pnas.0606578103.

5

Bridging Defects in Chronic Spinal Cord Injury Using Peripheral Nerve Grafts: From Basic Science to Clinical Experience

Sherif M. Amr

Abstract

Nerve grafting of the injured spinal cord should pursue a sixfold attack: lysing the fibrosis/gliosis to an extent that allows settling of the basal lamina preventing meanwhile collapse of the neural tissue matrix; supplying the tissue matrix with a suitable scaffold, on which the basal lamina can settle; basal lamina synthesis; seeding the basal lamina with cell adhesion molecules; providing the axonal growth cone with neurite outgrowth promoting factors that allow its distal progression; supplying the axonal growth cone with neurotrophic factors that power its continued growth. In addition to this, the intrinsic properties of the neurons should be stimulated, possibly through modulating the function of astrocytes by heparin, aspirin and other factors. Nerve side grafting of the cord increases the incidence of nerve regeneration by applying additional grafts extending from the side of the donor end of the cord to the side of the recipient end. Also, it allows the surgeon to enhance regeneration through a partially regenerated cord. During surgery, after establishment of CSF circulation, a long-lasting indwelling catheter has to be inserted for postoperative drug and cell delivery. This allows for continual lysis of the gliosis by chondroitinase ABC, sialidase and other factors.

Keywords: spinal cord injury, nerve grafting, indwelling intrathecal catheter implantation, lysis of the gliosis, chondroitinase ABC

1. Introduction

Since 1903, when Tello and Cajal demonstrated that the central nervous system (CNS) could regenerate [1, 2], experimental neuroscience has advanced our knowledge repairing the injured spinal cord. Several cellular transplantation strategies have been recommended with some clinical success [3–6]. Clinically, however, the injured spinal cord is usually extensively gliotic, cystic, even disrupted, necessitating bridging the injury zone first before contemplating cellular transplantation. Placing peripheral nerve grafts to bridge the injury zone has been successful experimentally [7–13], yet only anecdotal clinical evidence supports it [14, 15]. In a review article on bridging spinal cord injuries, Fawcett [16] commented on this disparity between experimental and clinical neuroscience: 'Sadly, we have yet to achieve a treatment that is licensed for this purpose in human patients'. The aim of this review is to enable clinicians to put the findings made by neuroscientists into clinical practice and to provide neuroscientists with upcoming ideas investigating the clinical issues physicians face.

2. Changing concepts of nerve grafting

2.1. Basic concepts of nerve grafting

Autogenous nerve grafting is the standard for repair of irreducible nerve gaps [17]. The basic principles of nerve grafting include the following (**Figure 1**):

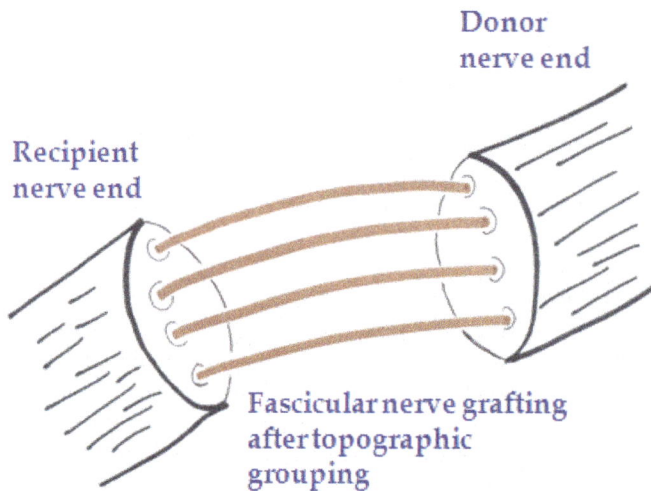

Figure 1. The basic principles of conventional end-to-end grafting include trimming both proximal and distal nerve ends up to healthy nerve fascicles; avoiding any tension at the repair site, avoiding any shearing stress at the repair site, fascicular grafting, end-to-end grafting suturing fascicles at proximal nerve ends to their counterparts at distal nerve ends after grouping them topographically, using small caliber sutures (9/0 or 10/0 sutures), and healthy vascular bed.

- trimming both proximal and distal nerve ends up to healthy nerve fascicles;

- avoiding any tension at the repair site, for even minimal tension, can end up with fibrosis, hampering progression of regeneration;

- avoiding any shearing stress at the repair site because this incites an inflammatory reaction ending up with fibrosis and hampering progression of regeneration;

- fascicular grafting because autogenous nerve grafts derive their nutrition from the extracellular matrix; using large diameter grafts instead of small diameter fascicles can produce central necrosis of the graft;

- end-to-end grafting suturing fascicles at proximal nerve ends to their counterparts at distal nerve ends after grouping them topographically, in order to avoid aberrant nerve sprouting;

- using small caliber sutures (9/0 or 10/0 sutures) because large caliber sutures may produce fibrosis;

- healthy vascular bed because a fibrotic bed may prevent progression of regeneration through the grafts.

In the absence of a proximal nerve end, such as in brachial plexus avulsions, nerve transfer (neurotisation) refers to using an expendable nearby donor nerve as a substitute, grafting it to the original recipient. The principles of nerve transfer include:

- donor nerve of high axonal load,

- single donor to single recipient to prevent cocontractions.

Autogenous grafts act as immunogenically inert scaffolds, providing appropriate neurotrophic factors and viable Schwann cells for axonal regeneration [17].

2.2. Molecular aspects of peripheral nerve regeneration

Advances in the understanding of molecular pathways and their physiological role have provided us with new insights as to the mechanism of axonal (peripheral nerve) regeneration [18, 19].

Fibrous tissue and chondroitin sulphate proteoglycans secreted by astrocytes provide the necessary scaffold for settling of the basal lamina and subsequent basement membrane synthesis. *Neurite outgrowth promoting factors* are basement membrane-related extracellular matrix proteins (such as laminin (LN), fibronectin (FN), heparin sulphate proteoglycans (HSP) and tenascin), which pave the proper path by supplying orientation and adhesiveness for axons. *Neurotrophic factors* are specific trophic agents that power peripheral nerve regeneration. They include (a) the neurotrophins (nerve growth factor (NGF), brain-derived neurotrophic factor (BDNF), neurotrophin-3 (NT-3) and neurotrophin-4/5(NT-4/5)); (b) the neurokines (ciliary neurotrophic factor (CNTF) and leukaemia inhibitory factor (LIF)); (c) the transforming growth factor (TGF)-b family (TGF-b1, TGF-b2, TGF-b3, glial cell line derived neurotrophic factor (GDNF)). *Schwann cells* secrete (a) cell adhesion molecules (CAMs), such as N-CAM, Ng-CAM/L1, N-cadherin and L2/HNK-1; (b) produce basement membrane that contains many extracellular matrix proteins, such as laminin (LN), fibronectin (FN), heparin sulphate proteoglycans (HSP) and tenascin; (c) secrete neurotrophic factors and their receptors. In addition to this, axonal regeneration is determined by trophic factors from activated perineural glial cells (astrocytes), trophic factors from efferent axons by anterograde transport, gene-induced trophic factors by intracrine or autocrine transport, trophic factors from retrograde target cell support, trophic factors from retroaxonal transport and trophic factors from recruited macrophages (secretory products, cytokines). Activated mesenchymal cells contribute to repair and vascularisation (**Figure 2**).

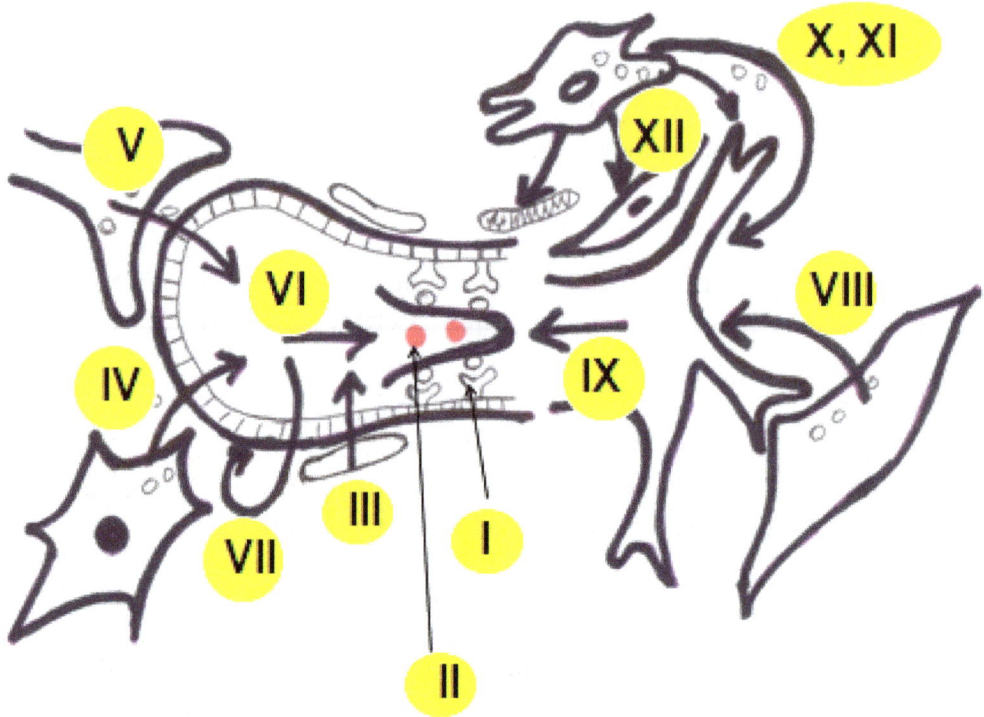

Figure 2. Molecular aspects of axonal regeneration. (I) *Neurite outgrowth promoting factors* [such as laminin (LN), fibronectin (FN), heparin sulphate proteoglycans (HSP) and tenascin] pave the proper path by supplying orientation and adhesiveness for axons. (II) *Neurotrophic factors* are the specific trophic agents that power peripheral nerve regeneration. They include (a) neurotrophins (NGF, BDNF, NT-4/5); (b) neurokines (CNTF, LIF); (c) (TGF)-β family (TGF-β1, TGF-β2, TGF-β3, GDNF). (III) *Schwann cells* secrete (a) cell adhesion molecules (CAMs), such as N-CAM, Ng-CAM/L1, N-cadherin, andL2/HNK-1; (b) basement membrane that contains many extracellular matrix proteins, such as laminin (LN), fibronectin (FN), heparin sulphate proteoglycans (HSP) and tenascin; (c) neurotrophic factors and their receptors. In addition to this, axonal regeneration is determined by trophic factors from activated perineural glial cells (astrocytes) (IV), trophic factors from efferents by anterograde transport (V), gene-induced trophic factors by intracrine (VI) or autocrine (VII) transport, trophic factors from retrograde target cell support (VIII), trophic factors from retroaxonal transport (IX), trophic factors from recruited macrophages (secretory products X, cytokines XI). Activated mesenchymal cells contribute to repair and vascularisation (XII). Among other molecules, heparin and aspirin modulate astrocytic function stimulating them to secrete axonal trophic factors (IV).

Based on the previous considerations, axonal sprouting and nerve grafting are based on a sixfold attack (**Figure 3**):

– lysing the fibrosis/gliosis in the injury zone to an extent that allows settling of the basal lamina preventing meanwhile collapse of the neural tissue matrix; or excision of the fibrotic segment and replacing it with nerve grafts;

– supplying the tissue matrix with a suitable scaffold, on which the basal lamina can settle,

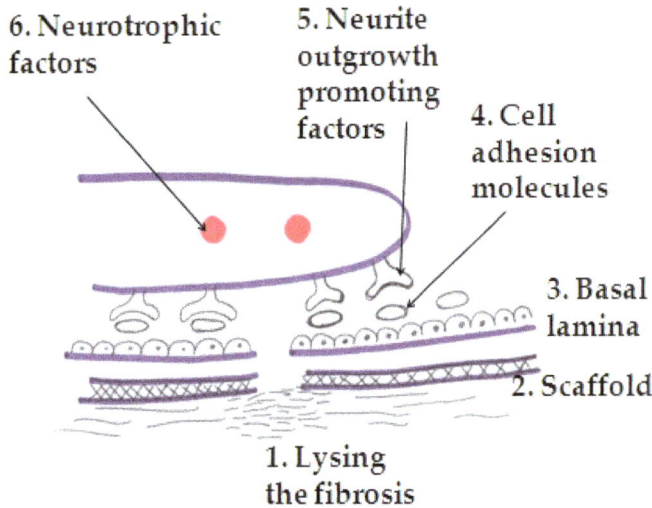

Figure 3. The sixfold attack: lysing the fibrosis/gliosis to an extent that allows settling of the basal lamina preventing meanwhile collapse of the neural tissue matrix; supplying the tissue matrix with a suitable scaffold, on which the basal lamina can settle; basal lamina synthesis; seeding the basal lamina with cell adhesion molecules; providing the axonal growth cone with neurite outgrowth promoting factors (FGF) that allow its distal progression; supplying the axonal growth cone with neurotrophic factors that allow its continued growth.

– basal lamina synthesis;

– seeding the basal lamina with cell adhesion molecules;

– providing the axonal growth cone with neurite outgrowth promoting factors that allow its distal progression;

– supplying the axonal growth cone with neurotrophic factors that power its continued growth.

2.3. Changing concepts of nerve grafting: side grafting

The previous conditions prevailing, if the side of a motor nerve is injured, the axonal growth cone may be enticed to grow off motor nerve side to the injured end of another motor nerve, the so-called recipient end to donor side coaptation. Described independently by Balance and Harris over a century ago (in 1903), interest in end-to-side coaptation has been rekindled by Viterbo et al. [17]. In its essence, it involves grafting donor side to recipient end after stimulating donor side collateral sprouting by mechanical trauma or axotomy (**Figure 4(a)**). An indirect application of it is increasing the incidence of nerve regeneration after conventional end-to-end grafting by applying additional grafts extending from the side of the donor end to the side of the recipient end [20] (**Figure 4(b)**). In nerve transfer, the latter technique allows the surgeon to use a single high axonal load donor for multiple recipients without producing cocontractions (e.g., major brachial plexus root to several peripheral nerves and caudal cord to cauda equina) [20] (**Figure 4(c)**). Also, partially regenerated nerves cannot be surgically cut and nerve grafted leading to loss of already regained function; the latter technique allows the surgeon to enhance regeneration through them (**Figure 4(d)**).

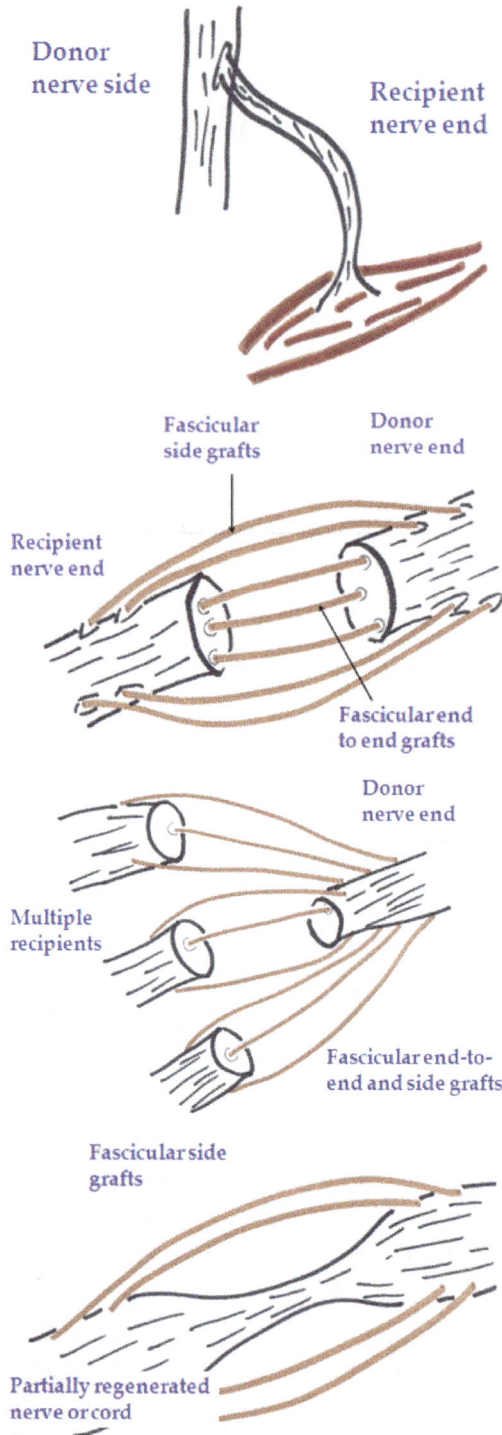

Figure 4. (a) End-to-side grafting involves grafting donor side to recipient end after stimulating donor side collateral sprouting by mechanical trauma or axotomy. (b) An indirect application of side grafting is increasing the incidence of nerve regeneration after conventional end-to-end grafting by applying additional grafts extending from the side of the donor end to the side of the recipient end. (c) Side grafting allows the surgeon to use a single high axonal load donor for multiple recipients without producing cocontractions. (d) Partially regenerated nerves cannot be surgically cut and nerve grafted sacrifying already regained function; side grafting allows the surgeon to enhance regeneration through them.

2.4. Mathematical modelling and channel-carrying capacity applied to nerve grafting: necessary concepts for subsequent computer-assisted fabrication of artificial nerve grafts

Can we manipulate the molecular mechanisms of the sixfold attack to increase neurite outgrowth into the side grafts? Manipulating molecular mechanisms is based on the sensitivity of the axonal growth cone to spatial molecular concentration gradients [21, 22]. In a study by Rosoff et al. [21], axonal growth has been shown to be enhanced by a steep nerve growth factor (NGF) spatial concentration gradient. There is a narrow range, however, between the lowest NGF concentration necessary for axonal growth stimulation and the highest NCF concentration beyond which axonal growth is competitively blocked. As the lower and upper limits of the concentration gradient should fall within this narrow range, the maximal distance for axonal growth cone progression guided by that gradient would be far less than the length of the neural defect. Utilising synthetic nerve graft scaffolds and observing the sixfold attack, axonal growth can be hypothetically made to bridge the whole length of the neural gap by seeding the scaffolds with multiple NGF spatial concentration gradients [22]. Neurite outgrowth has been modelled as a non-linear partial differential equation, that is solved by an iterative mathematical process suitable for numerical analysis and for subsequent computer-assisted fabrication of artificial nerve grafts [22]. By diffusion, these NGF spatial concentration gradients might also enhance axonal growth within the adjacent natural nerve side grafts.

Alternatively, and also to increase neurite outgrowth into the side grafts and decrease aberrant neural sprouting, multiple microspheres embedding chemical attractive and repulsive cues and placed along nerve side grafts may be used to guide axonal growth [23]. Preliminary experiments conducted with embryonic rat hippocampal neurons and calcium alginate microspheres have been encouraging [24]. A mathematical model has been developed based on the diffusion gradient of the implanted microspheres; a genetic algorithm has been used to study its proper spatial implementation [23].

A more accurate mathematical model for axonal growth cone progression has been provided based on sensory pinch test data [25]. Disadvantages of this model, however, include the assumptions that the initial delay is the major cause of variability, and that delay to scarring of the neural bed lies within the initial delay and that the regeneration rate is linear (constant).

Can we quantify the molecular mechanisms of the sixfold attack so that nearly 100% of all axons sprouting from the proximal spinal cord reach the distal spinal cord through the side grafts and simultaneously minimise the probability of aberrant neural sprouting to nearly 0%? Unless incorporated in information theory, which is a theory based on mathematical probability [26, 27], the mathematical models mentioned above do not provide a numerical solution for this problem. This is imperative, however, for subsequent computer-assisted fabrication of artificial nerve grafts. The Shannon-Hartley channel-carrying capacity principle, a central concept in information theory, refers to the intrinsic property of any information channel to accept all information from the donor and transmit it noiseless to the recipient. Applied to nerve grafting, the channel-carrying capacity of a nerve graft scaffold is its ability to transmit all axons sprouting from the proximal cord to the distal cord and simultaneously minimise the probability of aberrant neural sprouting.

3. Peripheral nerve grafting of the injured spinal cord as an application of the concept of side grafting and the sixfold attack

3.1. Technical aspects of peripheral nerve grafting and repair of the injured spinal cord

An indirect application of side grafting, as mentioned previously, is, first, increasing the incidence of nerve regeneration after conventional end-to-end grafting by applying addition-al grafts extending from the side of the donor end to the side of the recipient end; and, second, preserving partially regenerated nerves which cannot be surgically cut and nerve grafted leading to loss of already regained function [20]. Both of these apply to the spinal cord; compared to its high axonal load, the cross-sectional area of the spinal cord is too small for efficient end-to-end grafting. In addition, some kind of regeneration may have occurred in a contused cord in a completely paraplegic patient; this may take the form of less than Grade 3 motor power improvement, which, according to ASIA standards, is not enough to be consid-ered motor or neurological level progression [28]. Third, side grafting produces less trauma to the spinal cord. In fact, the glial tissue secreted by astrocytes provides the necessary supporting tissue for axons and neurons [2, 29]. In side grafting, fine pial incisions are used. This process is far less traumatic than freshening of the cord ends during end-to-end graft-ing, a procedure which would lead to excessive glial tissue secretion and subsequent block-ing of regeneration.

3.2. Donor nerves

Clinically, the sural nerve is the most commonly used donor nerve, other suitable donor nerves include the medial and lateral cutaneous nerves of the forearm, dorsal cutaneous branch of the ulnar nerve, superficial and deep peroneal nerves, intercostal nerves, and the posterior and lateral cutaneous nerves of the thigh [17].

Pre-degenerated (segments of nerve cut and left in situ for 7–10 days prior to harvesting) peripheral nerves are infiltrated by regenerating axons to a greater extent (both in number and distance) than freshly cut and harvested nerves [30]. The use of pre-degenerated nerves has been contested by other authors, however [31].

3.3. Experimental applications of side grafting

Based on the work of David and Aguayo [5, 7], numerous studies have confirmed axonal outgrowth after nerve grafting of the injured spinal cord [30, 32–38]; axons growing within peripheral nerve grafts have not only retained their physiological properties [39] but have synapsed with neurons near the point of central nervous system re-entry as well [40].

3.4. Re-evaluation of the use of peripheral nerve grafts to bridge spinal cord defects

Nerve grafts supply the injured spinal cord with five factors of the sixfold attack: a suitable scaffold, on which the basal lamina can settle; basal laminae; cell adhesion molecules; neurite outgrowth promoting factors; and neurotrophic factors. Nevertheless, the use of peripheral nerve grafts has been challenged [5, 16, 35, 41, 42]. According to experimental observation, damaged spinal cord axons might grow from the cranial cord into peripheral nerve grafts but would not leave them to enter the caudal cord [5]. Schwann cells might even promote gliosis [16, 41].

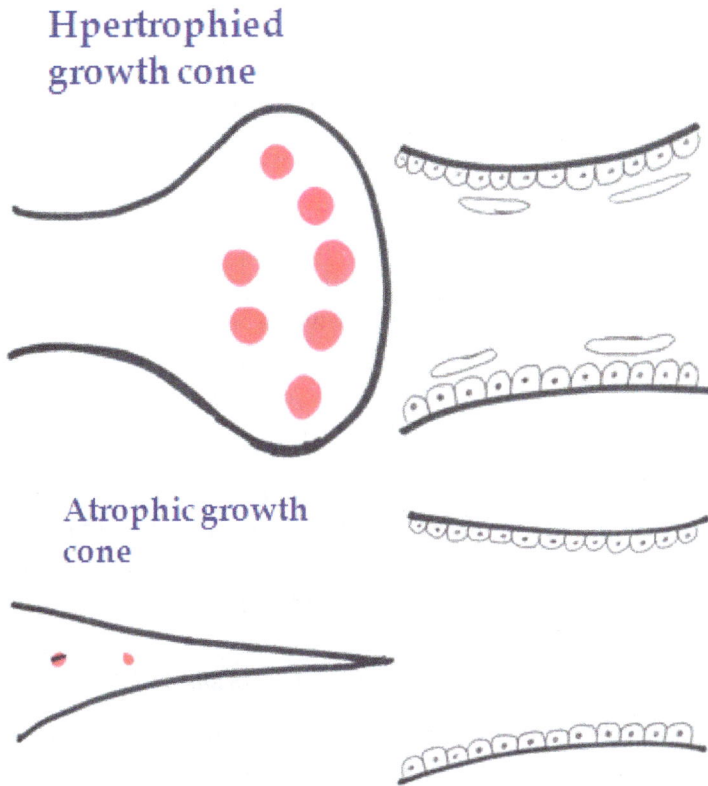

Hpertrophied growth cone

Atrophic growth cone

Figure 5. (a) Excessive fibrosis in the presence of neurotophic factors and adequate neuron growth potential leads to hypertrophy of both donor and recipient ends of the damaged neural tissue (excessive neuroma formation; dystrophic growth cones). (b) Excessive fibrosis in the absence of neurotophic factors and adequate neuron growth potential leads to atrophy of both donor and recipient ends of the damaged neural tissue (atrophic neuroma formation; atrophic growth cones).

It might be assumed that failure of growth cone progression is due to missing of the sixth factor in the sixfold attack (lysing the fibrosis/gliosis to an extent that allows settling of the basal lamina preventing meanwhile collapse of the neural tissue matrix). However, failure of axons to regenerate following peripheral nerve grafting may also result from intrinsic properties of the neurons and the absence of neurotrophic factors [43–46]. These considerations help us assess neural tissue during surgery. Excessive fibrosis in the presence of neurotophic factors and adequate neuron growth potential leads to hypertrophy of both donor and recipient ends of the damaged neural tissue (excessive neuroma formation and dystrophic growth cones) [47, 48] (**Figure 5(a)**), whereas excessive fibrosis in the absence of neurotophic factors and adequate neuron growth potential leads to atrophy of both donor and recipient ends of the damaged neural tissue (atrophic neuroma formation; atrophic growth cones) (**Figure 5(b)**). In conclusion, in addition to the sixfold attack, the intrinsic properties of the neurons should be stimulated to produce neurites.

4. Lysing the gliosis in conjunction with nerve grafting

4.1. The gliosis: blocking of regeneration mechanically and through the activation of RhoA

Injured axons encounter a series of inhibitory factors that are non-permissive for growth [4, 29, 41, 49]. These include myelin inhibitors (Nogo-A ,MAG108 (myelin-associated glycoprotein) and OMgp109 (oligodendrocyte myelin glycoprotein)); chondroitin sulphate proteoglycans (neurocan, versican, aggrecan, brevican, phosphacan and NG2); and semaphorins and ephrins. Upregulated in response to spinal cord injury [50–52], they act not only by mechanical blocking of neural regeneration but by inhibiting axon outgrowth neuronal receptors and subsequent activation of signalling pathways known to be involved in the activation of RhoA and the rise in intracellular calcium.

4.2. Lysing the gliosis by chondroitinase ABC

Chondroitinase ABC cleaves the inhibitory chondroitin sulphate glycosaminoglycan chains from the core protein, reducing the inhibition by chondroitin sulphate proteoglycans [53, 54]. Houle et al. [55] have demonstrated CNS axons regenerating through a peripheral nerve graft and entering the caudal spinal cord following chondroitinase ABC treatment.

4.2.1. Chondroitinase ABC in combination with growth factors and scaffolds

Combined with glial-derived neurotrophic factor (GDNF) delivery, chondroitinase ABC promotes axon extension through peripheral nerve bridges [50, 56]. Combined with growth factors, chondroitinase ABC enhances the activation and oligodendrocyte differentiation of endogenous precursor cells after spinal cord injury and attenuates astrogliosis. When added to polycaprolactone or poly (acrylonitrile)/poly(vinyl chloride) (PAN/PVC) scaffolds, chondroitinase ABC allows regenerating axons to exit the distal end of the scaffold and continue on to distal targets [57–60].

4.2.2. Chondroitinase ABC in combination with cell therapies

Chondroitinase ABC has improved recovery of function in synergy with mesenchymal stromal cells [D43], or a Schwann cell bridge and olfactory ensheathing cells or in combination with transplanted neural precursor cells and a growth factor (GF) cocktail containing EGF, FGF2 and platelet-derived growth factor (PDGF)-AA [61, 62].

4.2.3. Thermostabilisation, delivery, dosage and complications of chondroitinase ABC: chondroitinase ABC might be a weak enzyme

Thermostabilisation of chondroitinase ABC with the sugar trehalose can reduce its temperature-dependent loss of activity [50, 63]. Delivery of chondroitinase ABC is predominantly intrathecal using osmotic minipumps [30, 55, 64]. Nevertheless, the enzyme can also be loaded into lipid microtubes or possibly poly (lactic-co-glycolic acid) (PLGA), providing a means for its gradual release over 1–2 weeks [65]. It can also be loaded into fibrin gel scaffolds before injecting it intrathecally; this ensures its continuous release for at least 3 weeks [66].

The effect of chondroitinase ABC is dose-dependent [67]. Injected intrathecally in acute injuries at a low dose (1 or 5 IUs), chondroitinase ABC may enhance axonal progression; injected at a high dose (50 IU), it may produce subarachnoid haemorrhage. In subacute or chronic injuries, low-dose injection produces no or limited functional recovery, whilst high-dose injection (50 or 100 IUs) produce lysis of the gliosis [68, 69].

Single-dose chondroitinase ABC is not considered enough. Therefore, multiple single injections at 0, 1, 2 and 4 weeks have been recommended [70]. Daily injections for 2 weeks at 0.06 Units per dose have also been recommended [71]. Four weeks of treatment have promoted recovery more than 2 weeks [72]. One way to ensure the continued release of chondroitinase ABC is neuron transfection with a vector containing the gene encoding chondroitinase ABC [73]. Another way is loading scaffolds with chondroitinase ABC.

Although chondroitinase ABC allows substantial structural plasticity in the spinal cord, it is not sufficient to enhance locomotor recovery unless combined with neural precursor cell transplantation and in vivo infusion of growth factors [74]. In a rat spinal cord injury model, Wilems et al. [62] have used fibrin scaffolds loaded with neurotrophic factors (item I), anti-inhibitory molecules (item II) and encapsulated embryonic stem-cell-derived progenitor motor neurons (pMNs) (item III). Fibrin scaffolds containing items I and II but not item III have had lower chondroitin sulphate proteoglycan levels compared to scaffolds containing items II and III. This shows the importance of combining neurotrophic factors with chondroitinase ABC and cellular transplants. Scaffolds containing item III, but not item II, have shown differentiation into neuronal cell types, axonal extension and the ability to integrate into host tissue. However, the combination of items II and III have led to reduced cell survival and increased macrophage infiltration. This shows that cellular transplants not only claim priority over chondroitinase ABC, but that chondroitinase ABC may be a weak enzyme as well. Because of this fact, a combination treatment of zymosan and chondroitinase ABC has been recommended [75]. Lastly, adipose-derived stem cell transplantation has been found to produce the same effect as chondroitinase ABC administration [76]. Thus, chondroitinase ABC might be a weak enzyme.

4.3. Sialidase as an alternative

In a rat model of spinal cord contusion injury the effects of sialidase (Vibrio cholerae) and chondroitinase ABC (ChABC, Proteus vulgaris) have been tested [77]. Immunohistochemistry has revealed that infused sialidase has acted robustly throughout the spinal cord grey and white matter, whereas ChABC activity has been more intense superficially. Sialidase treatment alone has resulted in improved behavioural and anatomical outcomes.

4.4. Anti-Nogo

Blocking myelin-associated inhibitors with Nogo-A monoclonal antibodies or with Nogo-receptor competitive agonist peptide, NEP1-40 has been shown to increase axonal regeneration [50]. Combination therapies, such as cross-linking the Nogo-66 receptor antibody into a hyaluronic acid hydrogel [50], a combination of methylprednisolone and NEP1-40 and Nogo-receptor vaccination combined with neural stem cell transplantation have improved neural fibre regeneration.

4.5. Rho inhibition

Many of the inhibitory signals described above (ephrins, Nogo) converge on the intracellular molecule Rho-A, which is a key mediator of actin depolymerisation and hence inhibition of axonal elongation. Blocking Rho-A with Rho inhibitor 'cethrin' might overcome its effect. A synthetic membrane-permeable peptide mimetic of the protein tyrosine phosphatase σ (PTPσ), wedge domain can bind to PTPσ and relieve chondroitin sulphate proteoglycan-mediated inhibition [78].

4.6. Reversing the inhibition of phosphoinositide 3-kinase (PI3K) by cell permeable phosphopeptide (PI3Kpep)

Phosphoinositide 3-kinase (PI3K) is a lipid kinase activated by axon growth promoting signals. Chondroitin sulphate proteoglycans inhibit phosphoinositide 3-kinase signalling in axons and growth cones, an effect that can be reversed by cell permeable phosphopeptide (PI3Kpep). The latter acts by R-Ras-PI3K signalling [79].

4.7. Rolipram

Increased intracellular levels of cyclic adenosine monophosphate (cAMP) and protein kinase A have been associated with CNS ability to overcome the gliosis [50]. Rolipram, a phosphodiesterase4 inhibitor, can increase intracellular cAMP levels [50].

4.8. Improving blood vessel formation

Improving blood vessel formation might reduce cell death and promote angiogenesis within the injury zone. Neural stem cells modified to express vascular endothelial growth factor have improved white matter sparing following thoracic contusion spinal cord injury [50]. Biomaterial poly-lactic-co-glycolic acid (PLGA) scaffolds loaded with neural stem cells and endothelial cells have shown increased vessel and neurofilament density at the injury centre [50].

5. Modulating astrocyte function enhances the intrinsic properties of neurons to stimulate neurite outgrowth into peripheral nerve grafts

In addition to the sixfold attack, the intrinsic properties of the neurons have to be stimulated to produce neurites. This can take place by modulating astrocyte function (**Figure 2**).

5.1. Endogenous inhibitors of axonal regeneration (intrinsic properties of neurons)

Endogenous inhibitors of axonal regeneration include the molecule phosphatase and tensin homologue (PTEN), loss of neuronal cAMP and deactivation/activation of certain transcription factors [46].

The molecule phosphatase and tensin homologue (PTEN) on chromosome 10 is a tumour suppressor. Its deletion has been shown to increase post-embryonic neural regeneration after injury. Its inhibition–mediated regeneration is partly mediated by the inhibitor of the mechanistic target of rapamycin (mTOR) pathway; it is also mediated by glycogen synthesis kinase GSK-3β.

When levels of cAMP at the growth cone are high, the effect on the growth cone is chemoattraction, whereas when they are low, the effect is chemorepulsion.

Certain transcription factors are positive regulators of axonal growth (e.g., members of the Krüppel-like factors (KLFs) present in retinal ganglion cells (RGCs); STAT3 a transcription factor, part of the JAK-STAT signaling pathway; members of the Jun and Fos families, components of the transcription factor AP-1 and ATF3). Other transcription factors are negative regulators of axonal growth. Nuclear factor IL-3 (NFIL3) represses CREB-mediated transcription and expression of regeneration-associated genes such as arginase and GAP-43.

It follows that combatting endogenous inhibitors of axonal regeneration include the following:

– Inactivation of GSK-3β by neurotrophins. This increases collapsin response mediator protein-2 (CRMP-2) stabilisation of microtubules and increases axon elongation in developing neurites.

– Local administration of taxol. Microtubules and actin microfilaments are critical for regeneration [80]. They potentiate the effect of GAP-43. Thus, local administration of taxol, a microtubule-stabilising agent, increases neurite outgrowth [81].

– Elevating cAMP levels by local injection of a phosphodiesterase inhibitor. This improves axonal regeneration.

– Conditioning lesions. Conditioning lesions [46] are based on the observation that double level nerve lesions regenerate better than single level nerve lesions. Thus sciatic nerve transection prior to a spinal cord lesion improves regeneration within the injured spinal cord.

– Cell adhesion molecules. Their synthesis is increased after peripheral nerve injury but not after CNS injury [82, 83]. Expression of cell adhesion molecules by neurons can be induced by virally mediated vectors or by injecting them into the CNS injury site [84, 85].

Many of these functions can be activated by modulating astrocyte function.

5.2. Astrocyte trophic effects on neurite outgrowth and neurogenesis

Astrocytes release a variety of trophic factors [86–88]. These trophic factors include nerve growth factor, basic fibroblast growth factor, transforming growth factor-β, platelet-derived growth factor, brain-derived neurotrophic factor, ciliary neurotrophic factor and others. Reactive astrocytes increase the expression of several of these, notably nerve growth factor, basic fibroblast growth factor, brain-derived neurotrophic factor and neuregulins, which can stimulate neurite outgrowth. Reactive astrocytes also overexpress neuropilin-1 and vascular endothelial growth factor, which act in concert to promote angiogenesis after cerebral ischemia. Hevin (SPARC-like protein 1), a synaptogenic protein released by astrocytes, forms a relay between a neurexin (pre-synaptic) and a neuroligin (post-synaptic); this relay is crucial for the synaptogenesis [89].

5.3. Modulating the function of astrocytes and heparin

5.3.1. Role of heparin in lysing the gliosis

Both unfractionated and low molecular weight heparins inhibit thrombin activation [90]. In addition, they have a fibrolytic (gliolytic) effect and can modulate astrocyte function.

Clinically, perineural application of condensed polytetrafluoroethylene-extractum cepae-heparin-allantoin gel during peripheral nerve surgery improves functional recovery [91]. The anti-fibrotic effects of heparin are well documented after flexor tendon surgery of the hand [92], in the resolution of intraperitoneal fibrosis [93, 94] and in improving various scar types [95].

Among other actions, heparan sulphate/heparin influences fibroblast growth factor responsible for cell proliferation, differentiation, signal transduction and angiogenesis [96, 97]. Heparin is known to inhibit fibroblast growth factor (FGF)-2-stimulated DNA synthesis as well as gene expression of FGF-2 and its receptor in AT2 pneumocytes [98]. Probably via syndecan-1, the presence of heparin at high concentrations reduces the activity of FGF-7, which is responsible for enhancement of keratinocytes migration and proliferation. Heparin enhances the action of FGF-1, which regulates the proliferation of fibroblasts, endothelial and epithelial cells, and influences angiogenesis via effect on the activity of endothelial cells. Heparin can enhance the stability of FGF-1 and might determine the formation of FGF1-FGFR (fibroblast growth factor receptor) active complex.

5.3.2. Possible role of heparin in modulating astrocyte function

Astrocyte stress response and trophic effects are mediated by the FGF family member, on which heparin exerts a profound influence [96, 99]. Fibroblast growth factor 1 (FGF1) has been shown to maintain the survival of neurons and induce neurite outgrowth [100]. Basic fibroblast growth factor (FGF-2) has been found to increase neuronal survival and neurite extension in foetal rat hippocampal neurons when bound to heparin substrates [101]. The length and sulphated position of heparin regulate FGF-2-dependent astrocytic transformation (stella-tion), native heparin significantly promoting FGF-2-dependent astrocytic transformation, whereas heparin hexasaccharide and 2-O-, 6-O- and N-desulphated heparins inhibit it [102]. Heparin affin regulatory peptide (HARP, pleiotrophin, heparin-binding growth-associated molecule) promotes neurite outgrowth and synaptic development. High levels of heparin affin regulatory peptide HARP mRNA and protein are induced in transformed astrocytes [103, 104]. Glypican-1 is a major high-affinity ligand of the Slit proteins, both of which are strongly upregulated in reactive astrocytes, suggesting their possible role in the inhibitory environ-ment preventing axonal regeneration after injury. Heparins inhibit glypican-Slit interactions [105, 106].

5.4. Possible role of aspirin in modulating astrocyte function

Ciliary neurotrophic factor (CNTF) is a promyelinating trophic factor. Acetylsalicylic acid (aspirin) increases mRNA and protein expression of CNTF in primary mouse and human astrocytes in a dose- and time-dependent manner. Aspirin-induced astroglial CNTF is also functionally active; supernatants of aspirin-treated astrocytes of wild type, but not Cntf null, mice increase myelin-associated proteins in oligodendrocytes and protected oligodendro-cytes from TNF-α insult [107].

5.5. Possible role of hyaluronic acid salts in modulating astrocyte function

The presence of high molecular weight hyaluronic acid (hyaluronic acid with limited degra-dation) after spinal cord injury decreases glial scarring. High molecular weight hyaluronic acid stabilised against degradation mitigates astrocyte activation in vitro and in vivo. Therefore, hyaluronic-acid-based hydrogel systems hold great potential for minimising undesired scarring as part of future repair strategies after spinal cord injury [108].

6. Combining peripheral nerve grafts with scaffolds: the scaffold as a drug release system

The defect within the spinal cord is too large to be bridged by nerve grafts alone; besides, the myelin sheath within them is inhibitory to axonal growth. The rationale for polymer im-plants is twofold, to replace a damaged area of the cord with just such a structural matrix [109] and to provide it with a synthetic scaffold, in which myelin is absent. Combining peripheral nerve grafts with scaffolds has gained more acceptance because of the importance of seeding the scaffolds with multiple nerve growth factor (NGF) spatial concentration gradients in order to promote axonal growth both within the scaffolds and the nerve grafts [22].

Biomaterial scaffolds in spinal cord injury have been reviewed by Madigan et al. [109] and Straley et al. [110]. Commonly used scaffolds include natural polymers (in vivo extracellular matrix polymers, polymers derived from blood, and polymers from marine life) and synthet-ic polymers (poly-hydroxy acid polymers and synthetic hydrogels). Examples for in vivo extracellular matrix polymers are collagen solutions and the glycosaminoglycan hyaluronic acid. Examples for polymers derived from blood are plasma-derived polymers, fibronectin and fibrin. Examples for polymers from marine life are agarose, alginate and chitosan. Synthetic polymers include poly-hydroxy acid polymers and synthetic hydrogels. Compared to natural polymers, they offer wider scope to design and control the characteristics of the material. Poly-hydroxy acid polymers are biodegradable materials based on polyesters of lactic and glycolic acid (PLA and PGA) and their co-polymer PLGA. Synthetic hydrogels are based on polyethylene glycol, a biodegradable synthetic polymer of ethylene oxide units. Poly(2-hydroxyethyl methacrylate) (pHEMA) compounds and pHEMA-co-methyl methacrylate (pHEMA-MMA) are used as spinal cord scaffolds.

Whatever macroengineering and microengineering procedures scaffolds are subjected to allow for axonal growth, this will not occur unless the scaffold is seeded with basal lamina and supplied with neurite outgrowth promoting factors and neurotrophic factors (**Figure 3**). These factors can be released from the scaffold material itself, from integrated micro- or nano-spheres or tubules of a different material, or by means of a scaffold's capacity to support a genetically modified cell line in vivo [58, 109, 110].

7. Augmentation of peripheral nerve grafts with cellular transplants

Nearly half of the spinal cord injuries occur at the thoracolumbar junction (D12-L1), the site of the conus medullaris. We could potentially nerve graft the spinal cord (part of the CNS) directly to the cauda equina (part of the peripheral nervous system) without resorting to cellular transplants to restitute the neuronal and astrocytic components of the CNS. There is mounting evidence, however, that cellular transplants potentiate the effect of other factors and might even recruit endogenous neural precursor cells [62, 76].

7.1. Types of cellular transplants used to augment peripheral nerve grafts

In a meta-analysis reviewing cellular transplantation strategies in spinal cord injury, Tetzlaff et al. [111], have come to the following conclusions. Schwann cells are the most extensively studied cell type. They are reported both to remyelinate-injured spinal cord axons and to form a permissive substrate for their regeneration [112]. However, compared to neural precursors such as oligodendrocyte precursors or neural precursor/stem cells, they provoke a more robust astrocytic reaction, resulting in less effective integration into the host spinal cord [113]. Olfactory ensheathing cells demonstrate good integration into host spinal cord [114]. However, there is no robust evidence of improvement after their transplantation [115]. They also appear to require adjuvant treatment to increase efficacy (e.g., Schwann cells, Matrigel, rolipram, cAMP and neurotrophic factors) [116,117]. Neural stem/progenitor cells appear to integrate well into the host spinal cord with improved outcomes [118]. They differentiate mostly into astroglial cells, less so oligodendrocytes seen but rarely into neurons [119]. Suspicion has been raised as to their role in axonal regeneration [120, 121]. Fate-restricted neural and glial precursor have the potential to remyelinate injured axons [122]. More evidence is needed, however, to confirm this observation [123]. Bone marrow stromal cells have some bridging capacity in sharp transaction models [124]. However, their integration in the injured spinal cord is very limited. There is no convincing differentiation into neural cells despite claims to the contrary [125]. They are reported to stimulate neurite outgrowth over neural proteogly-cans, myelin-associated glycoprotein and Nogo-A [126, 127].

7.2. Cellular transplants in combination strategy

Because of the previous controversies, the use of a combination strategy including Schwann cells has been recommended by Bunge [128]. The following combination strategy has been suggested [128]: Schwann cells, neuroprotective agents and growth factors administered in various ways, such as, olfactory ensheathing cell (OEC) implantation, chondroitinase addition or elevation of cyclic AMP. A targeted approach has been proposed by Kadoya et al. [43]. It includes the following: a peripheral conditioning lesion (bilateral sciatic nerve crush), mesenchymal stem cell transplantation mixed with neurotrophin-3 (NT-3) and creating a neurotrophic factor gradient by injection of lentivirus expressing neurotrophin-3 (NT-3) just proximal to the site of the lesion.

7.3. Number of cellular transplant injections

A third unresolved issue is the number of injections that the patient has to receive. Mackay-Sim et al. [129] have used a single intraoperative injection. Multiple injections have been recorded by other authors [130, 131].

7.4. Inducing mobilisation of neural precursor cells

Stem cell transplantation has the potential to recruit endogenous neural stem cells [132]. Neural stem cells exist in the mammalian developing and adult nervous system (mainly in the hippocamous and subventricular area). Multiple cell-intrinsic regulators coordinate neural stem cell maintenance, self-renewal and migration into injured areas. Essential intracellular regulators include the orphan nuclear receptor TLX, the high-mobility-group DNA binding protein Sox2, the basic helix-loop-helix transcription factor Hes, the tumour suppressor gene Pten, the membrane-associated protein Numb and its cytoplasmic homolog Numblike. Manipulating these factors among others [133–135] by injecting them through indwelling catheters might induce mobilisation of neural stem cells to the injured spinal cord area.

8. Clinical application

8.1. Pre-operative assessment (neurological and radiographic evaluation)

Patients should be evaluated pre-operatively and at monthly intervals. Motor power and sensation should be evaluated using ASIA standards [28]. Confounding factors during motor power evaluation include fake muscle contractions produced by movements of the trunk and cocontractions between abdominal muscles and different muscle groups. Optional elements of ASIA neurologic impairment assessment should be included because the abdominal muscles and medial hamstrings are the first muscles to regain power.

Radiographic evaluation should include plain anteroposterior and lateral radiographs and pre-operative magnetic resonance imaging (MRI). The injury zone on the MRI is determined by the superior and inferior extents of the gliosis; nerve grafts have to be extended beyond the injury zone [136] (**Figure 6**).

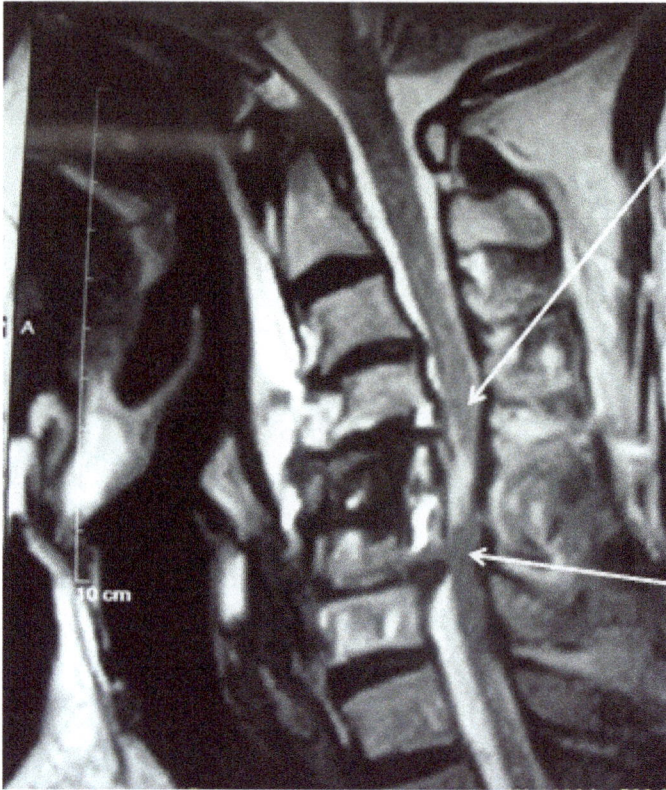

Figure 6. Cervical vertebral C5,6 fracture dislocation in a quadriplegic patient; the gliosis extends from the inferior border of cervical vertebra C4 to the superior border of cervical vertebra C6. The injury zone on the MRI is determined by the superior and inferior extents of the gliosis; nerve grafts have to be extended beyond the injury zone.

8.2. Timing of grafting

Spinal cord injury is considered chronic months to years after injury [6]. At this stage, the primary and secondary injuries have ceased. As the zone of gliosis may extend superiorly or inferiorly during the secondary injury phase, the patient should be operated upon at least 2 months after the injury, i.e., when it has become chronic.

Improvement is also independent of the time delay between the date of injury and the date of definitive surgery. This is supported by the observations made by Li and Raisman [137], who have noted that sprouts from cut corticospinal axons persist despite the presence of astrocytic scarring in long-term lesions of the adult rat spinal cord.

8.3. Operative technique, establishment of CSF circulation and establishment of a continuous drug delivery system (indwelling catheter implantation for post-operative drug and cell administration)

After exploring the injured cord through a posterior spinal laminectomy incision, sural nerves are side-grafted to the cord, especially on its ventral aspect [20, 138] (**Figures 7**(**a** and **b**) and **8**). The cord graft construct invariably adheres to the dura preventing CSF circulation. The latter is important for nutrient, cell and growth factor transport [139, 140]. To prevent the cord adhering to the dura, it has become the author's practice to wrap the cord graft construct with a silicone membrane (**Figure 9**). In fact, silicone chambers or tubes have been used as scaffolds for peripheral nerve regeneration [141–143]. Interest to use them as scaffolds for cellular growth has been rekindled [144, 145]. They have been modified physically to increase porosity or coated to allow for growth of mesenchymal stem cells [146–148] or even to allow neuron-like differentiation of mesenchymal stem cells [149]. They have been modified physically to increase porosity or chemically (with hyaluronic acid and hyaluronic acid--collagen conjugate) to allow for growth of neural cells [150, 151] or to inhibit glial tissue formation [152, 153]. To establish a continuous drug and cell delivery system, an indwelling percutaneous catheter is placed in the interstitium between the membrane and the dura; the dura is finally closed (**Figure 9**). **Figure 10** is a schematic drawing of the hypothetical spinal cord-graft-scaffold-catheter construct.

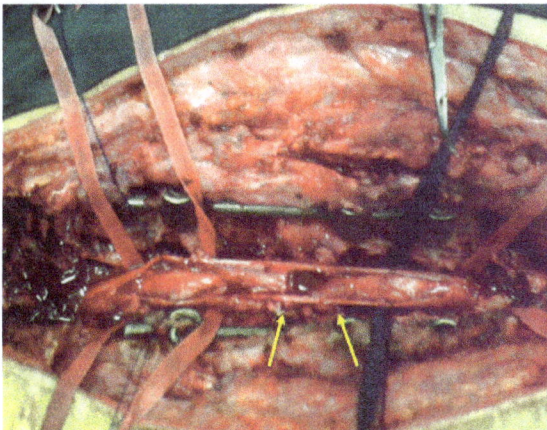

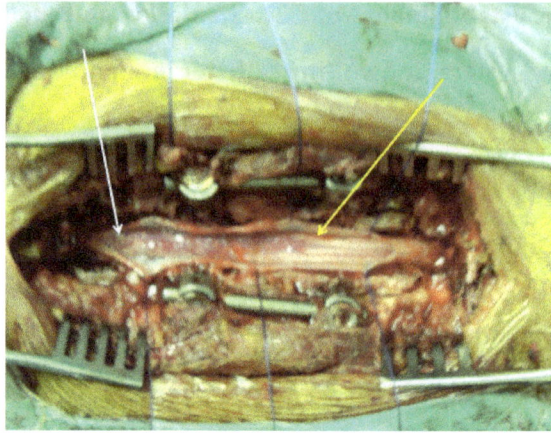

Figure 7. (a) Through a midline dorsal incision, a formal laminectomy is performed preserving the facet joints and pedicles. The dura is exposed. The dura is incised longitudinally and held with stay sutures exposing the cord lesion. The yellow arrows points to the defect in the cord. (b) Spinal cord lesion without defect but with a completely gliotic segment in a paraplegic patient suffering from a dorsolumbar fracture dislocation. The gliotic segment extends from the cord (white arrow) up to the cauda equine (yellow arrow).

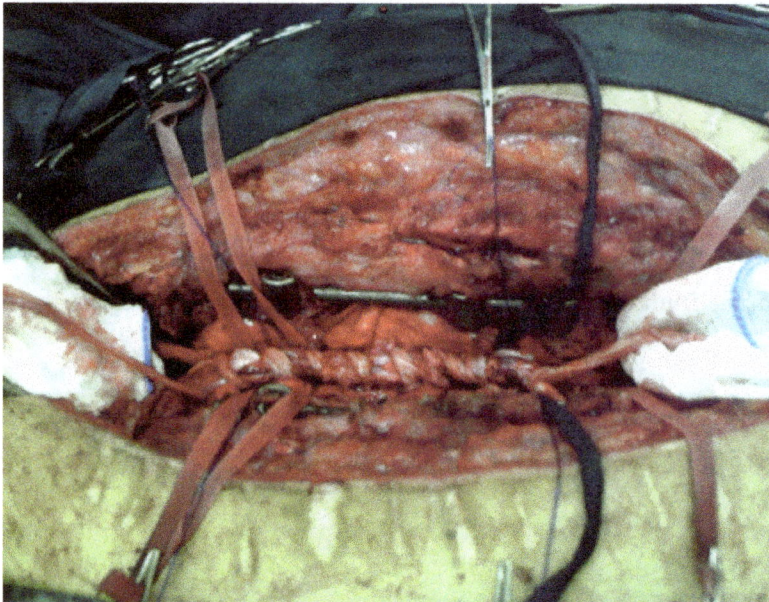

Figure 8. Sural nerve grafts having been side-grafted to the cord.

Dura mater

Silicone membrane

Spinal cord

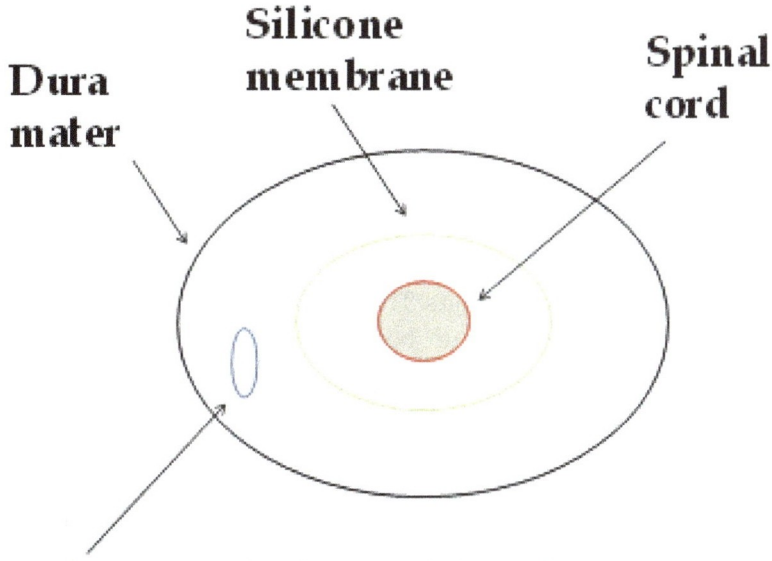

Catheter in the interstitium between the silicone membrane surrounding the cord and the dura

Figure 9. To prevent the cord adhering to the dura, it has become the author's practice to wrap the cord graft construct with a silicone membrane. To establish a continuous drug and cell delivery system, an indwelling catheter is placed in the interstitium between the membrane and the dura; the dura is finally closed.

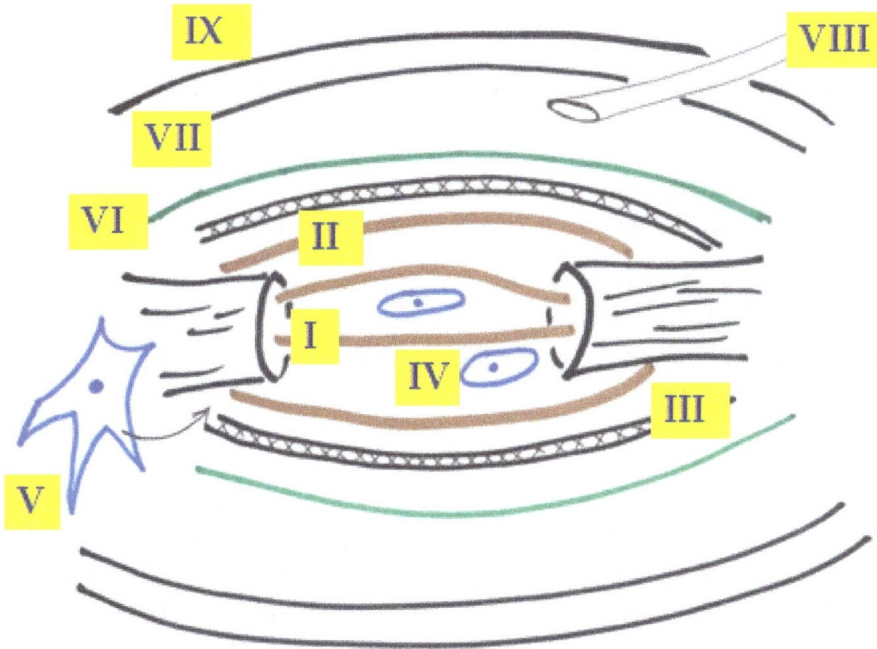

Figure 10. A schematic drawing of the hypothetical spinal cord-graft-scaffold-catheter construct: (I) end-to-end grafts; (II) side grafts; (III) synthetic scaffolds; (IV) cellular transplants; (V) modulated astrocytes; (VI) silicone membrane; (VII) dura mater; (VIII) indwelling catheter for post-operative delivery of neurolyzing agents (chondroitinase ABC, heparin), neurotrophic factors, neurite outgrowth promoting factors, injectable scaffolds and cellular transplants; (IX) skin.

8.4. Post-operative drug and cellular transplant administration through the catheter

The catheter can be used for post-operative administration of growth factors, neurolyzing agents, cellular transplants or even scaffolds. The author's practice has been as follows. Starting from the fifth post-operative day calcium heparin (5000 IU) is injected every second day through the catheter. Chondroitinase ABC (5 IU, Sigma) is dissolved in 2 cc normal saline and injected on a weekly basis.

8.5. Catheter-related complications: keeping the indwelling catheter for 18 months or more around the spinal cord as a means of establishing a continuous spinal drug delivery system

Catheter-related complications include tension headache, meningitis, fibrous track forma-tion, catheter slippage, difficult catheter insertion and catheter blockage. Fibrous track formation is noted by increased pressure on injection through the catheter, associated with increased serosanguinous discharge from the catheter skin exit site due to drug extrusion. Tension headache can be avoided by decreasing the volume of injection; meningitis and early catheter blockage and slippage are avoided by proper catheter care. Complications associat-ed with fibrous track formation, such as difficult catheter insertion, late catheter blockage and slippage (during months 9–18) can only be avoided by inserting the catheter in the interstiti-um between the silicone membrane and the dura. In this way, the catheter need not be exchanged over 18 months.

8.6. Author's clinical experience with heparin and chondroitinase ABC: its clinical safety and limitations

Delayed wound healing and sinus formation is related to repeated calheparin injection. Its incidence decreases when calheparin is administered every other day.

A vasovagal reaction occurs, when chondroitinase ABC is rapidly injected intrathecally. Its manifestations are cough, hypotension, general irritability and spinal cord irritability mani-fested by lower limb twitches. A vasovagal reaction does not occur, when the enzyme is injected extradurally or slowly intrathecally.

8.7. Results of surgery

In a clinical study [14], the right and left antero-lateral quadrant of the cord at T7-8 levels have been nerve grafted to homolateral L2-4 lumbar ventral roots. Eight months after surgery, voluntary contractions of bilateral adductors and of the left quadriceps have been observed.

Similar improvements have been observed in another study [15] after nerve side-grafting and augmentation by single-stage mesenchymal cell transplantation. Improvement has been hampered by cocontractions between abdominal muscles and different muscle groups. It has also been hampered by spasticity

In a not yet published study, the author has observed that repeated heparin, chondroitinase ABC and cellular transplant injection through an indwelling catheter placed in the interstitium between the membrane and the dura has led to the disappearance of cocontractions between abdominal muscles and different muscle groups. All patients have had pre-operative bouts of a moderate dull aching pain in the abdomen, back and both legs caused by adherence of the cord to the dura and the bony spinal canal. It has been completely resolved by inserting the silicone barrier membrane in the interstitium between the spinal cord and the dura.

Studies using cellular transplantation alone in spinal cord injuries have reported similar motor and sensory score improvement [154–157]. In all these studies, spontaneous or treatment-induced anatomical neural plasticity as well as the adaptive reorganisation of the neural pathways occurring after injury and acting to restore some of the lost function have to be taken into consideration [4].

8.8. False positive results

On evaluating results of surgery after grafting the cord to the cauda equina in thoracolumbar lesions, it should be noted that false positive results could be obtained from intercostal nerves (peripheral nerves) regenerating into the cauda equina (peripheral nerves) via nerve grafts (**Figure 11**).

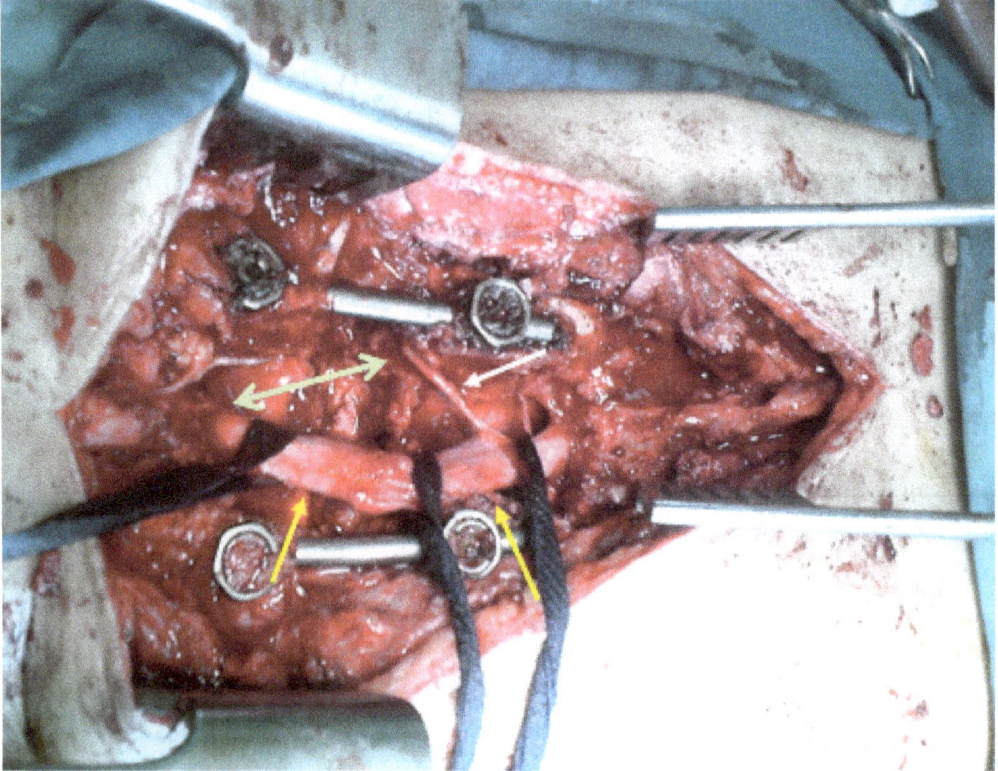

Figure 11. In thoracolumbar lesions, false positive results could be obtained from intercostal nerves (peripheral nerves) at the cranial cord (white arrow) regenerating into to the caua equina (peripheral nerves) (yellow arrow) via nerve grafts.

9. Post-operative target organ derived trophic support

Target organ derived neurotrophic factors, the so-called neurotrophins (nerve growth factor(NGF), brain-derived neurotrophic factor (BDNF), neurotrophin-3(NT-3) and neurotrophin-4/5(NT-4/5)), are transported by retrograde axonal via an endosomal mechanism involving dyneins [158, 159]. Neurotrophins contribute a lot to axonal progression; in the injured spinal cord, this stimulus is lost. After grafting the spinal cord, an important question is whether this stimulus can be restituted by injecting neurotrophins into target organs post-operatively, or whether axonal progression into specific nerves can be restituted by injecting neurotrophins into the specific muscles supplied by them. Experimental evidence points to this [158, 159]. By the same token, it can be questioned whether other neurotrophic factors and neurolyzing agents can be similarly injected into target muscles. Both in vitro and in vivo local infusion of fibroblastic growth factors (FGFs) have been found to rescue motoneuron death induced by spinal cord injury [160]. However, evidence for retrograde axonal transport of heparin-binding growth factors is lacking [161].

10. Conclusions

We have outlined current experimental and clinical experience applying nerve side grafts to the injured spinal cord. Nerve side grafting increases the incidence of nerve regeneration by applying additional grafts extending from the side of the donor end of the cord to the side of the recipient end. A partially regenerated cord cannot be surgically cut and end grafted; nerve side grafting can enhance regeneration through it without incriminating already regained function. Nevertheless, side grafting will fail, unless the gliosis is counteracted or lysed by chondroitinase ABC, sialidase, anti-Nogo, Rho inhibitors and other factors. Side grafting will also fail unless neurons are stimulated to produce neurites. Modulating the function of astrocytes by heparin, aspirin and other factors is one method to stimulate the intrinsic properties of the neurons to produce neurites. Side grafting should be augmented by artificial scaffolds and cellular transplants. Clinically, to prevent the cord adhering to the dura and re-establish CSF circulation, it has become the author's practice to wrap the cord graft construct with a silicone membrane. To establish a continuous drug and cell delivery system, an indwelling catheter is placed in the interstitium between the membrane and the dura; the dura is finally closed. Post-operative injection of paralysed muscles with neurotrophic factors stimulates neurite outgrowth by target-organ-derived neurotrophic support.

Author details

Sherif M. Amr*

Address all correspondence to: sherifamrh@hotmail.com

The Department of Orthopaedics and Traumatology, Cairo University, Cairo, Egypt

References

[1] DeFelipe J, Jones EG: Cajal's degeneration and regeneration of the nervous system (May RM, translator). New York: Oxford University Press, 1991.

[2] Raisman G: A promising therapeutic approach to spinal cord repair. J R Soc Med 2003;96(6):259–261.

[3] Samadikuchaksaraei A: An overview of tissue engineering approaches for management of spinal cord injuries. J Neuroeng Rehabil 2007;4:15.

[4] Bradbury EJ, McMahon SB. Spinal cord repair strategies: why do they work? Nat Rev Neurosci 2006;7:644–653.

[5] Reier PJ: Cellular transplantation strategies for spinal cord injury and translational neurobiology. Neurorx 2004 October;1(4):424–451.

[6] Hyun JK, Kim HW. Clinical and experimental advances in regeneration of spinal cord injury. J Tissue Eng. 2010 Nov 2; Vol. 2010 : 1–20: Article ID 650857. doi: 10.4061/2010/650857. PubMed PMID: 21350645; PubMed Central PMCID: PMC3042682.

[7] David S, Aguayo AJ: Axonal elongation into peripheral nervous system 'bridges' after central nervous system injury in adult rats. Science 1981;214:931–933.

[8] Tuszynski MH, Petersen DA, Ray J, Baird A, Nakahara Y, Gage FH: Fibroblasts genetically modified to produce nerve growth factor induce robust neuritic ingrowth after grafting to the spinal cord. Exp Neurol 1994;126:1–14.

[9] Guenard V, Aebischer P, Bunge RP: The astrocyte inhibition of peripheral nerve regeneration is reversed by Schwann cells. Exp Neurol 1994;126:44–60.

[10] Oudega M, Varon S, Hagg T: Regeneration of adult rat sensory axons into intraspinal nerve grafts: promoting effects of conditioning lesion and graft predegeneration. Exp Neurol 1994;129:194–206.

[11] Liu S, Kadi K, Boisset N, Lacroix C, Said G, Tadie M: Reinnervation of denervated lumbar ventral roots and their target muscle by thoracic spinal motoneurons via an implanted nerve autograft in adult rats after spinal cord injury. J Neurosci Res 1999 Jun 1;56(5):506–517.

[12] Liu S, Aghakhani N, Boisset N, Said G, Tadie M: Innervation of the caudal denervated ventral roots and their target muscles by the rostral spinal motoneurons after implanting a nerve autograft in spinal cord-injured adult marmosets. J Neurosurg 2001 Jan;94(1 Suppl):82–90.

[13] Dam-Hieu P, Liu S, Choudhri T, Said G, Tadie M: Regeneration of primary sensory axons into the adult rat spinal cord via a peripheral nerve graft bridging the lumbar dorsal roots to the dorsal column. J Neurosci Res 2002 May 1;68(3):293–304.

[14] Tadie M, Liu S, Robert R, Guiheneuc P, Pereon Y, Perrouin-Verbe B, Mathe JF: Partial return of motor function in paralyzed legs after surgical bypass of the lesion site by nerve autografts three years after spinal cord injury. J Neurotrauma 2002 Aug;19(8): 909–916.

[15] Amr SM, Gouda A, Koptan WT, Galal AA, Abdel-Fattah DS, Rashed LA, Atta HM, Abdel-Aziz MT: Bridging defects in chronic spinal cord injury using peripheral nerve grafts combined with a chitosan-laminin scaffold and enhancing regeneration through them by cotransplantation with bone-marrow derived mesenchymal stem cells; a series of 14 patients. J Spinal Cord Medicine 2014;37(1):54–71

[16] Fawcett JW: Bridging spinal cord injuries. J Biol 2008;7:25.

[17] Ray WZ: Mackinnon SE. Management of nerve gaps: autografts, allografts, nerve transfers, and end-to-side neurorrhaphy. Exp Neurol 2010 May ;223(1):77–85. doi: 10.1016/j.expneurol.2009.03.031.

[18] Frostick SP, Yin Q, Kemp G: Schwann cells, neurotrophic factors, and peripheral nerve regeneration. Microsurgery 1998;18:397–405.

[19] Blottner D, Baumgarten HG: Neurotrophy and regeneration in vivo. Acta Anat 1994;150:235–245.

[20] Amr SM, Moharram AN: Repair of brachial plexus lesions by end-to-side side-to-side grafting neurorrhaphy: experience based on 11 cases. Microsurgery 2005, 25(2):126–146.

[21] Rosoff WJ, Urbach JS, Esrick MA, McAllister RG, Richards LJ, Goodhill GJ. A new chemotaxis assay shows the extreme sensitivity of axons to molecular gradients. Nat Neurosci 2004;7(6):678–682. Epub 2004 May 25. Erratum in: Nat Neurosci. 2004;7(7): 785.

[22] Tse TH, Chan BP, Chan CM, Lam J: Mathematical modeling of guided neurite extension in an engineered conduit with multiple concentration gradients of nerve growth factor (NGF). Ann Biomed Eng 2007;35(9):1561–1572. Epub 2007 May 23.

[23] Ciofani G, Sergi PN, Carpaneto J, Micera S. A hybrid approach for the control of axonal outgrowth: preliminary simulation results. Med Biol Eng Comput 2011;49(2):163–170. doi: 10.1007/s11517-010-0687-x. Epub 2010 Oct 6. PubMed PMID: 20924708.

[24] Ciofani G, Raffa V, Menciassi A, Micera S, Dario P: A drug delivery system based on alginate microspheres: mass-transport test and in vitro validation. Biomed Microdevices 2007;9:395–403.

[25] Holmquist B, Kanje M, Kerns JM, Danielsen N. A mathematical model for regeneration rate and initial delay following surgical repair of peripheral nerves. J Neurosci Methods. 1993 Jun;Vol.48(1–2):27–33. PubMed PMID: 8377520.

[26] Cover TM, Thomas JA: Elements of Information Theory, 2nd ed. Hoboken, New Jersey: John Wiley & Sons, Inc., 2006.

[27] Effenberger F. A Primer on Information Theory, with Applications to Neuroscience. In: Rakocevic G., Djukic T., Filipovic N., Milutinović V. (editors) Computational Medicine in Data Mining and Modeling. New York: Springer 2013.

[28] Standards for Neurological Classification of Spinal Injury. American Spinal Injury Association (ASIA) Illinois: Chicago, 1996.

[29] Harel NY, Strittmatter SM: Can regenerating axons recapitulate developmental guidance during recovery from spinal cord injury? Nat Rev Neurosci 2006;7:603–616.

[30] Côté MP, Amin AA, Tom VJ, Houle JD: Peripheral nerve grafts support regeneration after spinal cord injury. Neurotherapeutics 2011;8(2):294–303.

[31] Hill CE, Brodak DM, Bartlett Bunge M: Dissociated predegenerated peripheralnerve transplants for spinal cord injury repair: a comprehensive assessment of their effects on regeneration and functional recovery compared to Schwann cell transplants. J Neurotrauma 2012;29(12):2226–2243. doi: 10.1089/neu.2012.2377. PubMed PMID: 22655857; PubMed Central PMCID: PMC3472680.

[32] Bray GM, Villegas-Perez MP, Vidal-Sanz M, Aguayo AJ: The use of peripheral nerve grafts to enhance neuronal survival, promote growth and permit terminal reconnections in the central nervous system of adult rats. J Exp Biol 1987;132:5–19.

[33] Bunge MB: Bridging areas of injury in the spinal cord. Neuroscientist 2001;7:325–339.

[34] Guzen FP, de Almeida Leme RJ, de Andrade MS, de Luca BA, Chadi G: Glial cell line-derived neurotrophic factor added to a sciatic nerve fragment grafted in a spinal cord gap ameliorates motor impairments in rats and increases local axonal growth. Restor Neurol Neurosci 2009;27(1):1–16.

[35] Cheng H, Cao Y, Olson L: Spinal cord repair in adult paraplegic rats partial restoration of hind limb function. Science 1996;273:510–513.

[36] Lee YS, Hsiao I, Lin VW: Peripheral nerve grafts and aFGF restore partial hindlimb function in adult paraplegic rats. J Neurotrauma 2002;19:1203–1216.

[37] Campos L, Meng Z, Hu G, Chiu DT, Ambron RT, Martin JH: Engineering novel spinal circuits to promote recovery after spinal injury. J Neurosci 2004;24:2090–2101.

[38] Gauthier P, Rega P, Lammari-Barreault N, Polentes J: Functional reconnections established by central respiratory neurons regenerating axons into a nerve graft bridging the respiratory centers to the cervical spinal cord. J Neurosci Res 2002;70:65–81.

[39] Decherchi P, Lammari-Barreault N, Gauthier P: Regeneration of respiratory pathways within spinal peripheral nerve grafts. Exp Neurol 1996;137:1–14.

[40] Aguayo AJ, Bray GM, Rasminsky MM, Zwimpfer T, Carter D, Vidal-Sanz M: Synaptic connections made by axons regenerating in the central nervous system of adult mammals. J Exp Biol 1990;153:199–224.

[41] Plant GW, Bates ML, Bunge MB: Inhibitory proteoglycan immunoreactivity is higher at the caudal than the rostral Schwann cell graft-transected spinal cord interface. Mol Cell Neurosci 2001;17:471–487.

[42] Thuret S, Moon LDF, Gage FH: Therapeutic interventions after spinal cord injury. Nat Rev Neurosci 2006;7:628–643.

[43] Kadoya K, Tsukada S, Lu P, Coppola G, Geschwind D, Filbin MT, Blesch A,Tuszynski MH: Combined intrinsic and extrinsic neuronal mechanisms facilitate bridging axonal regeneration one year after spinal cord injury. Neuron. 2009;64(2):165–172.

doi: 10.1016/j.neuron.2009.09.016. PubMed PMID: 19874785; PubMedCentral PMCID: PMC2773653.

[44] Neumann S, Bradke F, Tessier-Lavigne M, Basbaum AI: Regeneration of sensory axons within the injured spinal cord induced by intraganglionic cAMP elevation. Neuron. 2002;34:885–893 [PubMed].

[45] Qiu J, Cai D, Dai H, McAtee M, Hoffman PN, Bregman BS, Filbin MT: Spinal axon regeneration induced by elevation of cyclic AMP. Neuron 2002;34:895–903 [PubMed].

[46] Ferguson TA, Son YJ: Extrinsic and intrinsic determinants of nerve regeneration. J Tissue Eng 2011;2(1):2041731411418392. doi: 10.1177/2041731411418392. Epub 2011 Sep 13. PubMed PMID: 22292105; PubMed Central PMCID: PMC3251917.

[47] Tom VJ, Steinmetz MP, Miller JH, Doller CM, Silver J: Studies on the development and behavior of the dystrophic growth cone, the hallmark of regeneration failure, in an in vitro model of the glial scar and after spinal cord injury. J Neurosci 2004;24(29):6531–6539. PubMed PMID: 15269264.

[48] Blits B, Carlstedt TP, Ruitenberg MJ, de Winter F, Hermens WT, Dijkhuizen PA, Claasens JW, Eggers R, Sluis R van der, Tenenbaum L, Boer GJ, Verhaagen J: Rescue and sprouting of motoneurons following ventral root avulsion and reimplantation combined with intraspinal adeno-associated viral vector-mediated expression of glial cell line-derived neurotrophic factor or brain-derived neurotrophic factor. Exp Neurol 2004;189(2):303–316.

[49] Yiu G, He Z: Glial inhibition of CNS axon regeneration. Nat Rev Neurosci 2006;7:617–627.

[50] McCreedy DA, Sakiyama-Elbert SE: Combination therapies in the CNS: engineering the environment. Neurosci Lett 2012;519(2):115–121. doi: 10.1016/j.neulet.2012.02.025. Epub 2012 Feb 17. Review. PMID: 22343313.

[51] Bradbury EJ, Carter LM: Manipulating the glial scar: chondroitinase ABC as a therapy for spinal cord injury. Brain Res Bull 2011;84:306316 [PubMed: 20620201].

[52] Galtrey CM, Fawcett JW: The role of chondroitin sulfate proteoglycans in regeneration and plasticity in the central nervous system. Brain Res Rev 2007;54:118 [PubMed: 17222456].

[53] Yamagata T, Saito H, Habuchi O, Suzuki S: Purification and properties of bacterial chondroitinases and chondrosulfatases. J Biol Chem 1968;243:15231535 [PubMed: 5647268].

[54] Bradbury EJ, Moon LD, Popat RJ, King VR, Bennett GS, Patel PN, Fawcett JW, McMahon SB: Chondroitinase ABC promotes functional recovery after spinal cord injury. Nature 2002;416:636–640 [PubMed: 11948352].

[55] Houle JD, Tom VJ, Mayes D, Wagoner G, Phillips N, Silver J: Combining an autologous peripheral nervous system "bridge" and matrix modification by chondroitinase

allows robust, functional regeneration beyond a hemisection lesion of the adult rat spinal cord. J Neurosci 2006;26(28):7405–7415.

[56] Tom VJ, Sandrow-Feinberg HR, Miller K, Santi L, Connors T, Lemay MA, Houle JD: Combining peripheral nerve grafts and chondroitinase promotes functional axonal regeneration in the chronically injured spinal cord. J Neurosci 2009;29:14881–14890 [PMC free article] [PubMed].

[57] Hwang DH, Kim HM, Kang YM, Joo IS, Cho CS, Yoon BW, Kim SU, Kim BG. Combination of multifaceted strategies to maximize the therapeutic benefits of neural stem cell transplantation for spinal cord repair. Cell Transplant. 2011;20(9):1361–1379. doi: 10.3727/096368910X557155. Epub 2011 Mar 7. PubMed PMID: 21396156.

[58] Kumar P, Choonara YE, Modi G, Naidoo D, Pillay V: Multifunctional therapeutic delivery strategies for effective neuro-regeneration following traumatic spinal cord injury. Curr Pharm Des 2015;21(12):1517–1528 [PubMed PMID: 25594407].

[59] Jain A, Kim YT, McKeon RJ, Bellamkonda RV: In situ gelling hydrogels for conformal repair of spinal cord defects, and local delivery of BDNF after spinal cord injury. Biomaterials 2006;27:497504 [PubMed: 16099038].

[60] Kreider BQ, Messing A, Doan H, Kim SU, Lisak RP, Pleasure DE. Enrichment of Schwann cell cultures from neonatal rat sciatic nerve by differential adhesion. Brain Res 1981;207:433444 [PubMed: 7008901].

[61] Fouad K, Schnell L, Bunge MB, Schwab ME, Liebscher T, Pearse DD. Combining Schwann cell bridges and olfactory-ensheathing glia grafts with chondroitinase promotes locomotor recovery after complete transection of the spinal cord. J Neurosci 2005;25:1169–1178 [PubMed].

[62] Wilems TS, Pardieck J, Iyer N, Sakiyama-Elbert SE: Combination therapy of stem cell derived neural progenitors and drug delivery of anti-inhibitory molecules for spinal cord injury. Acta Biomater 2015. pii: S1742–7061(15)30112–4. doi: 10.1016/j.actbio. 2015.09.018. [Epub ahead of print]

[63] Lee H, McKeon RJ, Bellamkonda RV. Sustained delivery of thermostabilized chABC enhances axonal sprouting and functional recovery after spinal cord injury. Proc Natl Acad Sci U S A. 2010 Feb 23;107(8):3340–3345. doi: 10.1073/pnas.0905437106. Epub 2009 Nov 2. PubMed PMID: 19884507; PubMed Central PMCID: PMC2840440.

[64] Tom VJ, Houlé JD: Intraspinal microinjection of chondroitinase ABC following injury promotes axonal regeneration out of a peripheral nerve graft bridge. Exp Neurol 2008;211(1):315–319.

[65] Wilems TS, Sakiyama-Elbert SE: Sustained dual drug delivery of anti-inhibitory molecules for treatment of spinal cord injury. J Control Release 2015;213:103–111. doi: 10.1016/j.jconrel.2015.06.031 [Epub ahead of print] [PubMed PMID: 26122130].

[66] Hyatt AJ, Wang D, Kwok JC, Fawcett JW, Martin KR: Controlled release of chondroitinase ABC from fibrin gel reduces the level of inhibitory glycosaminoglycan chains in

lesioned spinal cord. J Control Release 2010;147(1):24–29. doi: 10.1016/j.jconrel. 2010.06.026.

[67] Hunanyan AS, García-Alías G, Alessi V, Levine JM, Fawcett JW, Mendell LM, Arvanian VL: Role of chondroitin sulfate proteoglycans in axonal conduction in Mammalian spinal cord. J Neurosci 2010;30(23):7761–7769. doi: 10.1523/JNEUROSCI.4659-09.2010.

[68] Cheng CH, Lin CT, Lee MJ, Tsai MJ, Huang WH, Huang MC, Lin YL, Chen CJ, Huang WC, Cheng H: Local delivery of high-dose chondroitinase ABC in the sub-acute stage promotes axonal outgrowth and functional recovery after complete spinal cord transection. PLoS One. 2015;10(9):e0138705. doi:10.1371/journal.pone.0138705. eCollection 2015.

[69] Shields LB, Zhang YP, Burke DA, Gray R, Shields CB: Benefit of chondroitinase ABC on sensory axon regeneration in a laceration model of spinal cord injury in the rat. Surg Neurol 2008;69(6):568–577; discussion 577. doi: 10.1016/j.surneu.2008.02.009.

[70] Iseda T, Okuda T, Kane-Goldsmith N, Mathew M, Ahmed S, Chang YW, Young W, Grumet M: Single, high-dose intraspinal injection of chondroitinase reduces glycosaminoglycans in injured spinal cord and promotes corticospinal axonal regrowth after hemisection but not contusion. J Neurotrauma 2008;25(4):334–349. doi: 10.1089/neu. 2007.0289.

[71] Caggiano AO, Zimber MP, Ganguly A, Blight AR, Gruskin EA: Chondroitinase ABCI improves locomotion and bladder function following contusion injury of the rat spinal cord. J Neurotrauma 2005;22(2):226–239.

[72] Mondello SE, Jefferson SC, Tester NJ, Howland DR: Impact of treatment duration and lesion size on effectiveness of chondroitinase treatment post-SCI. Exp Neurol 2015;267:64–77. doi: 10.1016/j.expneurol.2015.02.028. Epub 2015 Feb 26.

[73] Ma Y, Liu M, Li Y: Secretion of bacterial chondroitinase ABC from bone marrow stromal cells by glycosylation site mutation: a promising approach for axon regeneration. Med Hypotheses 2011;77(5):914–916. doi: 10.1016/j.mehy.2011.08.010. Epub 2011 Aug 31.

[74] Kumar P, Choonara YE, Modi G, Naidoo D, Pillay V(1): Multifunctional therapeutic delivery strategies for effective neuro-regeneration following traumatic spinal cord injury. Curr Pharm Des 2015;21(12):1517–1528.

[75] Steinmetz MP, Horn KP, Tom VJ, Miller JH, Busch SA, Nair D, Silver DJ, Silver J: Chronic enhancement of the intrinsic growth capacity of sensory neurons combined with the degradation of inhibitory proteoglycans allows functional regeneration of sensory axons through the dorsal root entry zone in the mammalian spinal cord. J Neurosci 2005;25(35):8066–8076.

[76] Sarveazad A, Bakhtiari M, Babahajian A, Janzade A, Fallah A, Moradi F, Soleimani M, Younesi M, Goudarzi F, Mohammad Taghi Joghataei: Comparison of human adipose-derived stem cells and chondroitinase ABC transplantation on locomotor recovery in

the contusion model of spinal cord injury in rats. Iran J Basic Med Sci 2014;17(9):685–693. PubMed PMID: 25691946; PubMed Central PMCID:PMC4322153.

[77] Mountney A, Zahner MR, Sturgill ER, Riley CJ, Aston JW, Oudega M, Schramm LP, Hurtado A, Schnaar RL: Sialidase, chondroitinase ABC, and combination therapy after spinal cord contusion injury. J Neurotrauma 2013;30(3):181–190. doi: 10.1089/neu.2012.2353

[78] Lang BT, Cregg JM, DePaul MA, Tran AP, Xu K, Dyck SM, Madalena KM, Brown BP, Weng YL, Li S, Karimi-Abdolrezaee S, Busch SA, Shen Y, Silver J: Modulation of the proteoglycan receptor PTPσ promotes recovery after spinal cord injury. Nature 2015;518(7539):404–408. doi: 10.1038/nature13974. Epub 2014 Dec 3. PubMed PMID: 25470046; PubMed Central PMCID: PMC4336236.

[79] Silver L, Michael JV, Goldfinger LE, Gallo G: Activation of PI3K and R-Ras signaling promotes the extension of sensory axons on inhibitory chondroitin sulfate proteoglycans. Dev Neurobiol 2014;74(9):918–933. doi: 10.1002/dneu.22174. Epub 2014 Mar 27.

[80] Tetzlaff W, Alexander SW, Miller FD, Bisby MA: Response of facial and rubrospinal neurons to axotomy: changes in mRNA expression for cytoskeletal proteins and GAP-43. J Neurosci 1991;11:2528–2544 [PubMed].

[81] Sengottuvel V, Leibinger M, Pfreimer M, Andreadaki A, Fischer D: Taxol facilitates axon regeneration in the mature CNS. J Neurosci 2011;31:2688–2699 [PubMed].

[82] Bates CA, Becker CG, Miotke JA, Meyer RL: Expression of polysialylated NCAM but not L1 or N-cadherin by regenerating adult mouse optic fibers in vitro. Exp Neurol 1999;155:128–139 [PubMed].

[83] Chaisuksunt V, Zhang Y, Anderson PN, et al: Axonal regeneration from CNS neurons in the cerebellum and brainstem of adult rats: correlation with the patterns of expression and distribution of messenger RNAs for L1, CHL1, c-jun and growth-associated protein-43. Neuroscience 2000;100:87–108 [PubMed].

[84] Chen J, Wu J, Apostolova I, et al: Adeno-associated virus-mediated L1 expression promotes functional recovery after spinal cord injury. Brain 2007;130:954–969 [PubMed].

[85] Roonprapunt C, Huang W, Grill R, et al: Soluble cell adhesion molecule L1-Fc promotes locomotor recovery in rats after spinal cord injury. J Neurotrauma 2003;20:871–882 [PubMed].

[86] Chen Y and Swanson RA: Astrocytes and brain injury. Rev Article J Cereb Blood Flow Metab 2003;23(2):137–149.

[87] Mohn TC, Koob AO: Adult astrogenesis and the etiology of cortical neurodegeneration. J Exp Neurosci 2015;9(s) 25–34. doi:10.4137/JEn.s25520.

[88] Hering TM, Beller JA, Calulot CM, Centers A, Snow DM: Proteoglycans of reactive rat cortical astrocyte cultures: abundance of N-unsubstituted glucosamine-enriched heparan sulfate. Matrix Biol 2015;41:8–18. doi: 10.1016/j.matbio.2014.11.006.

[89] Yates D: Synaptogenesis. Asynaptic bridge. Nat Rev Neurosci 2016;17,135. doi:10.1038/nrn.2016.12 Published online 11 February 2016.

[90] Harter K, Levine M, Henderson SO: Anticoagulation drug therapy: a review. West J Emerg Med 2015;16(1):11–17. doi: 10.5811/westjem.2014.12.22933. Epub 2015 Jan 12. Review. PubMed PMID: 25671002; PubMed Central PMCID: PMC4307693.

[91] Kahraman A, Kahveci R: Evaluating the effect of polytetrafluoroethylene and extractum cepae-heparin-allantoin gel in peripheral nerve injuries in a rat model. Plast Surg (Oakv) 2015 Spring;23(1):9–14. PubMed PMID: 25821766; PubMed Central PMCID: PMC4364148.

[92] Akbari H, Rahimi AA, Ghavami Y, Mousavi SJ, Fatemi MJ. Effect of heparin on postoperative adhesion in flexor tendon surgery of the hand. J Hand Microsurg 2015;7(2):244–249. Epub 2015 Aug 26. PubMed PMID: 26578825; PubMed Central PMCID: PMC4642480.

[93] Aydoseli A, Tahta A, Aras Y, Sabancı A, Keskin M, Balik E, Onder S, Sencer A, Izgi N: Use of antifibrotics to prevent ventriculoperitoneal shunt complications due to intra-abdominal fibrosis: experimental study in a rat model. J Neurol Surg A Cent Eur Neurosurg 2015;76(3):219–223. doi: 10.1055/s-0034-1389369. Epub 2015 Mar 26. PubMed PMID: 25811104.

[94] Alonso Jde M, Rodrigues KA, Yamada AL, Watanabe MJ, Alves AL, Rodrigues CA, Hussni CA: Peritoneal reactivity evaluation in horses subjected to experimental small colon enterotomy and treated with subcutaneous heparin. Vet Med Int 2014;2014:385392. doi: 10.1155/2014/385392. Epub 2014 Nov 11. PubMed PMID: 25436172; PubMed Central PMCID: PMC4243600.

[95] Ho WS, Ying SY, Chan PC, Chan HH: Use of onion extract, heparin, allantoin gel in prevention of scarring in chinese patients having laser removal of tattoos: a prospective randomized controlled trial. Dermatol Surg 2006;32(7):891–896. PubMed PMID: 16875470.

[96] Billings PC, Pacifici M: Interactions of signaling proteins, growth factors and other proteins with heparan sulfate: mechanisms and mysteries. Connect Tissue Res 2015;56(4):272–280. doi: 10.3109/03008207.2015.1045066.

[97] Olczyk P, Mencner Ł, Komosinska-Vassev K: Diverse roles of heparan sulfate and heparin in wound repair. Biomed Res Int 2015;2015:549417. doi: 10.1155/2015/549417. Epub 2015 Jul 7. Review. PubMed PMID: 26236728; PubMed Central PMCID: PMC4508384.

[98] Newman DR, Li CM, Simmons R, Khosla J, Sannes PL: Heparin affects signaling pathways stimulated by fibroblast growth factor-1 and -2 in type II cells. Am J Physiol

Lung Cell Mol Physiol 2004;287(1):L191–L200. Epub 2004 Feb 13. PubMed PMID: 14966081.

[99]   Santos-Silva A, Fairless R, Frame MC, Montague P, Smith GM, Toft A, Riddell JS, Barnett SC: FGF/heparin differentially regulates Schwann cell and olfactory ensheathing cell interactions with astrocytes: a role in astrocytosis. J Neurosci 2007;27(27):7154–7167.

[100] Yi-Chao Hsu, Su-Liang Chen, Dan-Yen Wang: Ing-Ming Chiu stem cell-based therapy in neural repair. Biomed J 2013;36:98–105.

[101] Walicke P, Cowan WM, Ueno N, Baird A, Guillemin R: Fibroblast growth factor promotes survival of dissociated hippocampal neurons and enhances neurite extension. Proc Natl Acad Sci U S A 1986;83(9):3012–3016.

[102] Nagayasu T, Miyata S, Hayashi N, Takano R, Kariya Y, Kamei K: Heparin structures in FGF-2-dependent morphological transformation of astrocytes. J Biomed Mater Res A 2005;74(3):374–380. PubMed PMID: 15973728.

[103] Poulsen FR, Lagord C, Courty J, Pedersen EB, Barritault D, Finsen B: Increased synthesis of heparin affin regulatory peptide in the perforant path lesioned mouse hippocampal formation. Exp Brain Res 2000;135(3):319–330. PubMed PMID: 11146810.

[104] Wanaka A, Carroll SL, Milbrandt J: Developmentally regulated expression of pleiotrophin, a novel heparin binding growth factor, in the nervous system of the rat. Brain Res Dev Brain Res 1993;72(1):133–144. PubMed PMID: 8453763.

[105] Hagino S, Iseki K, Mori T, Zhang Y, Sakai N, Yokoya S, Hikake T, Kikuchi S, Wanaka A: Expression pattern of glypican-1 mRNA after brain injury in mice. Neurosci Lett 2003;349(1):29–32. PubMed PMID: 12946579.

[106] Lau E, Margolis RU: Inhibitors of slit protein interactions with the heparin sulphate proteoglycan glypican-1: potential agents for the treatment of spinal cord injury. Clin Exp Pharmacol Physiol 2010;37(4):417–421. doi: 10.1111/j.1440-1681.2009.05318.x.

[107] Modi KK, Sendtner M, Pahan K: Up-regulation of ciliary neurotrophic factor in astrocytes by aspirin: implications for remyelination in multiple sclerosis. J Biol Chem 2013;288(25):18533–18545. doi: 10.1074/jbc.M112.447268.

[108] Khaing ZZ, Milman BD, Vanscoy JE, Seidlits SK, Grill RJ, Schmidt CE: High molecular weight hyaluronic acid limits astrocyte activation and scar formation after spinal cord injury. J Neural Eng 2011;8(4):046033. doi: 10.1088/1741-2560/8/4/046033.

[109] Madigan NN, McMahon S, O'Brien T, Yaszemski MJ, Windebank AJ: Current tissue engineering and novel therapeutic approaches to axonal regeneration following spinal cord injury using polymer scaffolds. Respir Physiol Neurobiol 2009;169(2):183–199. doi: 10.1016/j.resp.2009.08.015. Epub 2009 Sep 6. Review. PubMed PMID: 19737633; PubMed Central PMCID: PMC2981799.

[110] Straley KS, Foo CW, Heilshorn SC: Biomaterial design strategies for the treatment of spinal cord injuries. J Neurotrauma 2010;27(1):1–19. doi: 10.1089/neu.2009.0948. Review. PubMed PMID: 19698073; PubMed Central PMCID: PMC2924783.

[111] Tetzlaff W, Okon EB, Karimi-Abdolrezaee S, Hill CE, Sparling JS, Plemel JR, Plunet WT, Tsai EC, Baptiste D, Smithson LJ, Kawaja MD, Fehlings MG, Kwon BK: A systematic review of cellular transplantation therapies for spinal cord injury. J Neurotrauma 2011;28(8):1611–1682. Epub 2010 Apr 20. Review.

[112] Duncan ID, Milward EA: Glial cell transplants: experimental therapies of myelin diseases. Brain Pathol 1995;5:301–310 [PubMed].

[113] Santos-Silva A, Fairless R, Frame MC, Montague P, Smith GM, Toft A, Riddell JS, Barnett SC: FGF/heparin differentially regulates Schwann cell and olfactory ensheathing cell interactions with astrocytes: a role in astrocytosis. J Neurosci 2007;27(27):7154–7167.

[114] Ramon-Cueto A, Plant GW, Avila J, Bunge MB: Long-distance axonal regeneration in the transected adult rat spinal cord is promoted by olfactory ensheathing glia transplants. J Neurosci 1998;18:3803–3815 [PubMed].

[115] Lu P, Yang H, Culbertson M, Graham L, Roskams AJ, Tuszynski MH: Olfactory ensheathing cells do not exhibit unique migratory or axonal growth-promoting properties after spinal cord injury. J Neurosci 2006;26:11120–11130 [PubMed].

[116] Pearse DD, Sanchez AR, Pereira FC, Andrade CM, Puzis R, Pressman Y, Golden K, Kitay BM, Blits B, Wood PM, Bunge MB: Transplantation of Schwann cells and/or olfactory ensheathing glia into the contused spinal cord: survival, migration, axon association, and functional recovery. Glia 2007;55:976–1000 [PubMed].

[117] Ruitenberg MJ, Plant GW, Hamers FP, Wortel J, Blits B, Dijkhuizen PA, Gispen WH, Boer GJ, Verhaagen J: Ex vivo adenoviral vector-mediated neurotrophin gene transfer to olfactory ensheathing glia: effects on rubrospinal tract regeneration, lesion size, and functional recovery after implantation in the injured rat spinal cord. J Neurosci 2003;23:7045–7058 [PubMed].

[118] Alexanian AR, Crowe MJ, Kurpad SN: Efficient differentiation and integration of lineage-restricted neural precursors in the traumatically injured adult cat spinal cord. J Neurosci Methods 2006;150:41–46 [PubMed].

[119] Cao QL, Zhang YP, Howard RM, Walters WM, Tsoulfas P, Whittemore SR: Pluripotent stem cells engrafted into the normal or lesioned adult rat spinal cord are restricted to a glial lineage. Exp Neurol 2001;167:48–58 [PubMed].

[120] Macias MY, Syring MB, Pizzi MA, Crowe MJ, Alexanian AR, Kurpad SN: Pain with no gain: allodynia following neural stem cell transplantation in spinal cord injury. Exp Neurol 2006;201:335–348 [PubMed].

[121] Jin Y, Bouyer J, Shumsky JS, Haas C, Fischer I: Transplantation of neural progenitor cells in chronic spinal cord injury. Neuroscience 2016;320:69–82. doi: 10.1016/j.neuroscience.2016.01.066. Epub 2016 Feb 4. PubMedPMID: 26852702.

[122] Bambakidis NC, Miller RH: Transplantation of oligodendrocyte precursors and sonic hedgehog results in improved function and white matter sparing in the spinal cords of adult rats after contusion. Spine J 2004;4:16–26 [PubMed].

[123] Cao QL, Howard RM, Dennison JB, Whittemore SR. Differentiation of engrafted neuronal-restricted precursor cells is inhibited in the traumatically injured spinal cord. Exp Neurol 2002;177:349–359 [PubMed].

[124] Ankeny DP, McTigue DM, Jakeman LB: Bone marrow transplants provide tissue protection and directional guidance for axons after contusive spinal cord injury in rats. Exp Neurol 2004;190:17–31 [PubMed].

[125] Yano S, Kuroda S, Lee JB, Shichinohe H, Seki T, Ikeda J, Nishimura G, Hida K, Tamura M, Iwasaki Y: In vivo fluorescence tracking of bone marrow stromal cells transplanted into a pneumatic injury model of rat spinal cord. J Neurotrauma 2005;22:907–918 [PubMed].

[126] Wright KT, Masri WE, Osman A, Roberts S, Trivedi J, Ashton BA, Johnson WE: The cell culture expansion of bone marrow stromal cells from humans with spinal cord injury: implications for future cell transplantation therapy. Spinal Cord 2008;46(12):811–817.

[127] Wright KT, El Masri W, Osman A, Roberts S, Chamberlain G, Ashton BA, Johnson WE: Bone marrow stromal cells stimulate neurite outgrowth over neural proteoglycans (CSPG), myelin associated glycoprotein and Nogo-A. Biochem Biophys Res Commun 2007;354(2):559–566.

[128] Bunge MB: Novel combination strategies to repair the injured mammalian spinal cord. J Spinal Cord Med 2008;31:262–269.

[129] Mackay-Sim A, Feron F, Cochrane J, Bassingthwaighte L, Bayliss C, Davies W, Fronek P, Gray C, Kerr G, Licina P, Nowitzke A, Perry C, Silburn PAS, Urquhart S, Geraghty T: Autologous olfactory ensheathing cell transplantation in human paraplegia: a 3-year clinical trial. Brain 2008;131:2376–2386.

[130] Li H, Wen Y, Luo Y, Lan X, Wang D, Sun Z, Hu L: [Transplantation of bone marrow mesenchymal stem cells into spinal cord injury: a comparison of delivery different times] [Article in Chinese] Zhongguo Xiu Fu Chong Jian Wai Ke Za Zhi 2010;24(2):180–184.

[131] Ichim TE, Solano F, Lara F, Paris E, Ugalde F, Rodriguez JP, Minev B, Bogin V, Ramos F, Woods EJ, Murphy MP, Patel AN, Harman RJ, Riordan NH: Feasibility of combination allogeneic stem celltherapy for spinal cord injury: a case report. Int Archives Med 2010;3:30.

[132] Sullivan R, Duncan K, Dailey T, Kaneko Y, Tajiri N, Borlongan CV: A possible new focus for stroke treatment—migrating stem cells. Expert Opin Biol Ther 2015;15(7):949–958. doi: 10.1517/14712598.2015.1043264.

[133] Klingener M, Chavali M, Aguirre A: N-cadherin promotes recruitment and migration of neural progenitor cells from the SVZ stem cell niche into demyelinated lesions. Int J Dev Neurosci 2015;47(Pt A):107. doi: 10.1016/j.ijdevneu.2015.04.292. PubMed PMID: 26531615.

[134] Kim HJ, Shaker MR, Cho B, Cho HM, Kim H, Kim JY, Sun W: Dynamin-related protein 1 controls the migration and neuronal differentiation of subventricular zone-derived neural progenitor cells. Sci Rep 2015;5:15962. doi: 10.1038/srep15962.

[135] Chen Q, Zhang M, Li Y, Xu D, Wang Y, Song A, Zhu B, Huang Y, Zheng JC: CXCR7 mediates neural progenitor cells migration to CXCL12 independent of CXCR4. Stem Cells 2015;33(8):2574–2585. doi: 10.1002/stem.2022. Epub 2015 May 13. PubMed PMID: 25833331.

[136] Potter K, Saifuddin A: MRI of chronic spinal cord injury. Br J Radiol 2003;76:347–352.

[137] Li Y, Raisman G: Sprouts from cut corticospinal axons persist in the presence of astrocytic scarring in long-term lesions of the adult rat spinal cord. Exp Neurol 1995;134:102–111.

[138] Amr SM, Essam AM, Abdel-Meguid AM, Kholeif AM, Moharram AN, El-Sadek RE: Direct cord implantation in brachial plexus avulsions: revised technique using a single stage combined anterior (first) posterior (second) approach and end-to-side side-to-side grafting neurorrhaphy. J Brachial Plex Peripher Nerve Inj 2009;4:8.

[139] Nakagomi T, Molnár Z, Nakano-Doi A, Taguchi A, Saino O, Kubo S, Clausen M, Yoshikawa H, Nakagomi N, Matsuyama T: Ischemia-induced neural stem/progenitor cells in the pia mater following cortical infarction. Stem Cells Dev 2011 Dec;20(12):2037–2051.

[140] Johanson C, Stopa E, Baird A, Sharma H: Traumatic brain injury and recovery mechanisms: peptide modulation of periventricular neurogenic regions by the choroid plexus-CSF nexus. J Neural Transm 2011;118(1):115–133. Epub 2010 Oct 10.

[141] Francel PC, Francel TJ, Mackinnon SE, Hertl C: Enhancing nerve regeneration across a silicone tube conduit by using interposed short-segment nerve grafts. J Neurosurg 1997;87(6):887–892. PubMed PMID: 9384400.

[142] Spector JG, Lee P, Derby A, Roufa DG: Comparison of rabbit facial nerve regeneration in nerve growth factor-containing silicone tubes to that in autologous neural grafts. Ann Otol Rhinol Laryngol 1995;104(11):875–885.PubMed PMID: 8534028.

[143] Le Beau JM, Powell HC, Ellisman MH: Node of Ranvier formation along fibres regenerating through silicone tube implants: a freeze-fracture and thin-section electron microscopic study. J Neurocytol 1987;16(3):347–358. PubMed PMID: 3612184.

[144] Peláez RJ, Afonso CN, Vega F, Recio-Sánchez G, Torres-Costa V, Manso-Silván M, García-Ruiz JP, Martín-Palma RJ: Laser fabrication of porous silicon-based platforms for cell culturing. J Biomed Mater Res B Appl Biomater 2013;101(8):1463–1468. doi: 10.1002/jbm.b.32966.

[145] Punzón-Quijorna E, Sánchez-Vaquero V, Muñoz-Noval A, Pérez-Roldán MJ, Martín-Palma RJ, Rossi F, Climent-Font A, Manso-Silván M, Ruiz JP, Torres-Costa V: Nanostructured porous silicon micropatterns as a tool forsubstrate-conditioned cell research. Nanoscale Res Lett 2012;7(1):396. PubMed PMID: 22799489; PubMed Central PMCID: PMC3458952.

[146] Collart-Dutilleul PY, Panayotov I, Secret E, Cunin F, Gergely C, Cuisinier F, Martin M: Initial stem cell adhesion on porous silicon surface: molecular architecture of actin cytoskeleton and filopodial growth. Nanoscale Res Lett 2014;9(1):564. doi: 10.1186/1556-276X-9-564. eCollection 2014. PubMed PMID: 25386101; PubMed Central PMCID: PMC4217708.

[147] Pandis C, Trujillo S, Matos J, Madeira S, Ródenas-Rochina J, Kripotou S, Kyritsis A, Mano JF, Gómez Ribelles JL: Porous polylactic acid-silica hybrids: preparation, characterization, and study of mesenchymal stem cell osteogenic differentiation. Macromol Biosci 2015;15(2):262–274. doi: 10.1002/mabi.201400339. Epub 2014 Oct 10. PubMed PMID: 25303745.

[148] Zhou P, Cheng X, Xia Y, Wang P, Zou K, Xu S, Du J: Organic/inorganic composite membranes based on poly(L-lactic-co-glycolic acid) and mesoporous silica for effective bone tissue engineering. ACS Appl Mater Interfaces 2014;6(23):20895–20903. doi: 10.1021/am505493j.

[149] Kim H, Kim I, Choi HJ, Kim SY, Yang EG: Neuron-like differentiation of mesenchymal stem cells on silicon nanowires. Nanoscale 2015;7(40):17131–17138. doi: 10.1039/c5nr05787f. PubMed PMID: 26422757.

[150] Ai H, Lvov YM, Mills DK, Jennings M, Alexander JS, Jones SA: Coating and selective deposition of nanofilm on silicone rubber for cell adhesion and growth. Cell Biochem Biophys 2003;38(2):103–114. PubMed PMID: 12777710.

[151] Yue Z, Liu X, Molino PJ, Wallace GG: Bio-functionalisation of polydimethylsiloxane with hyaluronic acid and hyaluronic acid--collagen conjugate for neural interfacing. Biomaterials 2011;32(21):4714–4724. doi: 10.1016/j.biomaterials.2011.03.032.

[152] Minev IR, Moshayedi P, Fawcett JW, Lacour SP: Interaction of glia with a compliant, microstructured silicone surface. Acta Biomater 2013;9(6):6936–6942. doi: 10.1016/j.actbio.2013.02.048. Epub 2013 Mar 14. PubMed PMID: 23499849.

[153] Patel KR, Tang H, Grever WE, Simon Ng KY, Xiang J, Keep RF, Cao T, McAllister JP II: Evaluation of polymer and self-assembled monolayer-coated silicone surfaces to reduce neural cell growth. Biomaterials 2006;27(8):1519–1526. Epub 2005 Sep 19.

[154] Huang H, Chen L, Wang H, Xiu B, Li B, Wang R, Zhang J, Zhang F, Gu Z, Li Y, Song Y, Hao W, Pang S, Sun J: Influence of patients' age on functional recovery after transplantation of olfactory ensheathing cells into injured spinal cord injury. Chin Med J (Engl) 2003,116:1488–1491.

[155] Lima C, Pratas-Vital J, Escada P, Hasse-Ferreira A, Capucho C, Peduzzi JD: Olfactory mucosa autografts in human spinal cord injury: a pilot clinical study. J Spinal Cord Med 2006;29:191–203; discussion 204–206.

[156] Park HC, Shim YS, Ha Y, Yoon SH, Park SR, Choi BH, Park HS: Treatment of complete spinal cord injury patients by autologous bone marrow cell transplantation and administration of granulocyte-macrophage colony stimulating factor. Tissue Eng 2005;11:913–922.

[157] Yoon SH, Shim YS, Park YH, Chung JK, Nam JH, Kim MO, Park HC, Park SR, Min BH, Kim EY, Choi BH, Park H, Ha Y: Complete spinal cord injury treatment using autologous bone marrow cell transplantation and bone marrow stimulation with granulocyte macrophage-colony stimulating factor: phase I/II clinical trial. Stem Cells 2007;25(8):2066–2073.

[158] Chowdary PD, Che DL, Cui B: Neurotrophin signaling via long-distance axonal transport. Annu Rev Phys Chem 2012;63:571–594. doi: 10.1146/annurev-phys-chem-032511-143704. Epub 2012 Jan 30. Review. PubMed PMID: 22404590.

[159] Chowdary PD, Che DL, Kaplan L, Chen O, Pu K, Bawendi M, Cui B: Nanoparticle-assisted optical tethering of endosomes reveals the cooperative function of dyneins in retrograde axonal transport. Sci Rep 2015;5:18059. doi: 10.1038/srep18059. PubMed PMID: 26656461; PubMed Central PMCID: PMC4674899.

[160] Dono R: Fibroblast growth factors as regulators of central nervous system development and function. Am J Physiol Regul Integr Comp Physiol 2003;284(4):R867–R881. Review. PubMed PMID: 12626354.

[161] Hendry IA, Belford DA: Lack of retrograde axonal transport of the heparin-binding growth factors by chick ciliary neurones. Int J Dev Neurosci 1991;9(3):243–250. PubMed PMID: 1718148.

6

Role of the Neuroinflammation in the Degree of Spinal Cord Injury: New Therapeutic Strategies

Irene Paterniti, Emanuela Esposito and
Salvatore Cuzzocrea

Abstract

A case of spinal cord injury (SCI) is defined as the occurrence of an acute traumatic lesion of neural elements in the spinal canal (spinal cord and cauda equina), resulting in temporary or permanent sensory and/or motor deficit. Most studies on traumatic SCI show a bimodal age distribution, with a first peak in young adulthood and a second peak in older adults. Spinal cord trauma activates a cascade of events that exacerbates the damage such as activation of inflammatory process that determinates cytokine and chemokine production and that generates reduction in functional recovery resulting in necrosis or apoptosis of neurons. However, the precise mechanism of SCI-induced inflammatory response remains not fully understood at present. Current strategy to treat damage to the spinal cord is limited, only the treatment with methylprednisolone (MP), if administered in excessive dose during the acute phase of the damage, could ameliorate patients with severe SCI. However, associated to the beneficial effects, there are growing evidence that high-dose of MP is correlated to increased risk of infections, pneumonia and gastrointestinal bleeding. Therefore, there is a necessity to develop new therapies to treat SCI; one of these is to selectively reduce inflammation that possess unique role in the processes of injury and recovery.

Keywords: Immune response, oxidative stress, spinal cord injury, inflammation, neuroprotection

1. Inflammation response after spinal cord injury

Spinal cord injury (SCI) is damage caused to the spinal cord that compromise the major functions of the spinal cord and remains actually the most important cause of mortality in the society. In addition to its cost to the individual, physically as well as the health care system and society financially, SCI has profound psychosocial effects that are devastating for patients, families and friends. SCI usually begins with a sudden, traumatic blow to the spine that fractures or dislocates vertebrae; long-term mechanical compression of the spinal cord gradually causes various pathologic changes in neural tissue. The pathophysiology of SCI comprises both primary and secondary mechanisms of injury; the "primary injury" refers to the forces that impart the primary mechanical insult to the spinal cord, which in its mildest form causes a cord concussion with brief transient neurologic deficits and in its most severe form causes complete and permanent paralysis. The primary damage to tissue is followed by a second phase of tissue degeneration that might occur over weeks or even months and further generate progressive destruction of the tissue surrounding the necrotic core that expands from the injury "epicenter" and is known as secondary injury, that is a persistence of some crucial events of the acute phase such as edema and apoptotic cell death as well as generation of oxidative stress, activation of immune system response and inflammation process. In particular we focus our attention on some mechanisms that occur after spinal cord injury such as on the involvement of the inflammation process and immune system response.

Inflammation is a physiological process that removes damaged stimuli and initiates the healing process; however, if it persists and if it is over-activated, then the inflammation becomes devastating; inflammation is a key element in the pathophysiology of some disorders such as chronic pain, neurodegenerative pathology, trauma and spinal cord injury [1–5]. Principal pro-inflammatory markers that are both cellular components, such as neutrophils, macrophages and T cells, and non-cellular components, such as cytokines, prostaglandins and complement, have been found in spinal cord tissue that received a mechanical insult. Following spinal cord trauma, the site of injury is penetrated by neutrophils, that determinate release of cytokines that may progressive damage local tissue and recruit other inflammatory cells [6]; moreover, monocytes/macrophages are released and locally activated in microglia, that subsequently invade the injured tissue [7]. The pro-inflammatory cytokines that are produced at the site of injury, such as tumor necrosis factor (TNF-α), interleukins and interferons, mediate the inflammatory response and can generate further tissue damage [8,9]. Furthermore, cytokines can induce the expression of cyclo-oxygenase (COX) 2 and thus promote the breakdown of arachidonic acid into pro-inflammatory prostanoids (prostaglandins, prostacyclin and thromboxanes) that mediate vascular permeability/resistance and platelet aggregation/adherance [10,11]. The involvement of the cyclo-oxygenases in the generation of these inflammatory mediators represents a potential target for intervention, because inhibitors of these enzymes are in widespread clinical use. Additionally, TNF-α contributes to the tissue injury induced by neutrophils by directly activating them [12,13] as well as by increasing the expression of such molecules as ICAM-1 and E-selectin, which cause the activated neutrophils to adhere to the surface of the endothelial cells; it has also been shown that the inhibition of neutrophil adhesion to the endothelial cell surface markedly reduces the severity of the SCI induced by compressive trauma [14]. These observations indicate that the interaction of activated neutrophils with the surface of the endothelial cells is another important mediator in the secondary tissue damage of the spinal cord.

1.1. Cytokine responses to inflammation

Cytokines are small and non-structural proteins with no amino acid sequence motif, their biological activities allow us in turn to group them into different classes: exit 18 cytokines called interleukin (IL), some of these promote inflammation and are named pro-inflammatory cytokines such as IL1β and IL1α, IL6, IL8 and TNF-α, whereas other cytokines suppress the activity of pro-inflammatory cytokines and are called anti-inflammatory cytokines such as IL-4, IL-10, TGFβ. The hypothesis that some cytokine functions primarily induce inflammation while others suppress inflammation is essential to cytokine biology and also to clinical medicine.

Cytokines are secreted by a variety of immune cells such as T-lymphocytes and macrophages, as well as b non-immune cells such as fibroblasts; the physiological effects mediated by cytokines comprise the stimulation or inhibition of cell growth, cytotoxicity/apoptosis, antiviral activity and inflammatory responses. The main function of cytokines is the regulation of T-cell differentiation from undifferentiated cells to T-helper 1 and 2, regulatory T cells, and T-helper 17 cells [15]. These regulatory proteins include ILs, interferons (IFNs) and TNFs. Many of these cytokines have already been shown to be produced by neurons or glia in central nervous system (CNS) disorders in which they are notably increased.

The cytokine class of inflammatory mediators is secreted by microglia and astrocytes and their production is increased in inflammatory states; moreover they act by modulating the intensity and duration of the immune response. Pro-inflammatory cytokines and chemokines up-regulate microbicidal activity of neutrophils, and they can be considered as additional immunomodulatory agents to treat serious or refractory infections in humans.

Through cytokines IL-1 the immune response is initiated, having a crucial role in the onset and expansion of a complex hormonal and cellular inflammatory cascade; the IL-1 family of cytokines includes IL-1α and IL-1β, which generate cell activation upon binding with specific membrane receptors and has been documented that IL-1 plays a role in neuronal degeneration. In astrocytes, IL-1 induces IL-6 production, stimulates iNOS activity [16], enhances neuronal acetylcholinesterase activity, microglial activation and additional IL-1 production, and astrocyte activation.

Another important pro-inflammatory cytokine is the IL-6, a multifunctional cytokine that plays an important role in host defence [17] and possesses main effects during the inflammatory response [18]. IL-6 is associated to the family of neuropoietin cytokine and it possesses direct and indirect neurotrophic effects on neurons [19]; moreover, IL-6 promotes astrogliosis [20], activates microglia [21], and stimulates the release of acute phase molecules.

1.2. Inflammatory mediator: crucial role of TNF-α

Through all the cytokines involved in the secondary damage, TNF-α plays a crucial role; in fact it releases shortly after injury, it can accumulate rapidly at the site of injury, and it is produced by a number of different cell populations, such as neutrophils, macrophages and microglia, astrocytes and T cells [22]. Several cell types are able to produce TNF-α, including macrophages after its activation, dendritic cells, monocytes, NK cells, CD4+ T cells, CD8+ T cells, microglia and astrocytes. Macrophages/monocytes are able to produce TNF-α in the acute phase of inflammation and this cytokines drives several range of signalling events within cells, leading to necrosis or apoptosis.

Several biological functions are ascribed to the TNF-α and for this reason the mechanism of action is somewhat complex; although it inhibits the growth of tumor cells and it has an enhancing effect on the proliferation of normal cells [23]. TNF-α takes part in septic shock, autoimmunity, and inflammatory disorders. The major role of TNF-α is explicated as mediator in resistance against infections; moreover, it was postulated that TNF plays a pathological role in a number of autoimmune pathology such as graft vs host rejection or rheumatoid arthritis. Moreover, TNF-α possesses potent pro-inflammatory effects that are associated to its capacity to generate endothelial cell adhesion molecules and subsequently support neutrophil adherence to vascular endothelium. Neutrophils are exquisite targets of TNF-α that is under certain conditions it strengthens their expression of adhesion molecules induces their degranulation and successive release of lysosomal enzymes, causing the production of highly reactive oxygen species. TNF-α induces the migration of neutrophils mediating the production of chemotactic factors, including IL-8; this testifies cytokine networking involvement in inflammatory cell recruitment and an active role in inflammation.

TNF-α works by binding and clustering high-affinity receptors that are present in a great numbers on most cell membranes [24], the ligand/receptor complex is easily internalised via clathrin-coated pits and ends up in secondary lysozymes where it is degraded. Interestingly, the binding of TNF-α to the 75 kDa TNFR-2 is not sufficient to reach cytotoxicity, but rather binding to the 55 kDa TNFR-1 is sufficient to reach TNF-α mediated cell killing. TNF-α exerts its effects by activating several secondary proteins that provoke a variety of responses within the cell such as activation of gene transcription and/or production of reactive oxygen or nitrogen radicals (e.g., NO). Activated proteins include Gprotein, transcription factors such as NF-κB and AP-1 and serine and cysteine proteases, known as caspases. Many members of the TNF receptor superfamily have intracellular "death domains" which represent protein interaction domains each consisting of 65–80 amino acids; these proteins participate in TNF-α mediated apoptosis process; many evidence demonstrated that TNF–TNFR interactions are implicated in the pathogenesis of CNS disorders such as EAE and MS. These interactions are able to monitor the disease outcome by modifying immune response and the interactions between CNS-resident cells and effector immune cells in the CNS.

However, recent studies showed a dual nature for TNF-α that it can be not only neurotoxic but also neuroprotective; a study conducted with transgenic mice for TNF-α receptors demonstrated that the mice lacking TNF-α showed more tissue loss and functional deficits compared to wild-type mice, implying that TNF-α mediated a neuroprotective effect [25]. The beneficial or deleterious effects of TNF-α dependent when it is being released and on cellular population that is acting on, the conflicting actions of TNF-α described above reflects a growing view of inflammation as a "dual-edged sword" having neurotoxic and neuroprotective properties [26].

Thus, comprehension of their profile, kinetics of expression and interactions between TNF-α ligands and their TNFRs on different CNS residents and infiltrating immune cells would aid to better design strategies to control neuroinflammation and CNS autoimmunity. Blockers of TNF-α have been acknowledged for human use in treating TNF-linked autoimmune and inflammatory disorders. Pathways downstream of receptor ligation supply critical points for interjection for planning new therapeutic strategies.

1.3. Microglia activation

Moreover, other important mediators of inflammation that respond rapidly to disturbances within the microenvironment by change in morphology are the microglia, the expression "activated microglia" is used to define cells that change their immunophenotype and their morphology after a specific stimuli; the principal role of microglia at the lesion site is a rapid phagocytosis of fragments and induction of apoptosis [27]. The different response of microglia *in vitro* suggests that these cells may elicit unique functional properties and consequently control the inflammatory response at the injury site. Microglial activation has been well-known in the spinal cord tissue that has received a trauma and has shown to occur from caudal to lumbar enlargement, based on that there are papers supporting the role of microglia in pain after injury and showing activation of microglia post-SCI.

Thus, we postulated that activated spinal microglia have a role in chronic pain after SCI.

Microglia activate the innate immune system and are key regulators of inflammatory processes in CNS pathologies such as trauma and neurodegenerative diseases participation in both acute and chronic phase of the inflammatory responses. Activated microglia secrete cytotoxic substances including various cytokines such as TNF-α, IL-1, reactive free radicals, and nitric oxide. However, the principal effects of microglia at the levels of the lesion core are probably rapid phagocytosis of debris rather than induction of apoptosis. Microglia when activated can cause neuronal and glial toxicity through the release of cytokines, free radicals, eicosanoids, activated neutrophils, and macrophages [28]. On the other hand, microglia activation leads to beneficial effects producing growth factors that are fundamental for neuronal and tissue restoration. Moreover, it has been demonstrated that transplantation of peripherally activated macrophages has beneficial effects on spinal cord regeneration.

1.4. Apoptosis

In the last decade the generation of apoptotic process after spinal cord trauma was also confirmed, apoptosis can be triggered by a variety of insults including cytokines, inflammatory injury, free radical damage, and excitotoxicity.

The apoptotic process after spinal cord trauma is activated in neurons, oligodendrocytes, microglia, and perhaps, astrocytes; apoptosis in microglia contributes to inflammatory secondary injury.

Two main pathways of apoptosis—extrinsic or receptor-dependent and intrinsic or receptor-independent—have been well characterized, and both appear to be active in SCI; the extrinsic or receptor-dependent pathway is mediated by Fas ligand and Fas receptor [29] and/or inducible nitric oxide synthase production by macrophages [30], while intrinsic or receptor-independent pathway is mediated via direct caspase-3 pro-enzyme activation [31] and/or mitochondrial damage, release of cytochrome c and activation of the inducer caspase-9, pathways of caspase-mediated apoptotic death [32].

Receptor-dependent apoptosis is evoked by extracellular signals, the most significant of which is TNF, so it is termed as "extrinsic" pathway; TNF is known to rapidly accumulate in the injured spinal cord, and activation of the Fas receptor of neurons, microglia, and oligodendrocytes induces a programmed sequence of caspase activation. Moreover, additional control of cell death/survival is provided by the balance between major pro-apoptotic proteins such as Bax, Bad, and Bid and anti-apoptotic proteins such as Bcl-XL and Bcl-2.

Apoptotic cells were reached in the grey matter after injury, starting from 1h with a proliferation during the other 8 h [33]. The number of apoptotic cells is increased at the site of injury and are related with axons degeneration [34].

Apoptotic process that is activated in the secondary injury in SCI has recently come under close study, and the precise contribution and potential therapeutic implications of apoptosis in SCI could be helpful to generate new therapeutic approach to treat the secondary events associated to spinal cord injury.

2. Inflammatory/immunologic response

The inflammatory and immunological response to injury within the CNS is different than that which is occurring in other tissues [35]. The inflammatory and immunologic responses to injury involve activation of innate immune cells that provide immediate defence against inflammatory stimuli and in turn help to recruit cells of the adaptive immune system (i.e., T- and B-lymphocytes). The activation of immune system is driven by interactions involving presentation of antigen and release of various inflammatory mediators [36]. Also, cells present at the injury site may sequester debris and carry CNS antigens to secondary lymphoid organs [37], where trigger lymphocyte activation. Recent studies done on mice showed that the number of activated T and B cells increases in the spleen and bone marrow within 24 hours of trauma [38].

2.1. Lymphocytes infiltration

T-lymphocytes are distributed in the intact spinal cord and gradually grow in number after trauma in parallel with the stimulation of microglia and influx of peripheral macrophages. Lymphocytes infiltrate the spinal cord tissue starting from 24 hours until 7 days after injury and return gradually back to normal levels in 4 to 5 weeks [14].

Under normal conditions, activated T cells can cross the Add Blood–brain barrier (BBB) and enter the CNS parenchyma. In contrast with other inflammatory cells enrolled after a trauma, the number of lymphocytes remains low [39]; however, T-lymphocytes play an important role in the CNS immune system, since on activation, T-lymphocytes may kill target cells and produce cytokines [40].

Once lymphocytes enter the lesion site, they persist indeterminately [38,41], whereas T and B cells increase at the lesion site at least 9 weeks post-injury [42,43], suggesting that cytokine/chemokine gradients exist chronically and regulate integrin expression on endothelia and cells [44,45]. These chemokine gradients and adhesion molecules represent molecular targets for manipulating the effects of intraspinal lymphocytes after SCI [46–48]; the progressive increase in lymphocyte numbers may also be justified by lymphocyte activation and proliferation within the injured centre of spinal cord.

Moreover, induction of immune response could be generated as impaired nerve transmission; increasing the production of pro-inflammatory cytokines in chronic phase of SCI could worsen the damage increasing the axonal injury and demyelination. Furthermore, there are evidences that autoreactive lymphocytes promote neuronal survival *in vivo* through activation not only of autoreactive T cell but also through activation of other non-CNS reactive T cells or B cells such as resident microglia and infiltrating macrophages.

Thus, because lymphocytes remain for long term at the site of the lesion; new strategy of treatment could orientate on these cells that possess a fundamental role in regulating degenerative and regenerative processes after injury.

3. Pharmacologic interventions for acute spinal cord injury

The temporal profile of the secondary injury cascade provides a window within which it is theoretically possible to reduce the pathophysiological processes; many of the current pharmacological and surgical strategies for the treatment of SCI are based on minimising secondary injury and preserving neurological function following trauma to the brain and spinal cord. Over the past couple of decades, a myriad of agents have been nominated as putative neuroprotective therapies, several of these have been tested in the pre-clinical and clinical studies.

The following section briefly highlights some of the most promising neuroprotective approaches that are being pursued.

3.1. Corticosteroids

In the last decade one of the most used approaches to treat patients with a severe SCI is the use of corticosteroids that possess a well-recognized anti-inflammatory properties reducing spinal cord edema. However, the exact mechanisms by which corticosteroids mediated neuroprotection are not yet completely understood but seems that they induce a reduction of inflammatory cytokines production, modulation of the inflammatory/immune cells, inhibition of lipid peroxidation and reduction of oxidative stress. In this regard, methylprednisolone (MP) appears to be particularly efficacious compared with other glucocorticoids. According to the National Acute Spinal Cord Injury Study 2 (NASCIS 2) protocol, MP is usually administered within 8 h after trauma in a high concentration of 30 mg/kg, followed by an infusion of 5.4 mg/kg/h for 23 hours [49,50]. MP is the only well-known pharmacological treatment of SCI injury patients; however, its administration has been shown to be controversial. Some toxic effects such as infection rates, pulmonary embolism, severe pneumonia and sepsis and even death secondary to respiratory complications appeared to be higher with steroid use.

The anti-inflammatory properties of MP are mediated by different mechanisms that are known as transrepression, this mechanism involves interference with pro-inflammatory transcription factor signalling (such as NF-κB) which is upstream of several inflammatory mediators including COX2, chemokines and cytokines.

Together with the minor functional improvement in humans and risk of adverse side effects, these studies highlighted the compelling need to develop better neuroprotective agents with more convincing efficacy.

3.2. Estrogen as a neuroprotective agent

At present, several effects have been associated to estrogen that acts with different mechanism of action [51]. Recently, the neuroprotective and anti-inflammatory effect of estrogen are of great interest; leukocyte adhesion and microglia activation are also sensitive to estrogen and show significantly decreased superoxide dismutase production and phagocytic activity when treated with estrogen *in vitro* [52].

Moreover, cell death is associated to decreases blood flow in spinal cord and estrogen are involved in increasing post-traumatic blood flow induced by ischemia [53] and TBI [54]. Thus, estrogen treatment has been related with increased expression of pro-apoptotic Bcl-2 in the spinal cord injured tissue, this anti-apoptotic increase in Bcl-2 may be mediated by Akt activation with downstream phosphorylation of cAMP response element binding protein (CREB) [55].

However, estrogen may also act on Add N-methyl-D-aspartate receptor (NMDA) receptors, indicating a potential to limit secondary cell death due to excitotoxicity [56].

3.3. Nuclear hormone receptors family: PPARs receptor

Other members of the nuclear hormone receptors family (NHRs) are now explored for their anti-inflammatory properties in experimental models, including SCI.

Peroxisome proliferator-activated receptors (PPARs) are part of the nuclear hormone receptor superfamily, upon ligand activation regulate gene expression and have been shown to be anti-inflammatory in different model of inflammatory pathology, including SCI. PPAR exists as three isoforms (α, β/δ and γ) that control many cellular functions including lipid metabolism, glucose absorption, cell growth and differentiation, and inflammation.

One mechanism involves direct interaction of PPAR with pro-inflammatory transcription factors, most importantly NFκB and AP-1, and the subsequent reduction of gene transcription. Pioglitazone and rosiglitazone are PPARγ agonists that are in common clinical use for type II diabetes. Beyond their metabolic effects, interest in PPAR γ ligand has grown due to their anti-inflammatory, neuroprotective, and even anti-neoplastic properties, suggesting its potential use after spinal cord trauma [57]. As such, PPAR agonists have already been clinically tested in other disorders with inflammatory pathology, such as Alzheimer's disease (AD), rheumatoid arthritis (RA), and ischemia reperfusion injury, but not in SCI yet. Moreover, in the last few years a great interest has been focused on other PPAR receptors agonist such as for PPARα and β/δ receptors. One of the first reports indicating that PPARα is involved in attenuating inflammation demonstrated that the eicosanoid LTB4 binds and activates PPARα [58]. Several studies on inflammatory cytokine produced in aged mice demonstrated an active interaction of PPARα with NFκB; in fact the oxidative stress in different tissue leads to active NFκB. Treatment with PPARα agonists were found to restore the alteration of oxidative mediators, to inhibit the activation of NFκB and to remove IL-6 and IL-12 produced [59,60].

These features were accompanied by enhanced functional motor recovery and reduced hyperalgesia.

Since PPAR agonists are currently used in medical treatment of diabetes, clinical studies for stroke and different CNS pathologies are to be expected. The knowledge about anti-inflammatory properties of PPAR ligands obtained from cell cultures and animal model of SCI demonstrate that PPARs signalling may be therapeutic targets after spinal cord injury.

4. Conclusion

Thus, recent researches are moving to develop new pharmacological approaches that may offer an effective neuroprotection after spinal cord injury. After spinal cord injury, inflammatory reactions account for a large proportion of the secondary damage to neurons and oligodendrocytes.

Promising research is being carried out to better understand the aspects of inflammation, lipid peroxidation and apoptotic cell death that may be the target of pharmacologic intervention.

Few agents have been studied demonstrating efficacy in animal models of spinal cord injury and may become appropriate for testing in the human setting in the near future.

Clearly, much effort has to be done to bring experimental strategies to clinical fruition, but they do represent promising potential interventions.

Thus, the current medical and surgical interventions for the acutely cord-injured patient attempt to minimize the inflammatory process that possess a crucial role in generating and maintaining secondary damage associated to injury and defend the neural cells that initially survived the mechanical injury.

Author details

Irene Paterniti, Emanuela Esposito* and Salvatore Cuzzocrea

*Address all correspondence to: eesposito@unime.it

Department of Chemical, Biological, Pharmaceutical and Environmental Sciences, University of Messina, Messina, Italy

References

[1] Giovannini MG, Scali C, Prosperi C, Bellucci A, Vannucchi MG, Rosi S, et al. Beta-amyloid-induced inflammation and cholinergic hypofunction in the rat brain in vivo: involvement of the p38MAPK pathway. Neurobiology of disease. 2002; 11(2): 257–74.

[2] Dauer W, Przedborski S. Parkinson's disease: mechanisms and models. Neuron. 2003; 39(6): 889–909.

[3] Tenorio G, Kulkarni A, Kerr BJ. Resident glial cell activation in response to perispinal inflammation leads to acute changes in nociceptive sensitivity: implications for the generation of neuropathic pain. Pain. 2013; 154(1): 71–81. doi:10.1016/j.pain.2012.09.008.

[4] Najjar S, Pearlman DM, Alper K, Najjar A, Devinsky O. Neuroinflammation and psychiatric illness. Journal of neuroinflammation. 2013; 10: 43. doi: 10.1186/1742-2094-10-43.

[5] Iadecola C, Anrather J. The immunology of stroke: from mechanisms to translation. Nature medicine. 2011; 17(7): 796–808. doi:10.1038/nm.2399.

[6] Popovich PG, Wei P, Stokes BT. Cellular inflammatory response after spinal cord injury in Sprague–Dawley and Lewis rats. The journal of comparative neurology. 1997; 377(3): 443–64.

[7] Dusart I, Schwab ME. Secondary cell death and the inflammatory reaction after dorsal hemisection of the rat spinal cord. The European journal of neuroscience. 1994; 6(5): 712–24.

[8] Bartholdi D, Schwab ME. Expression of pro-inflammatory cytokine and chemokine mRNA upon experimental spinal cord injury in mouse: an in situ hybridization study. The European journal of neuroscience. 1997; 9(7): 1422–38.

[9] Klusman I, Schwab ME. Effects of pro-inflammatory cytokines in experimental spinal cord injury. Brain research. 1997; 762(1–2): 173–84.

[10] Tonai T, Taketani Y, Ueda N, Nishisho T, Ohmoto Y, Sakata Y, et al. Possible involvement of interleukin-1 in cyclooxygenase-2 induction after spinal cord injury in rats. Journal of neurochemistry. 1999; 72(1): 302–9.

[11] Dubois RN, Abramson SB, Crofford L, Gupta RA, Simon LS, Van De Putte LB, et al. Cyclooxygenase in biology and disease. FASEB journal : official publication of the Federation of American Societies for Experimental Biology. 1998; 12(12): 1063–73.

[12] Genovese T, Mazzon E, Di Paola R, Cannavo G, Muia C, Bramanti P, et al. Role of endogenous ligands for the peroxisome proliferators activated receptors alpha in the secondary damage in experimental spinal cord trauma. Experimental neurology. 2005; 194(1): 267–78. doi:10.1016/j.expneurol.2005.03.003.

[13] Paterniti I, Genovese T, Crisafulli C, Mazzon E, Di Paola R, Galuppo M, et al. Treatment with green tea extract attenuates secondary inflammatory response in an experimental model of spinal cord trauma. Naunyn-Schmiedeberg's archives of pharmacology. 2009; 380(2): 179–92. doi:10.1007/s00210-009-0414-z.

[14] Taoka Y, Okajima K. Role of leukocytes in spinal cord injury in rats. Journal of neurotrauma. 2000; 17(3): 219–29.

[15] Steinman L. A brief history of T(H)17, the first major revision in the T(H)1/T(H)2 hypothesis of T cell-mediated tissue damage. Nature medicine. 2007; 13(2): 139–45. doi: 10.1038/nm1551.

[16] Hausmann ON. Post-traumatic inflammation following spinal cord injury. Spinal cord. 2003; 41(7): 369–78. doi:10.1038/sj.sc.3101483.

[17] Okada S, Nakamura M, Mikami Y, Shimazaki T, Mihara M, Ohsugi Y, et al. Blockade of interleukin-6 receptor suppresses reactive astrogliosis and ameliorates functional recovery in experimental spinal cord injury. Journal of neuroscience research. 2004; 76(2): 265–76. doi:10.1002/jnr.20044.

[18] Roxburgh CS, McMillan DC. Therapeutics targeting innate immune/inflammatory responses through the interleukin-6/JAK/STAT signal transduction pathway in patients with cancer. Translational research: the journal of laboratory and clinical medicine. 2016; 167(1): 61–6. doi:10.1016/j.trsl.2015.08.013.

[19] Teng FY, Tang BL. Axonal regeneration in adult CNS neurons-signaling molecules and pathways. Journal of neurochemistry. 2006; 96(6): 1501–8. doi:10.1111/j. 1471-4159.2006.03663.x.

[20] Morales I, Farias G, Maccioni RB. Neuroimmunomodulation in the pathogenesis of Alzheimer's disease. Neuroimmunomodulation. 2010; 17(3): 202–4. doi: 10.1159/000258724.

[21] Inoue K. Microglial activation by purines and pyrimidines. Glia. 2002; 40(2): 156–63. doi:10.1002/glia.10150.

[22] Yan P, Li Q, Kim GM, Xu J, Hsu CY, Xu XM. Cellular localization of tumor necrosis factor-alpha following acute spinal cord injury in adult rats. Journal of neurotrauma. 2001; 18(5): 563–8. doi:10.1089/089771501300227369.

[23] Mandi Y, Endresz V, Krenacs L, Regely K, Degre M, Beladi I. Tumor necrosis factor production by human granulocytes. International archives of allergy and applied immunology. 1991; 96(2): 102–6.

[24] Loetscher H, Gentz R, Zulauf M, Lustig A, Tabuchi H, Schlaeger EJ, et al. Recombinant 55-kDa tumor necrosis factor (TNF) receptor. Stoichiometry of binding to TNF alpha and TNF beta and inhibition of TNF activity. The Journal of biological chemistry. 1991; 266(27): 18324–9.

[25] Kim GM, Xu J, Xu J, Song SK, Yan P, Ku G, et al. Tumor necrosis factor receptor deletion reduces nuclear factor-kappaB activation, cellular inhibitor of apoptosis protein 2 expression, and functional recovery after traumatic spinal cord injury. The journal of neuroscience : the official journal of the society for neuroscience. 2001; 21(17): 6617–25.

[26] Bethea JR. Spinal cord injury-induced inflammation: a dual-edged sword. Progress in brain research. 2000; 128: 33–42. doi:10.1016/S0079-6123(00)28005-9.

[27] Shuman SL, Bresnahan JC, Beattie MS. Apoptosis of microglia and oligodendrocytes after spinal cord contusion in rats. Journal of neuroscience research. 1997; 50(5): 798–808.

[28] Schwartz M. Autoimmune involvement in CNS trauma is beneficial if well controlled. Progress in brain research. 2000; 128: 259–63. doi:10.1016/S0079-6123(00)28023-0.

[29] Leskovar A, Moriarty LJ, Turek JJ, Schoenlein IA, Borgens RB. The macrophage in acute neural injury: changes in cell numbers over time and levels of cytokine production in mammalian central and peripheral nervous systems. The journal of experimental biology. 2000; 203(Pt 12): 1783–95.

[30] Satake K, Matsuyama Y, Kamiya M, Kawakami H, Iwata H, Adachi K, et al. Nitric oxide via macrophage iNOS induces apoptosis following traumatic spinal cord injury. Brain research molecular brain research. 2000; 85(1–2): 114–22.

[31] Citron BA, Arnold PM, Sebastian C, Qin F, Malladi S, Ameenuddin S, et al. Rapid upregulation of caspase-3 in rat spinal cord after injury: mRNA, protein, and cellular localization correlates with apoptotic cell death. Experimental neurology. 2000; 166(2): 213–26. doi:10.1006/exnr.2000.7523.

[32] Hartley CJ, Reddy AK, Madala S, Martin-McNulty B, Vergona R, Sullivan ME, et al. Hemodynamic changes in apolipoprotein E-knockout mice. American journal of physiology-heart and circulatory physiology. 2000; 279(5): H2326–34.

[33] Zurita M, Vaquero J, Zurita I. Presence and significance of CD-95 (Fas/APO1) expression after spinal cord injury. Journal of neurosurgery. 2001; 94(2 Suppl): 257–64.

[34] Casha S, Yu WR, Fehlings MG. Oligodendroglial apoptosis occurs along degenerating axons and is associated with FAS and p75 expression following spinal cord injury in the rat. Neuroscience. 2001; 103(1): 203–18.

[35] Schwartz M, Moalem G, Leibowitz-Amit R, Cohen IR. Innate and adaptive immune responses can be beneficial for CNS repair. Trends in neurosciences. 1999; 22(7): 295–9.

[36] Ling C, Sandor M, Fabry Z. In situ processing and distribution of intracerebrally injected OVA in the CNS. Journal of neuroimmunology. 2003; 141(1–2): 90–8.

[37] Karman J, Ling C, Sandor M, Fabry Z. Initiation of immune responses in brain is promoted by local dendritic cells. Journal of immunology. 2004; 173(4): 2353–61.

[38] Ankeny DP, Lucin KM, Sanders VM, McGaughy VM, Popovich PG. Spinal cord injury triggers systemic autoimmunity: evidence for chronic B lymphocyte activation and lupus-like autoantibody synthesis. Journal of neurochemistry. 2006; 99(4): 1073–87. doi: 10.1111/j.1471-4159.2006.04147.x.

[39] Schnell L, Fearn S, Klassen H, Schwab ME, Perry VH. Acute inflammatory responses to mechanical lesions in the CNS: differences between brain and spinal cord. The European journal of neuroscience. 1999; 11(10): 3648–58.

[40] Kierdorf K, Wang Y, Neumann H. Immune-mediated CNS damage. Results and problems in cell differentiation. 2010; 51: 173–96. doi:10.1007/400_2008_15.

[41] Sroga JM, Jones TB, Kigerl KA, McGaughy VM, Popovich PG. Rats and mice exhibit distinct inflammatory reactions after spinal cord injury. The journal of comparative neurology. 2003; 462(2): 223–40. doi:10.1002/cne.10736.

[42] Bilgen M, Dogan B, Narayana PA. In vivo assessment of blood-spinal cord barrier permeability: serial dynamic contrast enhanced MRI of spinal cord injury. Magnetic resonance imaging. 2002; 20(4): 337–41.

[43] Whetstone WD, Hsu JY, Eisenberg M, Werb Z, Noble-Haeusslein LJ. Blood-spinal cord barrier after spinal cord injury: relation to revascularization and wound healing. Journal of neuroscience research. 2003; 74(2): 227–39. doi:10.1002/jnr.10759.

[44] Lee YL, Shih K, Bao P, Ghirnikar RS, Eng LF. Cytokine chemokine expression in contused rat spinal cord. Neurochemistry international. 2000; 36(4–5): 417–25.

[45] Babcock AA, Kuziel WA, Rivest S, Owens T. Chemokine expression by glial cells directs leukocytes to sites of axonal injury in the CNS. The journal of neuroscience: the official journal of the society for neuroscience. 2003; 23(21): 7922–30.

[46] Bao F, Chen Y, Dekaban GA, Weaver LC. Early anti-inflammatory treatment reduces lipid peroxidation and protein nitration after spinal cord injury in rats. Journal of neurochemistry. 2004; 88(6): 1335–44.

[47] Eng LF, Lee YL. Response of chemokine antagonists to inflammation in injured spinal cord. Neurochemical research. 2003; 28(1): 95–100.

[48] Gonzalez R, Glaser J, Liu MT, Lane TE, Keirstead HS. Reducing inflammation decreases secondary degeneration and functional deficit after spinal cord injury. Experimental neurology. 2003; 184(1): 456–63.

[49] Bracken MB. Methylprednisolone in the management of acute spinal cord injuries. The medical journal of Australia. 1990; 153(6): 368.

[50] Bracken MB, Shepard MJ, Collins WF, Holford TR, Young W, Baskin DS, et al. A randomized, controlled trial of methylprednisolone or naloxone in the treatment of acute spinal cord injury. Results of the Second National Acute Spinal Cord Injury Study.

The New England journal of medicine. 1990; 322(20): 1405–11. doi:10.1056/NEJM199005173222001.

[51] Sribnick EA, Wingrave JM, Matzelle DD, Ray SK, Banik NL. Estrogen as a neuroprotective agent in the treatment of spinal cord injury. Annals of the New York Academy of Sciences. 2003; 993: 125–33; discussion 59–60.

[52] Bruce-Keller AJ, Keeling JL, Keller JN, Huang FF, Camondola S, Mattson MP. Antiinflammatory effects of estrogen on microglial activation. Endocrinology. 2000; 141(10): 3646–56. doi:10.1210/endo.141.10.7693.

[53] He Z, He YJ, Day AL, Simpkins JW. Proestrus levels of estradiol during transient global cerebral ischemia improves the histological outcome of the hippocampal CA1 region: perfusion-dependent and independent mechanisms. Journal of the neurological sciences. 2002; 193(2): 79–87.

[54] Roof RL, Hall ED. Estrogen-related gender difference in survival rate and cortical blood flow after impact-acceleration head injury in rats. Journal of neurotrauma. 2000; 17(12): 1155–69. doi:10.1089/neu.2000.17.1155.

[55] Honda K, Shimohama S, Sawada H, Kihara T, Nakamizo T, Shibasaki H, et al. Nongenomic antiapoptotic signal transduction by estrogen in cultured cortical neurons. Journal of neuroscience research. 2001; 64(5): 466–75.

[56] Nilsen J, Chen S, Brinton RD. Dual action of estrogen on glutamate-induced calcium signaling: mechanisms requiring interaction between estrogen receptors and src/mitogen activated protein kinase pathway. Brain research. 2002; 930(1–2): 216–34.

[57] Cuzzocrea S. Peroxisome proliferator-activated receptors gamma ligands and ischemia and reperfusion injury. Vascular pharmacology. 2004; 41(6): 187–95. doi:10.1016/j.vph.2004.10.004.

[58] Devchand PR, Keller H, Peters JM, Vazquez M, Gonzalez FJ, Wahli W. The PPAR alpha-leukotriene B4 pathway to inflammation control. Nature. 1996; 384(6604): 39–43. doi:10.1038/384039a0.

[59] Esposito E, Cuzzocrea S. Palmitoylethanolamide is a new possible pharmacological treatment for the inflammation associated with trauma. Mini reviews in medicinal chemistry. 2013; 13(2): 237–55.

[60] Esposito E, Cuzzocrea S. Targeting the peroxisome proliferator-activated receptors (PPARs) in spinal cord injury. Expert opinion on therapeutic targets. 2011; 15(8): 943–59. doi:10.1517/14728222.2011.581231.

Spastic Paraplegias Due to Non-Traumatic Spinal Cord Disorders

Haruo Shimazaki

Abstract

Spinal cord disorders are induced by diseases of various categories: infectious, inflammatory, degenerative, genetic, traumatic, and so on. These diseases involve spastic paraplegia or tetraplegia, abnormal sensation, bladder and anal dysfunction, etc. This chapter describes the medical etiologies and treatments for spastic paraplegias. I will mention diagnostic and therapeutic aspects of spastic paraplegias due to non-traumatic spinal cord disorders. I will describe my cases who suffered from amyotrophic lateral sclerosis (ALS), hereditary spastic paraplegia (HSP), HTLV-1 associated myelopathy (HAM), and multiple sclerosis (MS). I also investigate the recent therapeutic strategies for spastic paraplegias. Spastic paraplegia is an intractable condition accompanied by many spinal cord disorders. Some therapeutic methods (intrathecal baclofen and botulinum toxin injection) have symptomatic effects. Rehabilitation and some devices are also effective for spasticity.

Keywords: adrenoleukodystrophy (ALD), amyotrophic lateral sclerosis (ALS), hereditary spastic paraplegia (HSP), HTLV-1 associated myelopathy (HAM), multiple sclerosis (MS), intrathecal baclofen, botulinum toxin, rehabilitation

1. Introduction

Spinal cord disorders are induced by diseases of various categories: infections [1] (e.g. herpes zoster or human T-cell lymphotropic virus type 1), inflammation (e.g. multiple sclerosis [2]), vascular diseases (e.g. spinal cord infarction [3]), degeneration (e.g. amyotrophic lateral sclerosis [4]), genetic diseases (e.g. hereditary spastic paraplegias [5]), metabolic disorders [6], trauma, etc. These diseases involve spastic paraplegia or tetraplegia, abnormal sensation, bladder and anal dysfunction, etc. This chapter describes the medical etiologies and treatments for spastic paraplegias. Diagnostic and therapeutic aspects of spastic paraplegias due to non-traumatic spinal cord disorders will be described. In this chapter, cases with X-linked adrenoleukodystrophy (X-ALD), amyotrophic lateral sclerosis (ALS), hereditary spastic paraplegia (HSP), HTLV-1-associated myelopathy (HAM), multiple sclerosis (MS) are introduced.

2. Adrenoleukodystrophy (X-ALD)

Adrenoleukodystrophy is an X-linked recessive disorder that affects the central nervous system white matter and the adrenal cortex [7, 8]. It is classified into several subtypes. The most frequent type is the childhood cerebral form, which initially resembles a behavior disorder and presents adrenal insufficiency, followed by mental impairment, cortical blindness, cortical deafness, spastic tetraplegia and convulsions. This form leads to a decerebrate state for a few years after onset. Whereas the adult forms are divided into adult cerebral, adrenomyeloneuropathy, and cerebellobrainstem. Here we present adult cerebral form case with cerebellar ataxia and spastic paraplegia.

A 53-year-old man was admitted to our hospital because of mental deterioration and gait disturbance. His uncle on his mother's side suffered from gait disturbance from 40 years of age. His total IQ according to Wechsler Adult Intelligence Score (WAIS)-III was 64. He showed emotional incontinence and attention deficit. Gingival pigmentation was noted. Neurological

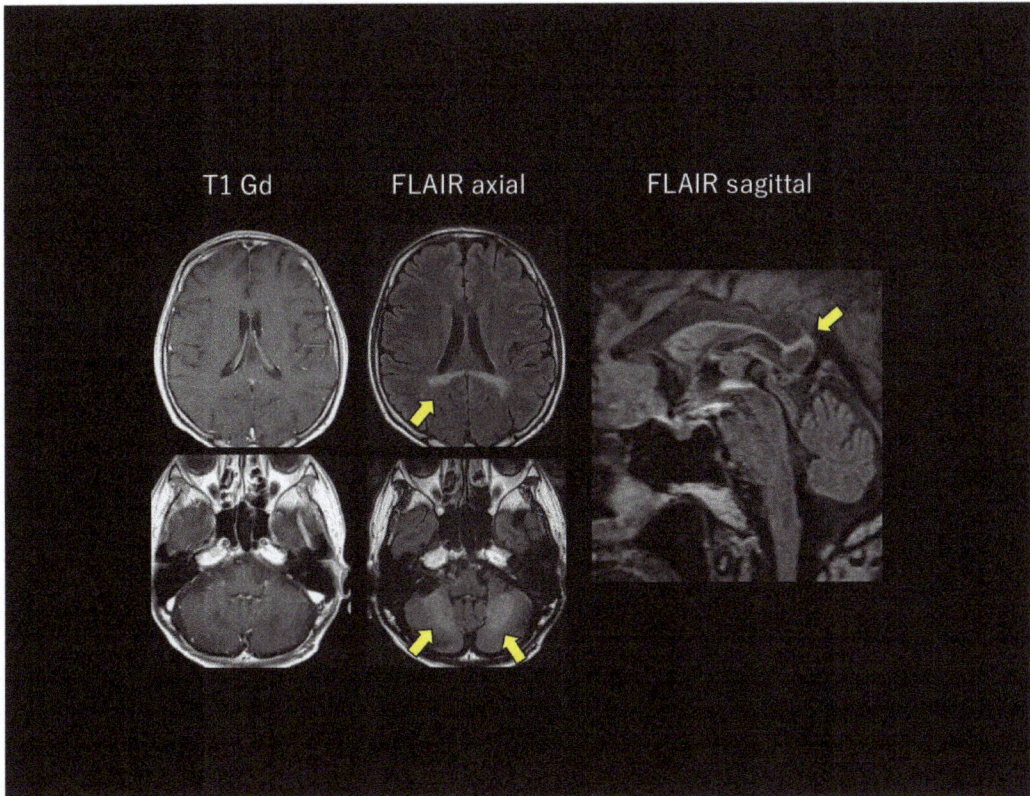

Figure 1. Brain MRI of the adrenoleukodystrophy patient. T1 gadolinium (Gd) enhance: no enhanced area in his brain. FLAIR axial: FLAIR hyperintensities in the cerebellar white matters and callosal body (arrow). FLAIR sagittal: FLAIR hyperintensities in the callosal body (arrow).

examination revealed saccadic eye movement, dysarthria, ataxia and spasticity of the bilateral feet, exaggerated deep tendon reflexes (DTRs), and bilateral positive Babinski signs. Blood examination disclosed elevation of very long chain fatty acids (C24:0/C22:0 2.09, C25:0/C22:0 0.080, and C26:0/C22:0 0.075) and ACTH (173 pg/ml). Brain MRI showed FLAIR hyperintensities in the cerebellar white matter and callosal body, whereas there was no gadolinium enhanced area (**Figure 1**). No atrophy or abnormal signals were observed on MRI of the spinal cord. Brain single photon emission computed tomography (SPECT) demonstrated cerebellar hypoperfusion. For an accurate diagnosis, gene analysis was performed by another institution, which revealed a non-synonymous missense variant of the *ABCD1* gene.

He was administered hydrocortisone and propiverine because of his adrenal insufficiency and frequent urination, and underwent physical rehabilitation (walking and balance exercise) for his leg spasticity and ataxia. We referred him to another hospital, and allogeneic hematopoietic stem cell transplantation was recommended [9, 10], but he denied this treatment.

3. Amyotrophic lateral sclerosis (ALS)

ALS is a fatal disorder characterized by muscle weakness and atrophy, and swallowing and respiratory disturbances [11]. The pathologic findings are upper (brain) and lower (spinal cord) motor neuron degenerations. In some ALS cases, spastic paraplegia can be a predominant symptom in the early stage of the disease. Here we present a case that showed spastic paraplegia as an initial phenotype.

A 60-year-old man was admitted to our hospital to alleviate his lower leg spasticity. Three years ago, he suffered from left leg discomfort and gait disturbance. Then the same sense of discomfort spread to his right foot. Neurological examination on admission showed marked leg spasticity with laterality and a spastic gait, exaggerated DTRs, and positive pathological reflexes. The brain and spinal cord MRI findings were normal. Motor evoked potentials suggested upper motor neuron disturbances.

We administered some muscle relaxants. He underwent gait rehabilitation and botulinum toxin injection to his lower legs. These therapies slightly improved the range of motion of knee and foot joints. But he refused intrathecal baclofen.

After 1 year, he noticed dysphagia and intrinsic hand muscle atrophy. Neurological reevaluation revealed bulbar signs and distal muscle weakness, these findings leading to a diagnosis of ALS. Although he underwent intermittent edaravone infusion therapy [12], his muscle weakness and atrophy gradually worsened and he became bedridden.

4. Hereditary spastic paraplegia (HSP)

HSP is a genetic neurodegenerative disorder that involves bilateral leg spasticity with additional features: mental impairment, peripheral neuropathy, cerebellar ataxia, retinal degeneration, etc. [5]. Its progression is slower than that of ALS. We have encountered and described several cases who suffered from HSPs. First, I present a SPG3A case. SPG3A is an autosomal dominant, early-onset pure spastic paraplegia caused by an *Atlastin1* (*ATL1*) gene mutation [13].

A 52-year-old man visited our clinic because of early-onset gait disturbance at age two (**Figure 2**, IV-7). He had been diagnosed as having cerebral palsy by a doctor at another hospital. He underwent bilateral Achilles tendon lengthening in his early childhood. His older brother suffered from late-onset gait disturbance (**Figure 2**, IV-6).

On examination, his gait was spastic. Muscle weakness and atrophy of his lower extremities were observed. Exaggerated DTRs except for a diminished Achilles tendon reflex and pathological reflexes of his legs were noted (**Table 1**). MRI of his brain revealed no abnormal findings, whereas his spinal cord was slightly atrophic. Serum HTLV-1 antibody was positive, but he refused a lumbar puncture. Whole-exome sequencing analysis allowed the diagnosis of SPG3A. He had a reported heterozygous missense mutation (c.1239T>C, p.F413L) of the *ATL1* gene [14] (**Figure 3**).

This mutation was not detected in DNA from his father (III-1) or older brother (IV-6). We prescribed muscle relaxants (tizanidine and dantrolene), but he could not continue to take them due to their side effects (nausea and sleepiness).

Next, I present a SPG11 case. SPG11 is an autosomal recessive, complicated SPG accompanied by mental impairment, peripheral neuropathy and a thin corpus callosum. This disease is caused by mutations of the *SPG11* gene encoding spatacsin protein [15].

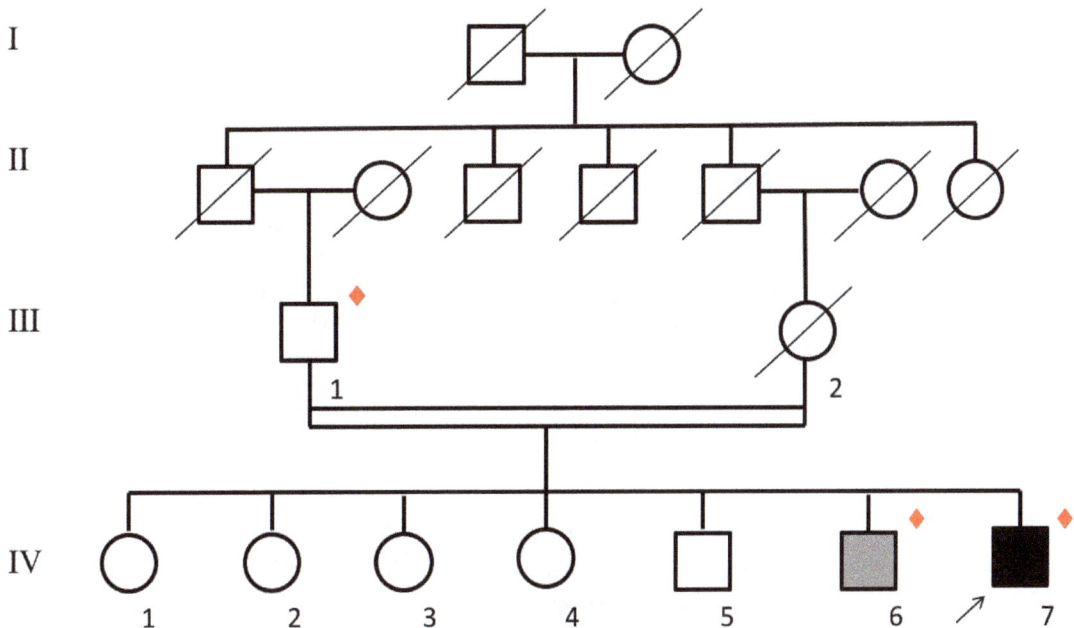

Figure 2. Family tree including the SPG3A/HAM cases. Proband (IV-7): SPG3A patient, HTLV-1 carrier. Older brother (IV-6): HAM patient. Father (III-1): Healthy HTLV-1 carrier. Diamonds indicate positive anti-HTLV-1 antibodies.

	IV-6 (HAM)	IV-7 (SPG3A)
Age at examination	54	52
Age at onset	42	2
DTR of legs	↑	PTR↑, ATR↓
Babinski reflex	+	+
Leg atrophy	−	+
Sensory disturbance	+	−
Spinal MRI	Normal	Mild atrophy

Table 1. Clinical symptoms of the HAM and SPG3A cases.

A 31-year-old man was admitted to our hospital because of standing difficulty and bilateral leg pain. He noticed gait disturbance at age 13. His gait disturbance gradually worsened and he became wheel-chair bound at age 23. He has mental impairment. On examination, exaggerated DTRs and marked spasticity with sustained clonus of both legs were observed. Brain MRI showed a thin corpus callosum. Genetic analysis disclosed compound heterozygous mutations of the *SPG11* gene [16]. We tried intrathecal low-dose baclofen administration, which dramatically alleviated his spasticity (from 4 to 2, modified Ashworth score) and pain with leg clonus. Then an intrathecal baclofen infusion pump was implanted by a neurosurgeon. He became almost free from leg clonus pain with intrathecal baclofen and the modified Ashworth score decreased to 2 or 3.

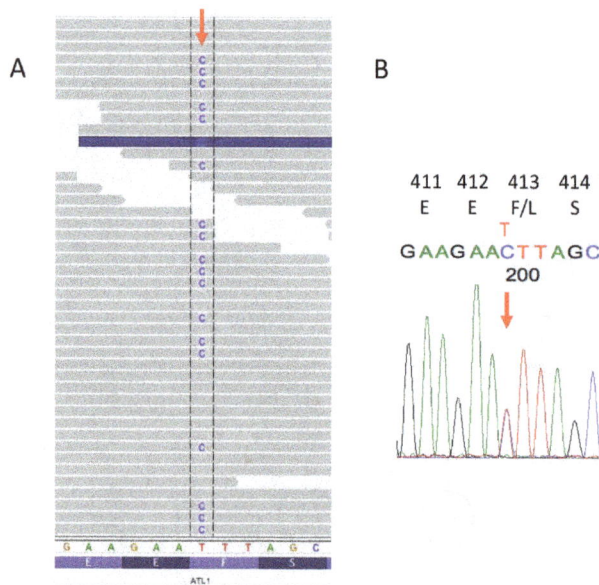

Figure 3. Gene analysis of the SPG3A patient. A. Whole-exome sequencing revealed the c.1239T>C (p.F413L) variant of the *Atlastin1* (*ATL1*) gene. B. Sanger sequencing confirmed the c.1239T>C (p.F413L) mutation of the *ATL1* gene.

5. Human T-lymphotropic virus type 1 (HTLV-1) associated myelopathy

HTLV-1 associated myelopathy (HAM) is a slowly progressive thoracic myelopathy characterized by spastic paraplegia with sensory and autonomic dysfunctions [17, 18]. There are many patients in the Kyushu district, the southwest part of Japan, because the prevalence rate of HTLV-1 carriers is high in Kyushu [18]. We found a HAM patient among the family members including a case of SPG3A (**Figure 2**, IV-6).

A 54-year-old man was admitted to our hospital for the further examination of gait disturbance. He first noticed the gait disturbance about 10 years ago. He walked without a heel and had urinary incontinence for 3 years. He pointed out increased deep tendon reflexes of his legs, a positive Babinski sign, and diminished deep sensation of the legs. On examination, increased leg spasticity was observed bilaterally (**Table 1**). Anti- HTLV-1 antibody was positive in both serum and cerebrospinal fluid (CSF). Serum from his healthy 91-year-old father (III-1, **Figure 2**) was also anti-HTLV-1 antibody positive, probably due to blood transfusion. Mild pleocytosis ($8/mm^3$), elevated neopterin (49 pmol/ml), and positive HTLV-1 proviral DNA were observed in his CSF. Whole-exome sequencing of his DNA did not identify pathogenic variants of the SPG3A and other SPG genes. We treated him with oral prednisolone [19], the symptoms did not worsen after that.

6. Multiple sclerosis (MS)

Multiple sclerosis (MS) is a neuroinflammatory disorder involving the spinal cord, optic nerve and brain, and is prevalent in young women. It takes relapse and remission courses. The characteristic finding is multiple lesions in the brain and spinal cord observed on MRI [20]. Neuromyelitis optica (NMO) is a similar disease to MS, but usually long cord lesions (>3 vertebral body) are observed on spinal MRI, and autoantibodies against aquaporin 4 are usually detected in patients' sera [21, 22].

A 47-year-old woman was admitted to our hospital because of gait disturbance, clumsiness and numbness of the bilateral hands. Neurological examination revealed leg spasticity, increased deep tendon reflexes of all extremities, extensor plantar responses and sensory disturbances of the bilateral upper extremities and trunk. Spinal MRI showed a central cord lesion at C2-C3 with mild enhancement (**Figure 4**). Multiple ovoid periventricular lesions were observed on brain MRI. However, clinically spasticity was presented in the clinical examination in the lower legs only. The anti-aquaporin 4 antibody was not detected in her serum. We started high-dose methylprednisolone pulse therapy and subsequently administered oral fingolimod for relapse prevention. Her symptoms gradually improved except for the leg spasticity. Then we tried to treat her with botulinum toxin injection to her legs and gait rehabilitation [2]. The modified Ashworth score for her legs improved from 3 to 2.

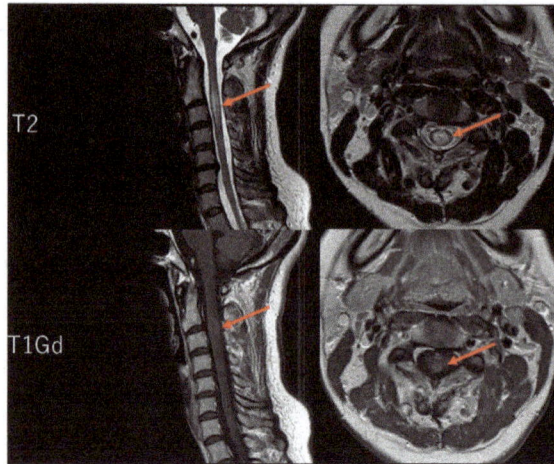

Figure 4. Spinal MRI of the multiple sclerosis patient. T2: T2 weighted image; central cord lesion in C2-C4 (arrow). T1 Gd: T1 weighted gadolinium enhancement; mild enhancement of C2-C3 lesion (arrow).

Acknowledgements

We greatly appreciate the *ABCD1* gene analysis by Professor Nobuyuki Shimozawa (Division of Genomics Research, Life Science Research Center, Gifu University).

Author details

Haruo Shimazaki

Address all correspondence to: hshimaza@jichi.ac.jp

Division of Neurology, Department of Internal Medicine, Jichi Medical University, Tochigi, Japan

References

[1] Cho TA, Vaitkevicius H. Infectious myelopathies. Continuum (Minneapolis, Minn.). 2012;**18**(6 Infectious Disease):1351-1373

[2] Patejdl R, Zettl UK. Spasticity in multiple sclerosis: Contribution of inflammation, auto-immune mediated neuronal damage and therapeutic interventions. Autoimmunity Reviews. 2017;**16**(9):925-936

[3] Romi F, Naess H. Spinal cord infarction in clinical neurology: A review of characteristics and long-term prognosis in comparison to cerebral infarction. European Neurology. 2016;**76**(3-4):95-98

[4] Fink JK. Progressive spastic paraparesis: Hereditary spastic paraplegia and its relation to primary and amyotrophic lateral sclerosis. Seminars in Neurology. 2001;**21**(2):199-207

[5] de Souza PV, de Rezende Pinto WB, de Rezende Batistella GN, Bortholin T, Oliveira AS. Hereditary spastic paraplegia: Clinical and genetic hallmarks. Cerebellum. 2017;**16**(2):525-551

[6] Hedera P. Hereditary and metabolic myelopathies. Handbook of Clinical Neurology. 2016;**136**:769-785

[7] Engelen M, Kemp S, Poll-The BT. X-linked adrenoleukodystrophy: Pathogenesis and treatment. Current Neurology and Neuroscience Reports. 2014;**14**(10):486

[8] Kemp S, Huffnagel IC, Linthorst GE, Wanders RJ, Engelen M. Adrenoleukodystrophy - Neuroendocrine pathogenesis and redefinition of natural history. Nature Reviews. Endocrinology. 2016;**12**(10):606-615

[9] Hitomi T, Mezaki T, Tomimoto H, Ikeda A, Shimohama S, Okazaki T, et al. Long-term effect of bone marrow transplantation in adult-onset adrenoleukodystrophy. European Journal of Neurology. 2005;**12**(10):807-810

[10] Kuhl JS, Suarez F, Gillett GT, Hemmati PG, Snowden JA, Stadler M, et al. Long-term outcomes of allogeneic haematopoietic stem cell transplantation for adult cerebral X-linked adrenoleukodystrophy. Brain. 2017;**140**(4):953-966

[11] Brown RH, Al-Chalabi A. Amyotrophic lateral sclerosis. The New England Journal of Medicine. 2017;**377**(2):162-172

[12] Group EM-AS. Safety and efficacy of edaravone in well defined patients with amyotrophic lateral sclerosis: A randomised, double-blind, placebo-controlled trial. Lancet Neurology. 2017;**16**(7):505-512

[13] Zhao X, Alvarado D, Rainier S, Lemons R, Hedera P, Weber CH, et al. Mutations in a newly identified GTPase gene cause autosomal dominant hereditary spastic paraplegia. Nature Genetics. 2001;**29**(3):326-331

[14] Durr A, Camuzat A, Colin E, Tallaksen C, Hannequin D, Coutinho P, et al. Atlastin1 mutations are frequent in young-onset autosomal dominant spastic paraplegia. Archives of Neurology. 2004;**61**(12):1867-1872

[15] Stevanin G, Santorelli FM, Azzedine H, Coutinho P, Chomilier J, Denora PS, et al. Mutations in SPG11, encoding spatacsin, are a major cause of spastic paraplegia with thin corpus callosum. Nature Genetics. 2007;**39**(3):366-372

[16] Shimazaki H, Nakajima T, Ando Y, et al. Intrathecal baclofen relieves leg pain in a case of SPG11. Neurological Therapeutics. 2014;**31**(5):622

[17] Osame M, Usuku K, Izumo S, Ijichi N, Amitani H, Igata A, et al. HTLV-I associated myelopathy, a new clinical entity. Lancet. 1986;**1**(8488):1031-1032

[18] Nakamura T, Matsuo T. Human T-lymphotropic virus type I-associated myelopathy. Brain and Nerve. 2015;**67**(7):845-858

[19] Coler-Reilly ALG, Sato T, Matsuzaki T, Nakagawa M, Niino M, Nagai M, et al. Effectiveness of daily prednisolone to slow progression of human T-lymphotropic virus type 1-associated myelopathy/tropical spastic paraparesis: A multicenter retrospective cohort study. Neurotherapeutics. 2017. DOI: 10.1007/s13311-017-0533-z

[20] Trapp BD, Nave KA. Multiple sclerosis: An immune or neurodegenerative disorder? Annual Review of Neuroscience. 2008;31:247-269

[21] Lennon VA, Wingerchuk DM, Kryzer TJ, Pittock SJ, Lucchinetti CF, Fujihara K, et al. A serum autoantibody marker of neuromyelitis optica: Distinction from multiple sclerosis. Lancet. 2004;364(9451):2106-2112

[22] Marignier R, Cobo Calvo A, Vukusic S. Neuromyelitis optica and neuromyelitis optica spectrum disorders. Current Opinion in Neurology. 2017;30(3):208-215

8

Protective Role of the Immune System in Spinal Cord Injury: Immunomodulation with Altered Peptide Ligands

Paola Suárez-Meade and Antonio Ibarra

Abstract

Spinal cord injury (SCI) is a phenomenon characterized by damage to the spinal cord and nerve roots, resulting in loss of physiological activity below the lesion. Injury to the spinal cord activates a cascade of cellular and molecular reactions in which the immune system plays an essential role, as there is an uncontrolled immune response that endows further damage to neural tissue. However, the activity of immune system at the site of injury can be modified in order to obtain a neuroprotective environment and promote SCI recovery. This strategy has been designed under the light of the innovative concept "protective autoimmunity" (PA) and can be stimulated with the use of altered peptide ligands (APL). Adequate immunomodulation with APL can be obtained with the peptide A91, which is a safe synthetic peptide derived from the myelin basic protein (MBP) that has proven to be effective in preclinical research. Immunization with A91 is carried out with the objective of preventing further damage and promoting neuroprotection. This peptide has direct influence over SCI secondary mechanisms such as inflammation, lipid peroxidation, and apoptosis. Preclinical results suggest that immunization with A91 could be an effective treatment in the clinical field, providing a better quality of life to SCI patients.

Keywords: spinal cord injury, protective autoimmunity, A91, altered peptide ligand, immunization

1. Introduction

Spinal cord injury (SCI) is perhaps one of the most devastating conditions as it results in a disruption of motor, sensory, and autonomic functions, leading to permanent neurological disability. According to the National Spinal Cord Injury Statistical Center (NSCISC), in 2014 over 276,000 people were suffering from SCI [1]. The incidence ranges over 12,500 new cases each year, with a prevalence of approximately 40 cases per million in the United States [2]. Epidemiological studies indicate that SCI has a higher incidence among male population, and people between 30 and 50 years old [3, 3]. Clinically, the most disabling outcomes of traumatic SCI are motor deficit and sensory loss. Nonetheless, due to autonomic dysfunction and depending on the level and severity of injury, SCI may also alter normal homeostasis and the respiratory, reproductive, urinary, and gastrointestinal systems [4–6]. Besides surgical intervention, the standard of care for SCI in several countries focuses on preventing shock and further damage with the use of methylprednisolone (MP), a synthetic glucocorticoid with anti-inflammatory properties. The National Acute Spinal Cord Injury Study (NASCIS) trials suggest that high-dose MP is effective for the management of acute SCI [5, 8]. However, further studies about NASCIS results indicate that the clinical benefits of the use of MP as a treatment for SCI are questionable [6, 10]. Acute MP therapy reduces cellular damage and secondary injury mechanisms but leads to risks of high-dose steroids [7]. For this reason, MP administration after SCI is still a controversial treatment, and it continues to be debated [8].

Another molecule that has been widely studied for the clinical treatment of SCI is Ganglioside, which is highly expressed in the cell membranes of the central nervous system (CNS). The synthetic form of this glycosphingolipid—monosialotetrahexosylganglioside (GM1)—was known for having anti-apoptotic, anti-excitotoxic, and neuroprotective properties [9, 14]. Therefore, several clinical trials were designed in order to test this drug on SCI [10]. In the most recent study, patients received NASCIS II doses of MP, and different doses of GM1 after the effect of MP was over. Although, GM1 treated patients presented a significant recovery, the beneficial effects related to the drug were inconsistent between different types of injuries and were lost during chronic SCI stages [11, 17]. These results suggest that GM1 has a limited effect and to the date, it is not an approved treatment for SCI [12].

Undoubtedly, the lack of an available treatment for SCI in the clinical field highlights the need to design new and safe therapies for injured patients. Nowadays, research is focused on targeting secondary SCI mechanisms with the objective of minimizing further damage, promoting regeneration and thus, improving functional recovery [13, 19]. One of the most important secondary injury mechanisms is the post-traumatic inflammatory response, which is roughly characterized by the presence of injury-dependent pro-inflammatory cytokines and infiltration of peripheral immune cells to the damaged area [14–22]. It was previously thought that the presence of this uncontrolled immune response in the CNS was harmful and pathological. However, other findings state a controversial theory: immune cells could play an essential role in neuroprotection and regeneration of the spinal cord after injury [15]. A better understanding of how inflammation mediates secondary injury suggests that suppressing all immune responses with the use of glucocorticoids is no longer a rational treatment approach. This information has led scientists to further investigate the beneficial effects of the immune system in several neurological conditions, including SCI [16]. Focusing on the beneficial mechanisms of the immune system after trauma has opened the doors for the design of a new therapeutic strategy. Nevertheless, some questions should first be answered. For instance, how can the immune system be modulated to attain a protective microenvironment? What are the immune-related elements capable of providing the required immune-modulation? And how are they able to provide recovery after SCI?

2. Spinal cord injury pathophysiology

Damage to the spinal cord (SC) causes anatomical and functional deficits to the CNS, that result in the appearance of several long-term medical comorbidities. SCI is characterized by two different pathophysiological phases: primary and secondary injury [17]. Initial trauma to the SC—known as primary injury—is caused by a compressive or contusive mechanism that results in gross anatomical tissue disruption, and immediate hemostatic self-defense events that produce further damage to CNS structures. Direct impact to the SC leads to vascular disturbances such as hemorrhage, ischemia, edema, and hypoperfusion, resulting in tissue necrosis [18]. Hemorrhage and edema formation can raise the risk of developing increased parenchymal pressure and produce more tissue damage [19]. Also, reactive gliosis, demyelination, and axonal loss are often caused by immediate trauma and sustained compression to neural tissue [20]. Depending upon primary injury characteristics, there could be greater tissue damage and worse functional outcomes. Therefore, during this phase, treatment should focus on hemorrhage control to avoid necrosis and early decompression to stabilize intrathecal pressure.

As a consequence of primary injury, there is a cascade of biological reactions that occur minutes after injury and last for several weeks known as secondary injury [21]. This phase is quite complex, as it consists of the development of mechanisms like loss of ATP-dependent cellular functions, ion homeostasis imbalance, excitotoxicity, oxidative stress, lipid peroxidation, inflammation, and apoptosis [22]. There are several secondary mechanisms that are strongly related to the ischemic event observed in SCI. Ischemia produces a depletion of the intracellular amount of ATP, leading to a reduction in the energy-dependent cell function that preserve ion homeostasis [23]. Therefore, the sodium-potassium pump cannot execute its physiological activity, resulting in an elevated potassium (K^+) efflux, and a high influx of sodium (Na^+), calcium (Ca^{2+}), and chloride (Cl^-) into the cell. This homeostasis imbalance alters normal ion concentrations within the intracellular and extracellular spaces, producing a sustained membrane depolarization and a release of excitatory amino acid (EAA) neurotransmitters [24]. The pathological effect related to an increased concentration of EAA neurotransmitters, such as glutamate and aspartate, is known as excitotoxicity. This secondary injury mechanism is characterized by an overstimulation of the NMDA, kainate and AMPA glutamate receptors, which causes massive intracellular Ca^{2+} concentrations, resulting in a pathological neuronal excitation and cell death [25, 32]. Glial cells—especially oligodendrocytes—are very sensitive to excitotoxic damage because of their high expression of ionotropic glutamate receptors [26]. That is why an excessive glutamate accumulation related to SCI can produce oligodendrocyte death, and consequent white matter demyelination [27]. Also, because of glutamate excitotoxicity, there is an increased production of free radicals by reactive microglia, which contribute to lipid peroxidation (LP), and mitochondrial dysfunction [28, 36]. Therefore, this sustained toxic microenvironment is postulated to be one of the most detrimental secondary injury mechanisms related to SCI.

Oxidative stress accompanies secondary injury damage, and is mainly characterized by an increased mitochondrial production of reactive oxygen species (ROS) and reactive nitrogen species (RNS) [29, 38]. The elevation in ROS and RNS concentration is closely related to the aforementioned high Ca^{2+} influx to the cells, as it stimulates free radical production [30]. Free radicals such as superoxide anion (O_2^-), nitric oxide (NO), and peroxynitrite ($ONOO^-$) create a toxic microenvironment by oxidizing nearby molecules producing neural energy failure, blood-brain barrier dysfunction, vascular reactivity, and potentiating inflammation [31, 41]. At high concentrations, these molecules can become cytotoxic and worsen secondary injury mechanisms [32]. Oxidative stress also influences excitotoxicity by exacerbating Ca^{2+} deregulation and thus, glutamate concentrations. The pathological production of ROS that arises after trauma causes oxidative damage, especially on lipids, originating LP. LP is characterized by producing a disruption in the normal structure of the polyunsaturated fatty acids in the cell membrane, such as arachidonic acid, and linoleic acid. In LP, the high concentration of free radicals, results in functional compromise and cell death [33, 43]. Also, structural damage to the cell membrane produces a reduction in the generation and transmission of the electrical potentials leading to synapse dysfunction [34]. Altogether these mechanisms potentiate apoptosis, which is a form of programmed cell death characterized by cell shrinkage, nuclear pyknosis, and chromatin aggregation in a stressful environment [35]. This deleterious event, (apoptosis) occurs after SCI by stimulation of the apoptosis-inducing factor (AIF) to the nucleus, or by direct mitochondrial disruption leading to a subsequent activation of caspase-3 signaling pathways [36, 47]. Evidence supports that secondary injury mechanisms contribute to delayed tissue damage, exacerbating damage, and limiting recovery after traumatic SCI.

2.1. Pathophysiological involvement of the immune system

The immune system has a pivotal and somehow controversial role within the pathophysiology of traumatic SCI. Immediately after trauma there is an activation of the inflammatory response that consists in the proliferation of resident microglia and astrocytes, a high concentration of pro-inflammatory molecules, and infiltration of peripheral immune cells to the site of injury (**Figure 1**). SCI induces the activation of a series of inflammatory stimuli leading to an increased concentration of cytokines and inflammatory cells that will determine the extent of secondary damage [37]. Evidence suggests that in the presence of an excitotoxic and inflammatory microenvironment, microglial cells differentiate into a M1 pro-inflammatory phenotype [38]. Under these conditions, activated microglia is capable of secreting interleukin 1β (IL-1β), IL-6, tumor necrosis factor-alpha (TNFα), and macrophage colony-stimulating factor (MCSF) which are pro-inflammatory in nature [39].

A high free radical and cytotoxic substances secretion is more evident when there is microglial activation starting at day one, and increasing at 7 days post-injury [40]. That is why the immune response is closely related to LP, as these cells are capable of boosting ROS and NO concentrations, favoring oxidative stress, cell membrane dysfunction and thus, apoptosis [41, 50]. At the same time, TNFα stimulates astrocyte proliferation and growth, leading to the formation of the glial scar within the chronic stages of SCI impeding axonal regeneration through the site of injury [42, 53]. Glial cells act immediately after trauma; they secrete pro-inflammatory molecules and promote inflammation, favoring the appearance of secondary injury mechanisms. In spite of the above mentioned deleterious effects, microglial—especially when differentiated into an M2 phenotype (IL-10 and TGF-beta)—and astrocyte activation could produce a beneficial effect through a high production of growth factors like brain derived neurotrophic factor (BDNF), and neurotrophin-3 (NT-3), essential for tissue repair [43]. Also, these cells are capable of expressing glutamate transporters that help reducing harmful

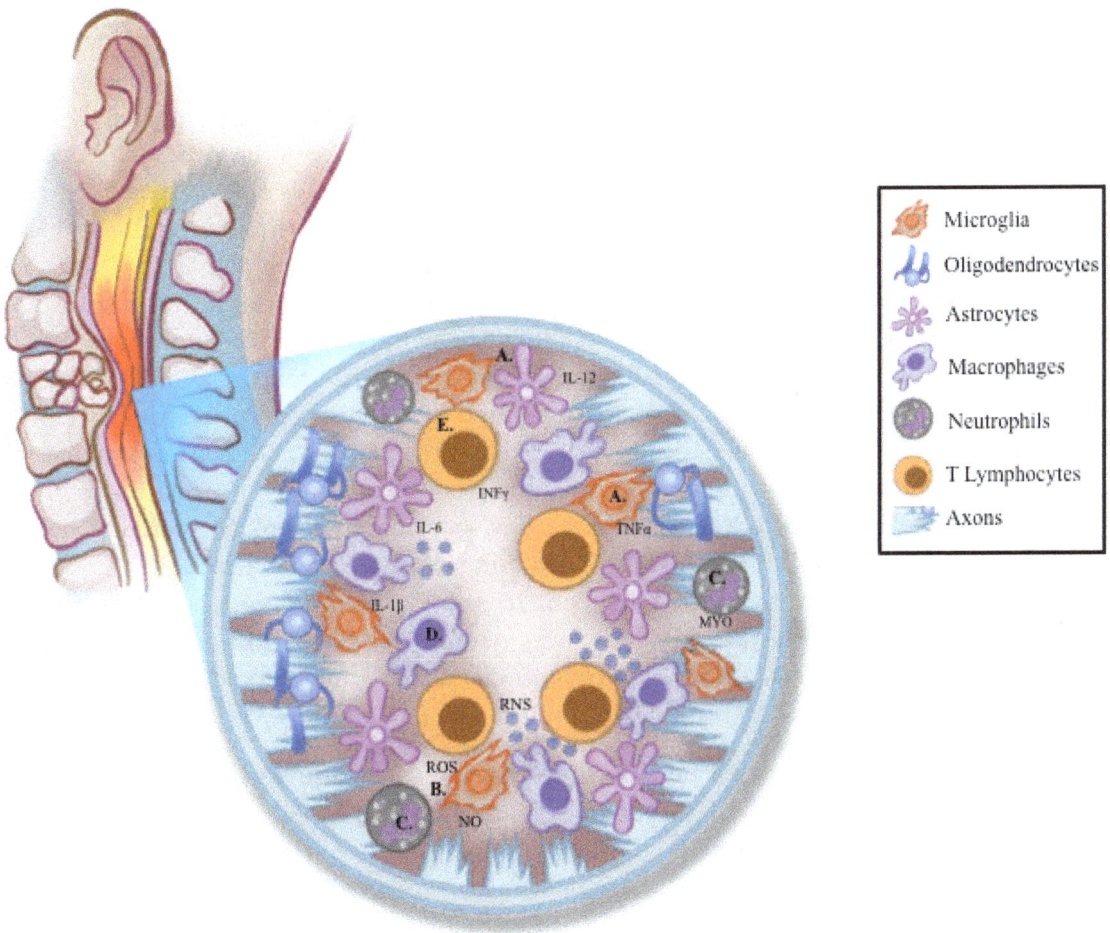

Figure 1. Cellular immune response in SCI. A. M1 microglial differentiation, astrocyte activation, and IL-1β, IL-6, and TNFα secretion. **B.** Increase in the concentration of ROS, NO, and RNS. **C.** Peripheral infiltration of neutrophils and myeloperoxidase secretion. **D.** Macrophages arise from peripheral tissue and activate the adaptive immune response. **E.** Infiltration of T-lymphocytes to the site of injury and INFγ secretion. Abbreviations: IL, interleukin; RNS, reactive nitrogen species; ROS, reactive oxygen species; NO, nitric oxide; TNFα, tumor necrosis factor-alpha; INFγ, interferon-gamma; MYO, myeloperoxidase.

concentrations, leading to a reduction in excitotoxicity [44]. Evidence suggests that even though the immune system is considered to be completely pathological in nature, it can also provide beneficial effects for SCI repair.

In normal conditions, inflammatory reaction leads the response to a pathological outcome, promoting damage and spinal cord degeneration. The severity of SCI determines the intensity of the inflammatory response and the glial reaction to SCI. Glial cells are well distributed within the CNS, and have the ability to proliferate and migrate to the site of injury. In response to injury there is a high glial secretion of cytokines and chemokines—such as IL-1, IL-6, and TNFα—that allows migration of peripheral immune cells [45]. TNFα stimulates the expression of adhesion molecules like endothelial intracellular adhesion molecule -1 (ICAM-1) and vascular cell adhesion molecule-1 (VCAM-1) altering the blood-brain barrier permeability and inducing a peripheral infiltration of immune cells to the CNS (**Figure 1**). Cell infiltration to the CNS is considered the principal factor for tissue disruption and sustained neural damage. The first peripheral cells to arrive at the site of injury are neutrophils [46]. These cells have the ability to phagocyte and clear debris, but they also secrete ROS and RNS, as well as other pathological proteolytic and oxidative enzymes like myeloperoxidase, producing greater tissue damage [47, 58]. At the same time, macrophages arise from resident microglia or from peripheral monocytes with the objective of removing cell debris and stimulating angiogenesis [48]. These cells play an essential role in the immune response, as they help in the activation and reclusion of the adaptive immune system cells. Microglia, astrocytes and dendritic cells may act as antigen-presenting cells (APC), leading to T lymphocyte activation, proliferation, and infiltration to the site of injury [49]. Lymphocytes recognize the signal and proliferate creating large numbers of clones, specific to the antigen being presented by the APC. At 3 days post-injury, there is an evident infiltration of T-cells to the CNS, these cells determine the intensity and continue on modulating the immune response to trauma [50]. In SCI, the presence of T-lymphocytes is considered detrimental as they secrete a Th1 cytokine profile including interferon gamma (IFNγ) [51, 63]. IFNγ is a pro-inflammatory cytokine capable of inducing free radical production, increasing IL-6, IL-12, IL-1β, and TNFα concentrations, and activating apoptotic-signaling pathways [52–65]. These events represent the immune activity within the acute phases of SCI and if it is not well controlled it could turn into a chronic and degenerative immune response.

When inflammation is modulated, i.e., we control the intensity of inflammatory response, the type, the action, and the arrival of immune cells, we could expect a change in the final outcome. With this regard, there is a strong evidence suggesting that lymphocytes could also have favorable activity, as they are capable of synthesizing several growth factors, like BDNF, NT3, and nerve growth factor (NGF) [53–68]. These molecules are known for being capable of promoting a protective and regenerative environment for CNS disorders [54].

To the date, it is clear that the immune response appearing after SCI could be pathological if it is not well controlled at the onset of SCI [55]. In a short period of time, this uncontrolled response leads to the extensive recognition of CNS peptides, proteins, lipids, or nucleic acids by the immune system [56]. This interaction between immune cells and CNS constituents—like the MBP—promotes the activation of lymphocytes and thereby, the possible development of an autoimmune response [57, 72, 73]. As a result, higher levels of demyelination are noted, leading to loss of sensitive and motor synapses. Also, several studies have identified that B cells secrete self-reactive antibodies and pro-inflammatory cytokines, promoting autoimmune activity [58, 75]. Therefore, the immune response elicited after SCI is considered to be one of the most important secondary injury mechanisms, as it plays an essential role in stimulating the appearance of a neurotoxic microenvironment after injury. However, further studies about the immune system and its relationship with CNS damage suggest that it is not completely pathological, as it has protective and regenerative properties [59–78].

3. Protective autoimmunity

The reactive immune response against self-constituents appearing after injury has been widely studied, as it can be an excellent target in the design of new therapies for SCI treatment. It was previously thought that the presence of immune activity was detrimental and it had to be suppressed [60–81]. However, more recent findings suggest that such response and the infiltration of peripheral immune cells to the site of injury is a phenomenon destined to protect and restore the CNS after trauma. The phenomenon capable of inducing this beneficial actions has been termed protective autoimmunity (PA) and is a mechanism in which the adaptive immune cells—especially lymphocytes that recognize self-constituents and potentiate an autoreactive response—help maintain tissue integrity in SCI. Researchers have demonstrated that PA is genetically encoded, and it is a physiological phenomenon linked to the inflammatory activity in the CNS, capable of providing protection in several neurodegenerative disorders [61, 83]. The immune system plays an essential role in tissue restoration, angiogenesis, and is capable of increasing functional recovery in CNS trauma [62]. However, in normal conditions the intense inflammatory response appearing after injury overshadows the beneficial effects of PA. For that reason, it was thought that boosting PA after injury could promote the beneficial instead of deleterious effects of the immune response to injury. In an attempt to test this hypothesis, researchers performed a passive transfer of T-cells specific to MBP, and demonstrated that it reduced tissue damage and improved motor recovery in rats with SCI [63, 86]. These studies suggested that the delayed adaptive immune response to injury and the low concentration of autoreactive T-cells are the reasons why PA is not evident, but a higher and earlier presence of these cells could potentiate the beneficial effects of PA over SCI.

Shortly after researchers envisioned that active immunization could elicit a higher proliferation and migration of autoreactive (antigen specific) T-cells to the CNS increasing the action of PA. Therefore, immunization with natural CNS components could help activate this response [64]. In line with this motion, several studies were performed indicating that, immunization with MBP can modulate the immune response, potentiate PA, and provide neuroprotection to the injured tissue [65, 88, 89]. In spite of the encouraging results, immune modulation with neural constituents increases the risk of developing an autoimmune disease such as experimental autoimmune encephalomyelitis (in rodents; EAE) or multiple sclerosis (in humans; MS) [66, 91]. For that reason, neural constituents were studied with the objective of creating a peptide capable of stimulating PA and reducing the risk of developing an autoimmune disease [67, 93]. These experiments led to the creation of altered peptide ligands (APL), which are synthetic peptides with changes in specific amino acid residues, critical for T-cell receptor (TCR) binding [68]. In the normal immune response, the MBP has agonist properties as it interacts with the TCR, leading to lymphocyte differentiation toward a Th1 phenotype [69, 96, 97]. With the objective of altering TCR recognition, a specific amino acid substitution makes APL become partial agonists or antagonists capable of deviating the immune response [70, 98]. That is why APL are able to cause lymphocyte anergy or their differentiation to an anti-inflammatory Th2 phenotype. This way, APL can alter the natural response of the immune system after SCI, by being able to change the whole Th1 (pro-inflammatory) cytokine profile toward a Th2 (anti-inflammatory) profile. Therefore, by altering the immune response, APL represent a good therapeutic approach for the treatment of SCI and other neurodegenerative diseases [71, 99].

3.1. Modulation of protective autoimmunity with the use of altered peptide ligands

A safe and effective way of increasing PA is through immunization with APL [72]. This strategy allows a change in the interaction with the TCR from an agonist to a partial agonist switching the response toward a Th2 cytokine pattern [73]. To create APL, identification of the essential residues of MBP for an acquired immune response to self-determinants was investigated. Evidence indicates that the amino acid sequence including the 87 to 99 residues is the most encephalitogenic portion of the MBP and that it is essential for TCR recognition [74, 102]. This amino acid sequence was fundamental for the creation of several APL and the evaluation of their effect over the immune response [75]. Altering the amino acid sequence by substituting each residue of the encephalitogenic region of the MBP with alanine, led to the discovery of this group of APL [76, 104]. While trying to identify an ideal peptide to promote PA, several APL derived from MBP encephalitogenic epitopes like G91, A96, or A97, along with A91 were tested as therapeutic strategies for CNS trauma. These peptides were capable of controlling the MBP peptide induced autoimmune reaction by altering the MBP specific T-cell responses [77]. Also, these APL demonstrated to be able of providing significant protection by reducing neuronal loss [78]. More importantly, they were limited the extent of the immune secondary injury mechanisms by inducing changes in the cytokine secretion profile of T-cells and enhanced the recovery of motor activity [79, 99, 103]. Studied APL showed different levels of neuroprotection, however, the conclusion of these conducted studies was that the APL A91 provided the best therapeutic effects without the risk of an autoimmune response [80].

Evidence has demonstrated that lysine at the position 91 is an essential residue of the MBP p87–99 for the development of a Th1 immune response. With this respect, it has been shown that when the amino acid 91 (lysine) is replaced with glycine (G91), the peptide which is non-encephalitogenic, regulates the proliferative response and modifies the cytokine secretion profile (toward a Th2 profile) of encephalitogenic MBP 87–99 reactive T-cells [81, 99, 103, 104]. The substitution of lysine at the position 91 for the amino acid alanine led to the creation of the APL: A91. This APL counteracts the production of pro-inflammatory cytokines, generating a microenvironment with anti-inflammatory features [82, 103, 104]. A91 (amino acid sequence:

VHFFANIVTPRTP) is a safe synthetic non-encephalitogenic peptide, capable of inhibiting the development of autoimmune disease while maintaining neuroprotection [83, 104]. This APL (A91) has proven to be an effective TCR partial agonist capable of modulating the immune response after CNS injury, and increasing the beneficial effects of PA. Immunization with A91 peptide down regulates Th1 activity and increases the levels of a Th2 cytokine pattern (IL-4 and IL-10) creating an anti-inflammatory microenvironment [84, 105, 106].

3.2. The altered peptide ligand A91 as a potential treatment for spinal cord injury

To increase neuroprotection, A91 was designed to boost PA and to act directly over secondary mechanisms in SCI. Immunization with A91 has been tested as a subcutaneous injection, which has resulted to be an effective and minimally invasive route of administration. The use of this strategy in preclinical studies indicates that active immunization with A91 with a single dose of 150–200 µg improves neurological recovery. It is important to note that in order to avoid the risk of an autoimmune disease while maintaining neuroprotection, immunization with myelin-associated antigens should be fully controlled. A study evaluating the dose and therapeutic window of A91 indicates that beneficial effect of this peptide lies between 10 minutes up to 72 hours after SCI [85]. Further studies also indicate that A91 could be considered as a prophylactic therapeutic vaccine since its administration before SCI could provide high levels of neuroprotection and motor recovery [86]. These results could be of relevant benefit as an approach to provide with prophylactic measures to patients sustaining invasive spinal surgery procedures.

On the other hand, with the objective of evaluating the effect of A91 immunization in the presence of the gold standard treatment for SCI (MP) another study was carried out. The results of this investigation indicated that when these two treatments were administered at the same time, the beneficial properties of A91 were abolished [87]. However, the extensive therapeutic time window of A91 enables immediate MP administration and immunization with A91 up to 48 hours later [88, 109]. This approach has given the possibility of rescuing the beneficial effects elicited by A91, as animals subjected to this combined strategy, present neuroprotection and a higher motor recovery. These results also allow envisioning the possible clinical application of this therapy with no risk of avoiding the therapeutic effects theoretically provided by MP. In the search of increasing the neuroprotective effect of A91, double immunization has also been evaluated [89]. However, unexpectedly a higher concentration of this peptide eliminates the beneficial aftermath of the therapy [90]. Studies in our laboratory have also demonstrated that A91 can be applied at different SCI stages and still be effective. Our investigation suggests that adequate immunization must be performed immediately after injury or during the acute phase [91, 109]. Moreover, studies including vaccination of A91 in chronic SCI are now being conducted, and results have demonstrated to be profitable (Unpublished data).

APL were designed to specifically target the immune-related secondary injury mechanisms in order to attain neuroprotection, promote regeneration, and thus improving motor and sensory recovery in SCI. In line with this, previous studies have shown that immunization with A91 peptide produces an adequate T-cell proliferation characterized by a Th2 phenotype, where the production of IL-4 and IL-10 is increased [92, 110]. Additionally, A91 specific T-cells are capable of producing BDNF, which could be linked directly with the functional recovery appearing after immunization [93]. This anti-inflammatory and permissive microenvironment controls the inflammatory response elicited by SCI, reducing some of the main harmful phenomena developed by inflammation. For instance, it has been demonstrated that A91-immunization is capable of inhibiting LP, which is closely related to the action of immune system and it is one of the most aggressive phenomena related to SCI [94]. LP is present immediately after injury reaching its maximum peak at 4–5 h and has a second increase between 24 hours and 5 days [95]. With this regard, a study conducted to evaluate the impact of A91-immunization on LP showed that A91 is able to reduce the concentration of ROS at the site of injury having a strong impact over the second peak of this phenomenon [96]. A further study indicated that A91-immunization counteracts the production of nitric oxide (NO) and down regulates the expression of the gene encoding for nitric oxide synthase (iNOS) [97]. These are some of the beneficial mechanisms that explain, at least in part, the effect of this strategy on LP.

Apoptotic cell death is another of the main destructive phenomena triggered after SCI. This phenomenon is activated by inflammatory cytokines, free radicals, excitotoxic agents, and increased levels of intracellular calcium [98]. After SCI, neurological recovery depends mainly on the extent of neuronal loss and the functionality of the residual neural tissue. Numerous studies have shown that many neurons die as a consequence of apoptosis. Therefore, regulating apoptotic cell death might play an important role in the neurological recovery following SCI [99, 116]. Recent investigations on the field found that immunizing with A91 decreases caspase-3 activity and TNFα concentrations, reducing the number of apoptotic cells, which is directly correlated with functional improvement after injury [100].

Altogether, the aforementioned observations provide clear evidence on the mechanisms by which A91-immunization exerts its beneficial effects. Besides reducing secondary injury mechanisms, A91 peptide has also proven to prevent tissue damage, as immunized animals presented a higher number of myelinated axons and survival of rubrospinal neurons compared to controls [101, 109, 110]. These results were consistent throughout several SCI preclinical studies. Also it was noted that motor recovery had a direct correlation with neuronal survival, myelin preservation, and apoptosis reduction in treated groups [102, 107, 109, 110, 114, 117, 118]. As a consequence of these encouraging results, we have envisioned the possibility of combining this strategy with others that have also shown beneficial effects [103, 117, unpublished data]. For that reason, A91-immunization was administered along with glutathione monoethyl ester (GSHE), which is an anti-oxidant capable of accelerating the immune response and providing neuroprotection [104, 117]. The results of this study showed that after a contusive or a compressive SCI, this combination induced better motor recovery, higher number of myelinated axons, and better rubrospinal neuron survival than immunization alone. These results open an interesting scenery for clinical studies.

Finally, in order to consider A91-immunization for being used at clinical settings, it is of relevance to contemplate vaccine safety. With this regard, immunizing with A91 shows no signs of autoimmune disease development, possibly due to its low affinity to major histocompatibility complex (MHC) molecules [105]. Furthermore to evaluate vaccine safety, the clinical appearance of treated animals was assessed, and no weight variation or other clinical data of EAE in immunized animals was detected [106]. A91 has proven to be effective in several studies conducted at different time points showing the stability of the vaccine in promoting recovery. Preclinical results of studies evaluating vaccine efficacy indicate that this therapy could be possibly applied to SCI patients and improve their recovery and quality of life.

4. Concluding statement

Injury to the spinal cord stimulates the appearance of innate and adaptive immune responses, which could participate in either the pathogenesis or healing responses to trauma. The immune system should not be suppressed; instead, it must be modulated to attain its beneficial effect. That is why the use of immunosuppressant drugs like MP in the clinical field no longer seems a rational treatment. As a physiological hemostatic self-defense mechanism, PA is an essential mechanism to be considered for the pathophysiology and treatment of SCI. Boosting PA with the use of APL is needed in order to increase the functional recovery in the immune related neurodegenerative diseases. In SCI, immunization with the APL A91 has proven to reduce part of the immune-related secondary injury mechanisms without the risk of developing an autoimmune response. Preclinical results suggest that this therapy could be an effective treatment for SCI recovery, as it is closely related to a higher motor improvement, which is the most evident deficit in SCI patients. However, further studies related to the use of APL in SCI are needed to translate this therapy to the clinical field. For instance, we have to ensure that immunization with this peptide does not cause any side effect (i.e. hypersensitivity or autoimmunity). Additionally, further experiments should be performed in order to find out the best adjuvant to be used in humans, even the investigation should be directed to elucidate if the use of adjuvants is really necessary. Finally, the dosing of the peptide as well as the schedule of administration at clinical settings should also be investigated.

Author details

Paola Suárez-Meade[1] and Antonio Ibarra[1,2*]

*Address all correspondence to: iantonio65@yahoo.com; jose.ibarra@anahuac.mx

1 Faculty of Health Sciences, Anáhuac University, Universidad Anáhuac Av. Huixquilucan Edo. Mexico, Mexico

2 CAMINA Research Project A.C. Mexico City, Mexico

References

[1] National Spinal Cord Injury Statistical Center, University of Alabama at Birmingham. 2015. Annual Statistical Report. Spinal cord injury facts and figures at glance. https://www.nscisc.uab.edu

[2] DeVivo MJ. Epidemiology of traumatic spinal cord injury: trends and future implications. Spinal Cord. 2012; 50: 365–372.

[3] Chiu WT, Lin HC, Lam C, Chu SF, Chiang YH, et al. Epidemiology of traumatic spinal cord injury: comparisons between developed and developing countries. Asia Pac J Public Health. 2015; 22 (1): 9–18.

[4] Karlsson AK. Autonomic dysfunction in spinal cord injury: clinical presentation of symptoms and signs. Prog Brain Res. 2006; 152: 1–8.

[5] Ibarra A, Rios-Hoyo A, Suarez-Meade P, Malagon E, Colin-Rodriguez A. Influence of the level, severity and phase of spinal cord injury on hematological and biochemical parameters. J Trauma Treat. 2014; 3 (4): 1–5.

[6] Hagen EM. Acute complications of spinal cord injuries. World J Orthop. 2015; 6 (1): 17–23.

[7] Bracken MB, Shepard MJ, Collins WF, Holford T, Young W, et al. A randomized, controlled trial of methylprednisolone or naloxone in the treatment of acute spinal-cord injury. Results of the Second National Acute Spinal Cord Injury Study. N Engl J Med. 1990; 332 (20): 1405–1411.

[8] Bracken M, Shepard MJ, Holford T, Leo-Summers L, Aldrich F, et al. Methylprednisolone or tirilazad mesylate administration after acute spinal cord injury: 1-year follow up. Results of the Third National Acute Spinal Cord Injury Randomized controlled Trial. J Neurosurg. 1998; 89 (5): 699–706.

[9] Hulbert J. Methylprednisolone for the treatment of acute spinal cord injury: point. Clin Neurosurg. 2014; 61 (1): 32–35.

[10] Hulbert J. Methylprednisolone for acute spinal cord injury: an inappropriate standard of care. J Neurosurg. 2000; (Spine 1) 93: 1–7.

[11] Rhen T, Cidlowski JA. Anti-inflammatory action of glucocorticoids—new mechanisms for old drugs. N Engl J Med. 2005; 353: 1711–1723.

[12] Ferrari G, Greene LA. Prevention of neuronal apoptotic death by neurotrophic agents and Ganglioside GM1: insights and speculations regarding a common mechanism. Perspect Dev Neurobiol. 1996; 3 (2): 93–100.

[13] Skaper SD, Leon A. Monosialogangliosides, neuroprotection, and neuronal repair processes. J Neurotrauma. 1992; 9 (Suppl 2): S507–516.

[14] Geisler FH, Dorsey FC, Coleman WP. Past and current clinical studies with GM-1 ganglioside in acute spinal cord injury. Ann Emerg Med. 1993; 22 (6): 104–1047.

[15] Geisler FH, Coleman WP, Grieco G, Poonian D, Sygen Study Group. Recruitment and early treatment in a multicenter study of acute spinal cord injury. Spine. 2001; 26 (Suppl 1): S58–67.

[16] Geisler FH, Coleman WP, Griego G, et al. Measurement and recovery patterns in a multicenter study of acute spinal cord injury. Spine. 2001; 26 (Suppl 1): S68–86.

[17] Geisler FH, Coleman WP, Griego G. The Sygen® Multicenter acute spinal cord injury study. Spine. 2001; 26 (Suppl 1): S87–98.

[18] Meurer WJ, Baran WG. Spinal cord injury neuroprotection and the promise of flexible adaptive clinical trials. World Neurosurg. 2014; 82: 3–4.

[19] Kabu S, Gao Y, Kwon BK, Labhasetwar V. Drug delivery, cell-based therapies, and tissue engineering approaches for spinal cord injury. J Control Release. 2015; 219: 141–154.

[20] Stammers AT, Liu J, Kwon BK. Expression of inflammatory cytokines following acute spinal cord injury in a rodent model. J Neurosci Res. 2012; 90: 782–790.

[21] Fleming JC, Norenberg MD, Ramsay DA, Dekaban GA, Marcillo AE, et al. The cellular inflammatory response in human spinal cords after injury. Brain. 2006; 129: 3249–3269.

[22] Karinathan N, Vanathi MB, Subrahmanyam VM, Rao JV. A review on response of immune system in spinal cord injury and therapeutic agents useful in treatment. Curr Pharm Biotechnol. 2015; 16 (1): 26–34.

[23] Schwartz M, Raposo C. Protective autoimmunity: a unifying model for the immune network involved in CNS Repair. Neuroscientist. 2014; 20 (4): 343–358.

[24] Mestre H, Ibarra A. Immunization with neural-derived peptides as a potential therapy in neurodegenerative diseases. Neurodegen Dis Proc Prev Prot Monit. 2011;519–540. ISBN: 978-953-307-485-6.

[25] Fehlings MG, Sekhon LHS. Cellular, ionic and biomolecular mechanisms of the injury process. In: Tator CH, Benzel EC, eds. Contemporary management of spinal cord injury: From Impact to rehabilitation. New York: American Association of Neurological Surgeons. 2000; 33–50.

[26] Mautes A, Weinzierl M, Donovan F, Noble L. Vascular events after spinal cord injury: contribution to secondary pathogenesis. Phys Ther. 2000; 80: 673–687.

[27] Leonard AV, Thornon E, Robert V. The relative contribution of edema and hemorrhage to raised intrathecal pressure after traumatic spinal cord injury. J Neurotrauma. 2015; 32 (6): 397–402.

[28] Rowland J, Hawryluk G, Kwon B, Fehlings M. Current status of acute spinal cord injury pathophysiology and emerging therapies: promise on the horizon. Neurosurg Focus. 2008; 25 (5): E2.

[29] Aidemise Oyinbo C. Secondary injury mechanisms in traumatic spinal cord injury: a nugget of this multiply cascade. Acta Neurobiol Exp. 2011; 71: 281–299.

[30] Xing C, Arai K, Lo EH, Hommel M. Pathophysiologic cascades in ischemic stroke. Int J Stroke. 2012; 7: 378–385.

[31] Mehta A, Prabhakar M, Kumar P, Deshmukh R, Sharma PL. Excitotoxicity: bridge to various triggers in neurodegenerative disorders. Eur J Pharmacol. 2013; 698: 6–18.

[32] Sattler R, Tymianski M. Molecular mechanisms of glutamate receptor-mediated excitotoxic neuronal cell death. Mol Neurobiol. 2001; 24: 107–129.

[33] Matute C, Domercq M, Sanchez-Gomez MV. Glutamate-mediated glial injury: mechanisms and clinical importance. Glia. 2006; 53: 212–224.

[34] Park E, Velumian A, Fehlings MG. The role of excitotoxicity in secondary mechanisms of spinal cord injury: a review with an emphasis on the implications for white matter degeneration. J. Neurotrauma. 2004; 21(6): 754–774.

[35] David S, Kroner A. Repertoire of microglial and macrophage responses after spinal cord injury. Nat Rev Neurosci. 2011; 12: 388–399.

[36] Azbill RD, Mu X, Bruce-Keller A, Mattson MP, Springer JE. Impaired mitochondrial function, oxidative stress and altered antioxidant enzyme activities following traumatic spinal cord injury. Brain Res. 1997; 765: 283–290.

[37] Cornelius C, Crupo R, Calabrese V, Graziano A, Milone P, et al. Traumatic brain injury: oxidative stress and neuroprotection. Antioxid Redox Signal. 2013; 19 (8): 836–853.

[38] Visavadiya PN, Patel SP, Venrooyen JL, Sullivan P, Rabchevsky A. Cellular and subcellular oxidative stress parameters following severe spinal cord injury. Redox Biol. 2016; 8: 59–67.

[39] Nathan C, Cunningham-Brussel A. Beyong oxidative stress: an immunologist's guide to reactive oxygen species. Net Rev Immunol. 2013; 13 (5): 349–361.

[40] Hall ED, Wang JA, Bosken JM, Singh IN. Lipid peroxidation in brain or spinal cord mitochondria after injury. J Bioenerg Biomembr. 2015. 48 (2): 169–174.

[41] Gilgun-Sherki Y, Rosenbaum Z, Melamed E, Offen D. Antioxidant therapy in acute central nervous system injury: current state. Pharmacol Rev. 2002; 54: 271–284.

[42] O'Connel KM, Littleton-Kearney MT. The role of free radicals in traumatic brain injury. Biol Res Nurs. 2012; 15 (3): 253–263.

[43] Farmer E, Mueller M. ROS-mediated lipid peroxidation and RES-activated signaling. Ann Rev Plant Biol. 2013; 64: 429–450.

[44] Ibarra A, Diaz-Ruiz A. Inhibition of lipid peroxidation by cyclosporin after spinal cord injury in rats. Humana Press. 2003: 283–298.

[45] Ekshyyan O, Aw TY. Apoptosis in acute and chronic neurological disorders. Front Biosci. 2004; 9: 1567–1576.

[46] Chun-Shu P, Loane DJ, Stoica BA, Shihong L, Hanscom M. Combined inhibition of cell death induced by apoptosis inducing factor and caspases provides additive neuroprotection in experimental traumatic brain injury. Neurobiol Dis. 2012; 46: 745–758.

[47] Springer JE, Azbill R, Knapp P. Activation of the caspase-3 apoptotic cascade in traumatic spinal cord injury. Nat Med. 1999; 5: 943–946.

[48] Stammers AT, Liu J, Kwon BK. Expression of inflammatory cytokines following acute spinal cord injury in a rodent model. J Neurosci Res. 2012; 90 (4): 782–790.

[49] Domercq M, Vázquez-Villoldo N, Matute C. Neurotransmitter signaling in the pathophysiology of microglia. Front Cell Neurosci. 2013; 49: 122–138.

[50] Hao C, Parney I, Roa W, Turner J, Petruk K, et al. Cytokine and cytokine receptor mRNA expression in human glioblastomas: evidence of Th1, Th2 and Th3 cytokine dysregulation. Acta Neuropathol. 2002; 103: 171–178.

[51] Hausmann ON. Post-traumatic inflammation following spinal cord injury. Spinal Cord. 2003; 41: 369–378.

[52] Dougherty KD, Dreyfus C, Black IB. Brain-derived neurotrophic factor in astrocytes, oligodendrocytes, and microglia/macrophages after spinal cord injury. Neurobiol Dis. 2000; 7 (6): 574–585.

[53] Camand E, Morel MP, Faissner A, Sotelo C, Dusart I. Long-term changes in the molecular composition of the glial scar and progressive increase of serotoninergic fibre sprouting after hemisection of the mouse spinal cord. Eur J Neurosci. 2004; 20 (5): 1161–1176.

[54] McPhail LT, Plunet WT, Partha D, Ramer M. The astrocytic barrier to axonal regeneration at the dorsal root entry zone is induced by rhizotomy. Eur J Neurosci. 2005; 21 (1): 267–270.

[55] Van Landeghem F, Stover JF, Bechmann I, Bruck W, Unterberg A, et al. Early expression of glutamate transporter proteins in ramified microglia after controlled cortical impact injury in the rat. Glia. 2201; 35 (3): 167–179.

[56] Esposito E, Cuzzocrea S. Anti-TNF therapy in the injured spinal cord. Trends Pharmacol Sci. 2011; 32 (2): 107–115.

[57] Neirinckx V, Coste C, Franzen R, Gothet A, Rogister B, et al. Neutrophil contribution to spinal cord injury and repair. J Neuroinflammation. 2014; 11: 150.

[58] Taoka Y, Okajima K, Uchiba M, Murakami K, Kushimoto S, Johno M. Role of neutrophils in spinal cord injury in the rat. Neuroscience. 1997; 79 (4): 1177–1182.

[59] Greenhalgh A, David S. Differences in the phagocytic response of microglia and pripheral macrophages after spinal cord injury and its effects on cell death. J Neurosci. 2014; 34 (18): 6316–6322.

[60] Popovich PG, Jones TB. Manipulating neuroinflammatory reactions in the injured spinal cord: back to basics. Trends Pharmacol Sci. 2003; 24 (1): 13–17.

[61] Triveldi A, Olivas A, Noble-Haeusslein L. Inflammation and spinal cord injury: infiltrating leukocytes as determinants of injury and repair processes. Clin Neurosci Res. 2006; 6: 283–292.

[62] Hu JG, Shi LL, Chen YJ, Xie XM, Zhang N, et al. Differential effects of myelin basic protein-activated Th1 and Th2 cells on the local immune microenvironment of injured spinal cord. Exp Neurol. 2016; 277: 190–201.

[63] Shaked I, Tchiresh D, Gersner R, Meiri G, Mordechai S, et al. Protective autoimmunity: interferon-γ enables microglia to remove glutamate without evoking inflammatory mediators. J Neurochem. 2005; 92: 997–1009.

[64] Mir M, Tolosa L, Asensio V, Llado J, Olmos G. Complementary roles of tumor necrosis factor alpha and interferón gamma in inducible microglial nitric oxide generation. J Neuroimmunol. 2008; 204 (1–4): 101–109.

[65] Esposito E, Cuzzocrea S. TNF-alpha as a therapeutic target in inflammatory diseases, ichemia-reperfusion injury and trauma. Curr Med Chem. 2009; 16 (24): 3152–3167.

[66] Stadelmann C, Kerschensteriner M, Misgeld T, Bruck W, Hohlfeld R, et al. BDNF and gp145trkB in multiple sclerosis brain lesions: neuroprotective interactions between immune and neuronal cells. Brain. 2002; 125: 75–85.

[67] Chen Q, Smith G, Shine D. Immune activation is required for NT-3-induced azonal plasticity in chronic spinal cord injury. Exp Neurol. 1008; 209 (2): 497–509.

[68] Stantambrogio L, Benedetti M, Chao M, Muzaffar R, Kulig K, et al. Nerve growth factor production by lymphocytes. J Immunol. 1994; 153: 4488–4495.

[69] Suarez-Meade P, Carvajal HG, Yasuhara T, Taijiri N, Date I, et al. Regenerative medicine for central nervous system disorders: role of therapeutic molecules in stem cell therapy. Brain Circul. 2015; 1 (2): 125–132.

[70] Saltzman JW, Battaglino RA, Stott HL, Morse LR. Neurotoxic or neuroprotective? Current controversies in SCI-induced autoimmunity. Curr Phys Med Rehabil Rep. 2013; 1: 174–177.

[71] Ankeny DP, Popovich PG. Mechanisms and implications of adaptive immune responses after traumatic spinal cord injury. Neuroscience. 2009; 158: 1112–1121.

[72] Schwab JM, Zhang Y, Kopp M, Brommer B, Popovich PG. The paradox of chronic neuroinflammation, systemic immune suppression, autoimmunity after traumatic chronic spinal cord injury. Exp Neurol. 2014; 258: 121–129.

[73] Zajarías-Fainsod D, Carrillo-Ruiz J, Mestre H, Grijalva I, Madrazo I, et al. Autoreactivity against myelin basic protein in patients with chronic paraplegia. Eur Spine J. 2012; 21: 964–970.

[74] Archelos JJ, Storch MK, Hartung HP. The role of B cells and autoantibodies in multiple sclerosis. Ann Neurol. 2000; 47 (6): 694–702.

[75] Fillatreau S, Sweenie CH, McGeachy MJ, Gray D, Anderton SM. B cells regulate autoimmunity by provision of IL-10. Nat Immunol. 2002; 3 (10): 944–950.

[76] Schwartz M, Kipnis J. Protective autoimmunity and neuroprotection in inflammatory and non-inflammatory neurodegenerative diseases. J Neurol Sci. 2005; 233 (1–2): 163–166.

[77] Schwartz M, Kipnis J. Protective autoimmunity: regulation and prospects for vaccination after brain and spinal cord injuries. Trends Mol Med. 2001; 7 (6): 252–258.

[78] Yoles E, Hauben E, Palqi O, Agranov E, Gothilf A, et al. Protective autoimmunity is a physiological response to CNS trauma. J Neurosci. 2001; 21 (11): 3740–3748.

[79] Hall E, Braughler M. Glucocorticoid mechanisms in acute spinal cord injury: a review and therapeutic rationales. Surg Neurol. 1982; 18 (5): 320–327.

[80] Schwartz M, Cohen I. Autoimmunity can benefit self-maintenance. Immunol Today. 2000; 21 (6): 265–268.

[81] Yoles E, Hauben E, Palgi O, Agranof E, Gothilf A, et al. Protective autoimmunity is a physiological response to CNS trauma. J Neurosci. 2001; 21 (11): 3740–3748.

[82] Kipnis J, Yoles E, Schori H, Hauben E, Shaked I, et al. Neuronal survival after CNS insult is determined by a genetically encoded autoimmune response. J Neurosci. 2001; 21: 4564–4571.

[83] Angelov DN, Waibel S, Guntinas-Lichius O, Lenzen M, Neiss WF, et al. Therapeutic vaccine for acute and chronic motor neuron diseases: implications for amyotrophic lateral sclerosis. PNAS. 2003; 100: 4790–4795.

[84] Schwartz M, Moalem G, Leibowitz-Amit R, Cohen I. Innate and adaptive immune responses can be beneficial for CNS repair. Trends Neurosci. 1999; 22: 295–299.

[85] Hauben E, Butovsky O, Nevo U, Yoles E, Moalem G, et al. Passive or active immunization with myelin basic protein promotes recovery from spinal cord contusion. J Neurosci. 2000; 10: 6421–6430.

[86] Kipnis J, Mizrahi T, Hauben E, Shaked I, Shevach E. Neuroprotective autoimmunity: naturally occurring CD4+CD25+ regulatory T cells suppress the ability to withstand injury to the central nervous system. PNAS. 2002; 99 (24): 15620–15625.

[87] Schwartz M, Raposo C. Protective autoimmunity: a unifying model for the immune network involved in CNS repair. Neuroscientist. 2014; 20 (4): 343–358.

[88] Barouch R, Schwartz M. Autoreactive T cells induce neurotrophin production by immune and neural cells in injured rat optic nerve: implications for protective auto-immunity. FASEB J. 2002; 16: 1304–1306.

[89] Aharoni R, Arnon R, Eilam R. Neurogenesis and neuroprotection induced by periph-eral immunomodulatory treatment of experimental autoimmune encephalomyelitis. J Neurosci. 2005; 25: 8217–8228.

[90] Sakai K, Sinha A, Mitchel D, Zamvil S, Rothbard J, et al. Involvement of distinct murine T-cell receptors in the autoimmune encephalitogenic response to nested epitopes of myelin basic protein. Proc Natl Acad Sci. 1988; 85: 8608–8612.

[91] Sakai K, Zamvil S, Mitchel DJ, Lim M, Rothbard J, et al. Characterization of a major encephalitogenic T cell epitope in SJL/J mice with synthetic oligopeptides of myelin basic protein. J Neuroimmunol. 1988; 19: 21–32.

[92] Nicholson L, Greer J, Sobel R, Lees M, Kuchroo V. An altered peptide ligand mediates immune deviation and prevents autoimmune encephalomyelitis. Immunity. 1995; 3: 397–405.

[93] Hauben E, Agranov E, Gothlif A, Nevo U, Cohen A, et al. Posttraumatic therapeutic vaccination with modified myelin self-antigen prevents complete paralysis while avoiding autoimmune disease. J Clin Invest. 2001; 108: 591–599.

[94] Winghagen A, Scholz C, Hollsberg P, Fukaura H, Sette A, et al. Modulation of cytokine patters of human autoreactive T cell cones by a single amino acid substitution of their peptide ligand. Immunity. 1995; 2: 373–380.

[95] Jameson S, Bevan M. T cell receptor antagonists and partial agonists. Immunity. 1995; 2 (1): 1–11.

[96] Nel A. T-cell activation through the antigen receptor. Part 1: signaling components, signaling pathways, and signal integration at the T-cell antigen receptor synapse. J Allergy Clin Immunol. 2002; 109 (5): 758–770.

[97] Evavold BD, Allen PM. Sparation of IL-4 production from Th cell proliferation by an altered T cell receptor ligand. Science. 1991; 252: 1308–1310.

[98] Hauben E, Ibarra A, Mizrahi T, Barouch R, Agranov E, et al. Vaccination with a Nogo-A-derived peptide after incomplete spinal cord injury promotes recovery via a T-cell mediated neuroprotective response: comparison with other myelin antigens. PNAS. 2001; 98 (26): 15173–15178.

[99] Nel AE, Slaughter N. T-Cell activation through the antigen receptor. Part 2: role of signaling cascades in T-cell differentiation, anergy, immune senescence, and development of immunotherapy. J Allergy Clin Immunol. 2002; 109 (6): 901–915.

[100] Yu M, Johnson J, Tuohy V. A predictable sequential determinant spreading cascade invariably accompanies progression of experimental autoimmune encephalomyelitis: a basis for peptide-specific therapy after onset of clinical disease. J Exp Med. 1996; 183: 1777–1788.

[101] Tuohy V, Yu M, Yin L, Kawczak J, Johnson J, et al. The epitope spreading cascade during progression of experimental autoimmune encephalomyelitis and multiple sclerosis. Immunol Rev. 1998; 164 (1): 93–100.

[102] Karin N, Mitchell D, Brocke S, Ling N, Steinman L. Reversal of experimental autoimmune encephalomyelitis by a soluble peptide variant of a myelin basic protein epitope: T cell receptor antagonism and reduction of interferon γ and tumor necrosis factor α production. J Exp Med. 1994; 180: 2227–2237.

[103] Gaur A, Boehme S, Chalmers D, Crowe P, Pahuja A. Amelioration of relapsing experimental autoimmune encephalomyelitis with altered myelin basic protein peptides involves different cellular mechanism. J Neuroimmunol. 1997; 74: 149–158.

[104] Willenbong D, Staykova M. Cytokines in the pathogenesis and therapy of autoimmune encephalomyelitis and multiple sclerosis. Adv Exp Med Biol. 2003; 520: 96–119.

[105] Martiñón S, García E, Gutierrez-Ospina G, Mestre H, Ibarra A. Development of protective autoimmunity by immunization with a neural derived peptide is ineffective in severe spinal cord injury. PLoS ONE. 2012; 7 (2): 1–7.

[106] Del rayo Garrido M, Silva-García R, García E, Martiñón S, Morales M, et al. Therapeutic window for combination therapy of A91 peptide and glutathione allows delayed treatment after spinal cord injury. Basic Clin Pharmacol Toxicol. 2013; 112: 314–318.

[107] Ibarra A, Sosa M, García E, Flores A, Cruz Y, et al. Prophylactic neuroprotection with A91 improves the outcome of spinal cord injured rats. Neurosci Lett. 2013; 554: 59–63.

[108] Ibarra A, Hauben E, Butovsky O, Schwartz M. The therapeutic window after spinal cord injury can accommodate T cell-based vaccination and methylprednisolone in rats. Eur J Neurosci. 2004; 19: 2985–2990.

[109] Martiñón S, García E, Flores N, González I, Ortega T. Vaccination with a neural-derived peptide plus administration of glutathione improves the performance of paraplegic rats. Eur J Neurosci. 2007; 26: 403–412.

[110] Ibarra A, García E, Flores N, Martiñón S, Reyes R. Immunization with neural-derived antigens inhibits lipid peroxidation after spinal cord injury. Neurosci Lett. 2010; 476: 62–65.

[111] Christie SD, Corneau B, Myers T, Sadi D, Purdy M, et al. Duration of lipid peroxidation after acute spinal cord injury in rats and the effect of methylprednisolone. J Neurosurg. 2008; 25 (5): E5.

[112] García E, Silva-García R, Mestre H, Flores N, Martiñón S. Immunization with A91 peptide or Copolymer-1 reduces the production of nitric oxide and inducible nitric oxide synthase gene expression after spinal cord injury. J Neurosci Res. 2012; 90: 656–663.

[113] Lou J, Lenke LG, Ludwig FJ, O'Brien MF. Apoptosis as a mechanism of neuronal cell death following acute experimental spinal cord injury. Spinal Cord. 1998; 36 (10): 683–690.

[114] Lee YJ, Choi SY, Oh TH, Yune TY. Estradiol inhibits apoptotic cell death of oligodendrocytes by inhibiting RhoA-JNK3 activation after spinal cord injury. Endocrinology. 2012; 153 (8): 3815–3827.

[115] Zhang N, Xu SJ, Chen WS, Yin Y, Wu YP. Inflammation and apoptosis in spinal cord injury. Indian J Med Res. 2012; 135 (3): 287–296.

[116] Rodríguez-Barrera R, Fernández-Presas A, García E, Flores-Romero A, Martiñón S, et al. Immunization with a neural-derived peptide protects the spinal cord from apoptosis after traumatic injury. Bio Med Res. 2013: 2013: 1–8.

[117] Hauben E, Ibarra A, Mizrahi T, Barouch R, Agranov E, et al. Vaccination with a Nogo-A-derived peptide after incomplete spinal-cord injury promotes recovery via a T-cell mediated neuroprotective response: comparison with other myelin antigens. PNAS. 2001; 98 (26): 15173–15178.

9

Penetrating Spinal Cord Injury

Moti M. Kramer, Asaf Acker and Nissim Ohana

Abstract

Penetrating spinal cord injury (SCI) is a relatively rare entity affecting mainly young males and military personnel worldwide. These injuries are the source of permanent disabilities to the affected patient and family and have substantial social and economic concerns. This chapter is an overview of the common penetrating spinal cord injuries, their incidence worldwide, causes, primary evaluation, and treatment including medical treatment and late definitive surgical treatment. It also describes common complications and strategies preventing secondary and collateral damage and disability.

Keywords: spinal cord injury, trauma, gunshot wound, paralysis, surgery, ATLS

1. Introduction

Spinal cord injury (SCI) and the lifelong disabilities associated with it are of a major concern to the society worldwide. Those injuries bear substantial personal and economic burden. Traumatic SCI is a subgroup of spinal cord injuries that affects mainly young males at their third decade of life, and its rate of incidence stays unchanged in the last three decades [1, 2]. Traumatic spinal cord injury can be divided into penetrating and blunt or non-penetrating injuries. Traumatic injuries have a steady incidence ranging from 12.1 to 57.8 cases per million annually [1, 2]. The most common etiologies are motor vehicle accident (MVA), falls from height, violence including gunshot injuries, and sport activities. Penetrating spinal injuries can be further divided into missile-penetrating spinal injury (gunshot, shrapnel, etc.) and non-missile-penetrating spinal injury (i.e., stabbing).

Penetrating gunshot injuries have been described as accounting for 17–21% of all spinal cord injuries [3]. Non-missile-penetrating spinal cord injuries are rare and account for less than 1.5%

of the total penetrating injuries [3]. The incidence of missile-penetrating SCI varies, and difference exists between its incidence in civilian population and military personnel population, where the latter is naturally more prevalent and influenced by eras of military conflicts [3].

2. Non-missile-penetrating spinal cord injury

Historically, the first non-missile-penetrating spinal cord injury (NMPSCI) was described by the Egyptians in 1700 BC. The Edwin-Smith papyrus was the first manual of military injuries in history and described different injuries and their proposed optimal treatment. Unlike other medical documents preserved from that era, the papyrus was based on medical procedures and not myths or prays [4]. In the second century AD, the Greek physician Galen reported his experiments on monkeys when a horizontal cut through their spine resulted in loss of sensation and motion below the level of the injury [5].

The largest series of NMPSCI was published by Lipschitz [6] with two case series in 1955–1967. Other smaller series were described in 1977 and 1995 [7, 8]. These publications came all from the same country (South Africa), both at an era of severe violence that unfortunately flooded the country.

Unlike in the rest of the world, in South Africa penetrating SCI is still responsible to about 60% of all SCI (spread evenly between NMPSCI and MPSCI). MVA, which is the most common cause of SCI in the rest of the world, accounts only for one-third of the cases in South Africa today [2].

Most of the affected victims of these injuries are young men in their second and third decades [2, 3]. Generally speaking, while in the past, NMPSI was rare in females, today the trend is changing, and over the past decades, it is seen more, especially in North America. Yet, about 80% of the affected victims of these injuries are males [2].

Knife is by far the most common assault weapon causing NMPSI. It accounts for 84% of the cases [9]. Other sharp objects such as screwdrivers, scissors, garden forks, and bicycle spokes were reported as the assaulting weapon for NMPSCI as well [9]. Even a pencil was reported as a stabbing object that caused NMPSCI [10].

Previous reports described a series of NMPSCI caused by acupuncture needles [11]. The World Health Organization published a systematic review of acupuncture-related adverse events in 2010, in which 44 cases of dural and arachnoid bleeding, causing severe adverse events and death (three cases), were reported [11].

Most non-missile-penetrating injuries happened when victims were stabbed from behind with the thoracic spine being the most common site (up to 63%), followed with cervical spine (up to 30%) [12]. A recent study examined that there are no differences in stab wounds to the neck, between military personnel (during combat) and civilians. This probably emphasizes the role of incidence in this type of injuries [13].

Victims are usually stabbed once, and the attacker usually withdrawals the stabbing object from the victim's body. However, in some cases the stabbing object brakes inside the body, and retained material occurs (**Figure 1A** and **B**). In the case of knives, the most common brakeage occurs at the handle or blade wedging a bone. The first one is usually very prominent from the victim's body and raises the dilemma of removing it at the scene [14].

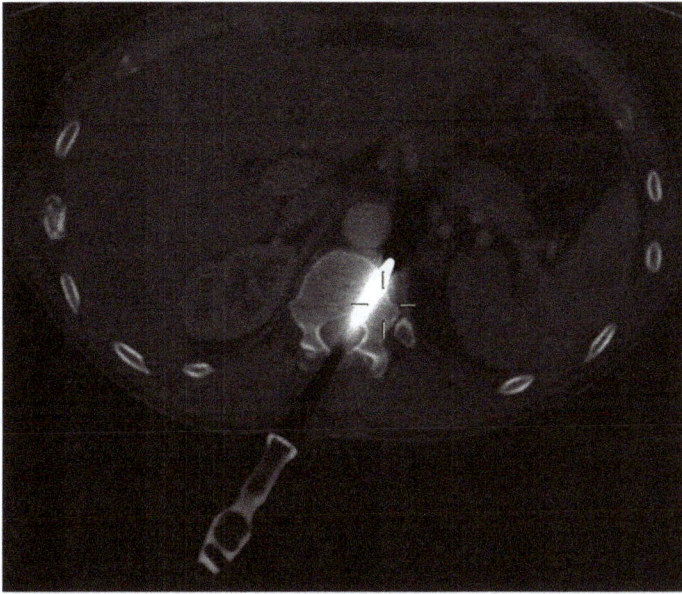

(a)

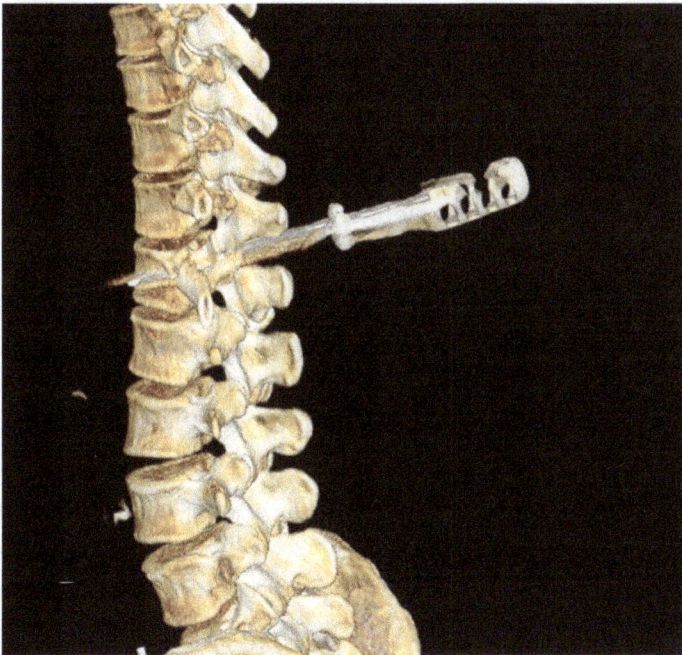

(b)

Figure 1. Axial CT scan (A) and 3D CT reconstruction (B) demonstrating a screwdriver going through the T12 vertebra, through the cord, and coming out adjacent to the aorta. The patient was fully alert on arrival with no neurological deficits. The screwdriver was removed in theater without complications, and the patient was discharged 2 days later.

The possible neurological deficit ranges from asymptomatic dural tears through different nerve root injuries, ranging from neurapraxia to neurothemesis and ending in the worst cases with complete or incomplete spinal cord injury.

The most common incomplete NMPSCI reported was the Brown-Sequard syndrome [15, 16]. This syndrome was first described by Charles-Édouard Brown-Séquard, in farmers cutting sugarcanes in Mauritius and sustaining hemisection of their spinal cord by long knives (1852) [17]. The syndrome is still the most common incomplete SCI [18].

Neurological injury to the spine may occur in two different mechanisms: immediate, through direct damage to neurological tissue, and delayed, following vascular injury to one of the feeding vessels in which a vessel that supplies the cord, most commonly the aorta or the Adamkiewicz perforant, is injured. The first one will cause most frequently an incomplete SCI, most commonly Brown-Sequard syndrome, while the last one is more likely to cause a complete SCI. The second pattern is the delayed onset which is caused most commonly from CSF leaks, edema, granuloma, scar formation, and infection. The delayed pattern can appear anytime from 2 years after the injury and up to 36 years as was described in a rare case of metal encrustation of a retained knife fragment in the spinal canal [19].

2.1. Primary evaluation: emergency department

All NMPSCI patients should be treated like other trauma victims according to the ATLS (Advanced Trauma Life Support) principles [20]. When the retained weapon is clearly prominent from the patient's body, the attention of the treating personnel tends to focus on it and distract them from acting according to the ATLS protocol. These injuries are sometimes less visible than it might be seen at first and may harbor other damages such as large vessels, heart, tracheal, or lung injuries that can affect hemodynamics, airway, and breathing and may be fatal. This is why any suspected patient should obtain an appropriate initial assessment and resuscitation before taking the next step. The initial assessment should not delay instance evacuation with minimal movements to the nearest hospital.

Extracting the penetrating object must not be done on site, not even at the emergency room, before obtaining proper imaging studies. These should include radiographs, sonography, and computerized tomography, according to the involved area. In case the patient is hemodynamically unstable and does not respond to initial resuscitation, an immediate transfer to the operating room with no further delay must take place.

NMPSCI always entails the risk of a retained foreign body material. It is well described in the literature [12, 21]. Patients presenting with delayed wound infections following stab wounds that were irrigated and primarily sutured without further evaluation were documented [22–24]. This is why many authors recommend routine imaging of any penetrating injury, even if only a skin or fascia discontinuity is observed, with no obvious damage.

2.2. Imaging

There are many imaging modalities that can be used to evaluate patients with NMPSCI. This includes plain radiographs, upper GI studies, ultrasound, computed tomography with or without contrast, and MRI. It must be remembered that imaging cannot replace clinical evaluation, judgment, or resuscitation. Imaging should be considered only in a hemodynamically stable patient.

2.2.1. Radiography

Enicker and his colleagues [12] published a large series of stab wounds that accounted for one-third of all SCI in their center. Forty-nine percent of these patients had retained foreign bodies where a knife blade was the most common object. Knife blades are easily identified by plain radiographs; however, the availability of CT scan in most ER in the developed world has shoved aside its role in cervical trauma. It still has a role in the evaluation of thoracic injury mainly for the evaluation of the associated lung injury and not for the demonstration of the foreign body.

2.2.2. Computed tomography

Computerized tomography is the mainstay in diagnosis of penetrating SCI. It is a fast and reliable modality that can scan any part of the body. It has the ability to demonstrate the thoracic or cervical column with the surrounding organs that may be involved in the injury. The main disadvantage of CT scan is its poor ability to demonstrate direct damage or pathologic changes of the neural tissue.

2.2.3. CTA

Saito and colleagues in their review [21] recommend CTA as the gold standard of imaging for penetrating SCI. It has all the advantages of CT plus the benefit of demonstrating blood vessels including extravasation, pseudoaneurysm, dissection, occlusion, and arteriovenous fistula. Angiography is still considered as the "gold standard" vascular imaging examination; however, CTA is gradually taking its place as an alternative. CTA has been proven to be as good as angiography and yet less invasive and faster which makes it suitable for diagnosis in such cases [21].

2.2.4. MRI

MRI is not used routinely as a diagnostic tool in these injuries. The main concern is potential migration of retained metal fragments that can further damage neurologic or other surrounding tissues. Other drawbacks are time, unavailability, and study quality in the presence of metal artifacts. On the contrary to its place in the acute setting, MRI has a major role in studying complications following the initial treatment. Patients who present with deteriorating neurological deficit, prolonged fever, CSF leak, or post-LP syndrome are expected to be further evaluated with an MRI.

2.2.5. Others

Other imaging studies may be used when clinical suspicion for specific collateral organ damage is raised. This may include sonography, Doppler, endoscopy, and barium contrast imaging studies. Those studies are not routinely used, and the need depends on the site of injury (thoracic vs. cervical), clinical examination, and the results of CTA. Sonography is a quick, noninvasive, and readily available tool; however, the technique is highly operator-dependent, and air from the injury, artifacts from retained metallic fragments, and hematoma can limit its interpretation.

2.3. Treatment

As mentioned above, initial treatment of these injuries should be treated as any other traumatic injury, by the ATLS guidelines. After securing airway breathing and circulation, the spine surgeon can address the NMPSCI. The management of regimen to date is still controversial, which is understandable given the low prevalence of these injuries. To date no guidelines exist as for the proper management plan, and the published series described are too small to dictate any clear conclusions.

Most authors agree that in cases of progressive neurological deficits, radiographic evidence of neural tissue compression, or persistent CSF leak, early intervention should be considered. In case of spinal canal penetration with no neurological deficit or CSF leak, surgery is not mandatory.

There is no clear evidence that removal of the retained foreign body will improve the neurological status. The literature describes conflicting reports where in some, foreign body removal improves neurological status and in others, neurological improvement was seen even with retained small fragments. Unfortunately, no RCT (randomized control trials) are available to guide us which option is better. Therefore, each case should be evaluated independently. One should judge the potential damage of extracting the penetrating object compared with the probability of late complications in case of leaving it in place.

In most cases, decompressive procedures, most commonly laminectomies, hemilaminectomies, and dural exploration, are the procedures of choice, mainly because the injury comes from the back. In other rarer cases, mainly in the cervical spine, anterior decompression is indicated.

Most NMPSCI are considered as stable spine injuries, and in an awake and alert patient without distracting injury, clearance of the spine can be done by clinical examination [11, 13, 14].

The surgical management of NMPSCI is a controversial topic [2, 6, 12, 14, 15]. This is more so in cases with a complete SCI but exist also in incomplete SCI.

The literature supports the fact that early surgical intervention for spinal cord injuries caused by low-velocity missile-penetrating injuries (bullets) does not improve the neurological status [1]. There is no clear-cut evidence regarding NMPSCI given the infrequency of these injuries. Case reports describe improvement of the neurological status following emergent or late surgical removal of the foreign body, in some cases even months after the injury [12, 19]. However, this improvement can occur without intervention as well, as reported by others [2] who recommended observation only, in most of their patients. Surgical intervention in NMPSCI may reduce late complications such as decreasing infection rate, cerebrospinal fluid fistula, and arachnoiditis. Delayed myelopathy has been described years following injury with a retained foreign body up to 36 years after the primary insult [12]. When there is rapid progression of neurological deficit or in case of incomplete SCI with radiographic evidence of cord compression (i.e., expanding hematoma, bony fragments, or a retained foreign body), it is a consensus to proceed with immediate surgical intervention.

Positioning a patient with a retained knife handle protruding from his upper back is a challenge. Intubation in an alert patient must be done on a lateral decubitus position, to avoid further damage. Fiber optic-assisted intubation is preferable in difficult cases.

Essential part of surgery is canal decompression. Ideally, it should be done from an uninjured part of the dura mater to the next uninjured space, one level distal and one proximal to the injured loci.

Direct repair of the dura in the immediate setting is controversial, especially in the thoracic spine. This area of the spine is the narrowest along the spinal column. Moreover, blood supply to this segment has been described as the watershed area. Direct repair of the dura mater in this zone raises concern of cord compression secondary to neural tissue swelling. This is why it was proposed by some authors to apply collagen matrix on the defect instead of primary closure. Others are more concerned with the risk of infection and thus repeal any use of sealing material [25].

2.4. Perioperative care

Intravenous administration of steroids in penetrating SCI has no role, and, moreover, it may raise the risk of infection [26, 27].

Preventive antibiotic treatment in the perioperative period is controversial. The incidence of meningitis following NMPSCI is very low [2]. However, the incidence of soft tissue infection around the stab wound is high. There are no evidences as to what is the recommended antibiotic therapy for these injuries; thus, no protocol was published. In the Lipschitz study [6], only 4 out of 252 patients developed meningitis and 2 developed superficial abscess. The authors did not describe whether these patients were treated with antibiotics around the surgery. They mentioned that antibiotics were prescribed to these six patients, only after sepsis was diagnosed. Our policy is to treat these patients empirically, like with open fractures, with a wide range of antibiotic therapies. When canal penetration is evident, we include CSF-penetrating agents such as third-generation cephalosporin, for 3 days.

2.5. Complications

Complications can be related to the spine injury itself or to the surrounding organs.

Spine-associated complications are continuous CSF leak; infection (less than 1% will develop chronic abscess and osteomyelitis) and rarely meningitis; chronic epidural granulation (sometimes will present as progressive myelopathy); and there are reports of arachnoiditis and syringomyelia. Retained foreign body reaction may present as late-onset myelopathy due to foreign body migration. Metal particles such as copper or silver may cause a marked inflammatory reaction, while nickel and lead particles can be a source of an intermediate reaction. Oxidation of metallic fragments and rust deposit were also described [28].

Extra-spinal complications are head injuries (5% of patients have low GCS on admission, and, hence, it may mask the diagnosis of SCI), vascular injury (most commonly, the carotid artery, but there are cases of injury to the vertebral artery as well) [29, 30], brachial plexus injury (it may superimpose cord injury), trachea and esophagus injury (the hypotheses is that these patients are too sick to survive), and thoracic organ injuries such as hemothorax, pneumothorax, and hemopneumothorax with a self-resolving emphysema. Less common injuries involve the major vessels, pericardium, and even the heart. Chylothorax and tear of the diaphragm were rarely described.

3. Missile-penetrating spinal cord injury

Missile-penetrating spinal cord injury (MPSCI) can be a devastating event and may cause severe and long-term morbidity and mortality. As in other SCI, these injuries have a substantial economic and psychosocial burden to patient, their family, and society.

MPSCI was first described in 1762 by a surgeon named Andre Louis that removed a bullet from the lumbar spine of a patient, who later on regained motion in his lower extremities [9].

Many famous fatalities of MPSCI are known throughout the history. Among them was Lord H. Nelson who was shot by a French sniper in the Trafalgar battle. The injury was to his shoulder, and he was described as experiencing immediate paraplegia. He died shortly after. Other known cases were the American presidents, J.A. Garfield and A. Lincoln. As a general rule, these injuries have a high rate of mortality and hence discouraged any treatment for many centuries [31]. Only at the end of World War II, surgeons started to treat it aggressively. Pool had reported [32] 57% marked neurological improvement with laminectomy compared with only 4.5% spontaneous improvement with previously untreated patients. Later, studies that were published following the Korea and Vietnam wars had shown no benefit of laminectomies in cases of complete and incomplete SCI. They concluded that surgery should be considered only in grossly contaminated wounds and for patients with progressive neurological deterioration [33–35].

MPSCI can be divided by the kind of the penetrating missile, that is to say, bullet vs. shrapnel or any other foreign body that penetrates, by blast, the patient body. Another way to classify these injuries is by the muzzle velocity of the shouting firearm: high versus low. The third option would be to classify them by the amount of penetrating particles—a solitary missile penetration versus multiple, usually combined with a blast injury. Segregation can also be done for civilian versus military injuries.

3.1. Epidemiology

Military MPSCI epidemiology depends greatly on military conflicts around the world. Like any other military injury inflicted, it is more common in areas of worldwide conflicts and less common in peaceful areas.

Civilian MPSCI are easy to quantify. This is now the third most common cause of spinal injury in civilian population accounting for one-fifth of all spine injuries after MVA and fall from height [36, 37]. They also account for 13–17% of all causes of spinal trauma [10, 38–41].

In both civilian and military injuries of the vast majority, more than 80% of affected victims are men, with the highest incidence at their third decade [42–46]. The most common involved level is the thoracic spine (approximately 50%), and the least is the lumbar spine [3, 37, 47–49]. The incidence of thoracic spine injuries tends to reduce in more developed armies with better personal protective equipment [50].

3.2. Ballistics

The term "ballistics" refers to the scientific analysis of projectile motion and is divided to three main stages:

- Internal ballistics refers to the projectile's behavior within the barrel of the firearm.
- External ballistics deals with the projectile's path and motion while in the air.
- Terminal ballistics describes what happens upon the impact with the target.

Wound ballistics is considered a subgroup of terminal ballistics and is the main concern of medical personnel [43, 51, 52]. Wound (terminal) ballistics, together with the characteristics of the damaged tissue and its reaction to the penetrating missile, dictate the severity of the injury and treatment strategy [53, 54].

Although surgeons are naturally mostly concerned with the terminal ballistics, understanding of the entire bullet course is crucial, since it has a direct effect on its introduction into the body and the extent of tissue damage.

3.2.1. Internal ballistics

All bullets are fired through a barrel, which is usually a tube of variable length with internal spiral grooving. The bullet is accelerated down the barrel to reach its final exit velocity due to high pressure expanding gases from the combustion of its propellant [55, 56]. During its path within the barrel, the bullet acquires its spin as it is engaged by the spiral grooves of the barrel. This spin is essential for the appropriate orientation of the bullet during its flight [57].

Bullets are usually classified as "high" or "low" velocity, which corresponds to the type of firearm they were shot from—a rifle or a pistol, respectively [58]. Low velocity usually refers to subsonic speed of about 350 m/s, while high velocity can reach up to 600–900 m/s [57].

The bullet itself, and most importantly—its mass, also influences wound ballistics, since the mass and velocity both comprise the well-known formula of kinetic energy = $1/2 \ mv^2$. Thus, a bullet fired from a handgun of 6.35 mm caliber, with a muzzle velocity of about 350 m/s and a mass of about 3.5 g, carries the energy of about 85 J. On the contrary, bullet fired from an assault rifle, such as the 7.62 mm caliber AK-47, with a mass of 8 g and muzzle velocity of about 800 m/sec, may reach the energy of about 2100 J—almost 25 times more than a handgun [59].

3.2.2. External ballistics

Once leaving the barrel, a bullet is subjected to several forces that might influence its energy-delivering capacity. First, it is affected by the escaping gases just as it is exiting the barrel

[60] that might destabilize it and thereafter to the drag forces as it traverses the air, which increases with rising velocity [51].

This combination of forces acting on the exiting bullet creates an overturning moment, which causes the bullet to diverge from its original line of trajectory. This divergence is called "yaw," and it is expressed by the angle between the bullet's axis and the velocity vector [36, 61]. Because of the bullet's spin, yawing results in complex spiral revolution of the tip about its center of mass. Eventually, if the distance the bullet travels is long enough, yawing becomes irreversible, and tumbling occurs—meaning the bullet advances base-forward [62, 63].

It is quite clear that as the distance between the firearm and the target is shortened, these are less so-called disturbances to the bullet's path, and hence it can deliver more energy upon the impact. Muzzle velocity decreases significantly after 45 m for most pistol bullets and after 100 m for rifle bullets [64]. Unfortunately, most civilian gunshot wounds (GSW) are inflicted from an average distance of only 10 m [65].

3.2.3. Terminal ballistics

Terminal ballistics is directly influenced by the internal and external ballistics, which delivered the bullet to meet its target in a certain condition. As discussed above, the energy entailed within the bullet upon the impact is the main characteristic that will influence its effect within the body and will determine the extent of the injury [66].

The other aspect that determines the amount of injury transferred to the body is the resistance to penetration of the body and the characteristics of the body surface and tissue. The ability of the body surface to resist penetration is influenced in turn by two factors—the presented area of the bullet, which increases with rising yaw up to a maximal impact surface when the yaw angle reaches 90°, and the bullet deformation upon impact, which has to do with its internal metal composition and structure [67].

As the bullet penetrates the skin, the energy transfer between the bullet and the tissue begins. As a result of the high level of resistance and drag that meets the bullet with its entrance, a high-pressure crushing effect develops in front of the bullet's tip, sometimes called the "shock wave," and together with the mechanical damage that occurs, while the bullet cuts through the tissue—these create one level of tissue damage [58, 68]. In contrast to the high pressure that develops in front of the bullet, as the bullet keeps on advancing, a vacuum is created in the back of the bullet, which in turn causes the tissue to collapse back.

This change of pressures causes the "cavitation" effect, which basically refers to the tissue's reaction to the very rapid change of pressures—the tissue first expands and then collapses back, leaving a tract within the tissue which is slightly larger in diameter than the bullet. The magnitude of the cavitation is directly related to the rate of energy transfer into the tissue and to the degree of yaw—the bigger the yaw, the bigger the cavitation [69].

The outer appearance of the body after the impact is not always suggestive of the true damage that lies within. With low-velocity handguns, the bullet usually does not cause cavitation, and the damage is usually due to the mechanical impact of the bullet. Sometimes, there is not even an exit wound and the bullet stays within the tissue. Alternatively, high-velocity rifles usually have an exit wound, and they leave behind them a distinct tract, usually very damaged and often contaminated because of the "suction" effect of the wound. One might find cloth fragments in a wound cavity [70].

3.3. Initial evaluation and management

As in any other trauma, MPSCI should be first treated according the ATLS principles [71]. This initial evaluation will reveal concomitant injuries. Rapid evacuation to a hospital is crucial. This is especially true for the military scenario, in which more than one injury is the rule. The Prehospital Trauma Life Support and the Military Trauma Life Support (PHTLS and the MTLS) emphasize the importance of rapid evacuation from the scene of injury. It recommends that only securing airway and breathing together with partial circulatory control (control external bleeding) are done at the scene, and, thus, instead of doing the whole "ABCDE" scheme, the team should perform stages A, B, and half C ("scoop and run").

After arrival to the hospital, these patients are initially evaluated in the trauma bay by a multidisciplinary team. Following initial resuscitations and stabilization, physical examination is undertaken. The sensitivity and specificity of this were shown to be high, in detecting spinal cord injury (100% and 87%, respectively) [72]. It should be emphasized that civilian and military scenarios are different. In the civilian, most injuries are inflicted by low-velocity weapons with a solitary injury and less comorbidity. The evacuation period is normally short, and most patients arrive conscious to the emergency room. Neurological examination in this setting is more feasible and accurate. The opposite is true for the military scenario where most injuries are of high-velocity nature, and usually there is more than one injury. Usually, since most of casualties have a longer period of evacuation, they are brought to the trauma bay intubated, and thus their neurologic assessment is limited. The clinician should rely mostly on the anamnestic report of the evacuation team that considering the circumstance might not always be accurate.

After securing airway, birthing, and circulation, and after an initial neurologic assessment was performed, the patient should be completely exposed to inspect the entire body. Documentation of the entry and exit wounds should be done. It should be kept in mind that in high-velocity weapons, more than one exit wound may be found. In a low-velocity weapon, no exit wound is usually the rule.

Treatment for associated injuries to other organs should be addressed.

Tetanus prophylaxis history should be inquired and treated accordingly. In cases of unknown immunization, tetanus immunoglobulin is required in addition to toxoid treatment.

Antibiotic treatment is usually given; however, no consensus for the type and duration of treatment exist. Evidence to support different antibiotic treatments in cases of organ perforation such as the larynx/esophagus in cervical injuries compared with abdominal viscera in thoracic injuries is low. There is, however, some evidence to support administration of a wide range of antibiotic treatments as prophylaxis [73]. Interestingly, a Cochrane review concluded that evidence exists for antibiotic treatment only for the first 24 h after initial debridement [74].

Most of the evidence exists for low-velocity injuries. There is less evidence guiding treatment recommendation in high-velocity injuries. We normally recommend empirically regimen of 3 days of prophylactic antibiotic which is discontinued if no sign of infection is observed.

3.4. Imaging

The mainstay of imaging for MPSCI is the CT scan. In some cases a retained metal fragment can be found in chest and pelvic X-ray routinely done in the trauma bay; however, these can provide limited information regarding concomitant injuries and spatial orientation.

3.4.1. CTA

CTA is usually available, is relatively quickly obtained, and gives sufficient information on other visceral injuries as well as bleeding. The only disadvantage is its inability to demonstrate neurological tissue with high accuracy. It should be reemphasized that an unstable patient should not be referred to CT prior to resuscitation and hemodynamic stabilization. In case of failure to achieve hemodynamic stability, patient should be taken to OR without any further delay. We routinely use CTA in any penetrating trauma as part of our protocol given the advantage of demonstrating major vessel injury and extravasation.

3.4.2. MRI

MRI has the ability to demonstrate neurologic tissue including direct and secondary injury. However, this is a time-consuming modality and probably not suitable for initial assessment in these scenarios. Some concern exists regarding retained metal fragment migration and further neurologic damage when performing the MRI. Copper and lead are the most common materials for bullet manufacturing. These materials are non-ferromagnetic and should not affect MRI [75]. The literature shows that MRI (up to 1.5 T) is safe to use in case of retained bullets [76–79]. Nevertheless, we recommend that the decision should be done on a case-to-case basis, especially if the penetrating missile is not a bullet.

3.4.3. Others

As mentioned above, other imaging studies may be used when clinical suspicion for specific collateral organ damage is raised.

3.5. Definitive treatment

Management of acute missile-penetrating SCI is multidisciplinary. The treatment is guided by many factors, but first and above all, the patient's respiratory and hemodynamic stability are defined by the ATLS guidelines. A hemodynamically unstable patient, whose primary resuscitation has failed, should be transferred immediately to angiography or surgery suite without further delay. In a stable patient, treatment should be guided by the presence of other factors such as neurological status, mechanical stability of the spine, CSF leak, risk for infection, and other systemic injuries.

3.5.1. Indication for surgery

There are no clear clinical guidelines to direct the treatment pathway in MPSCI, and hence each case should be treated individually. Some issues, however, should be considered:

Wound care: in high-velocity GSW, an extensive wound debridement and lavage should be performed in the OR given the expected large infected cavity and "wound suction effect" inserting debris into the wound [8, 45, 80]. A low-velocity, civilian-inflicted GSW (gunshot wound) can be treated locally in the ER and observed.

Loss of neurologic function: progressive loss of neurologic function with radiographic evidence of neural tissue compression either by hematoma, bone fragment, or foreign body is an absolute indication for surgery [81–85]. There is no doubt that the initial neurological status will dictate the fate of the patient's neurological function [84]. There is only minor evidence that demonstrate neurological improvement following early (24–48 h) intervention. This is especially true if the insult occurs in the cauda equine area [82, 83, 86]. However, there is more evidence to show that there is no improvement following surgery, especially if the injury occurs between the levels of T1–T11 and definitely in complete injuries due to high-velocity GSW [49, 62]. In low-velocity civilian injuries, these types of injuries might have better prognosis, depending on what was the initial clinical presentation.

Despite the above details, some subgroups of patients may benefit from surgical intervention, even in the presence of a complete or nonprogressing injury. This includes complete injuries of the cervical spine where a potential recovery of an affected level is anticipated or when the injury raises a mechanical issue that might be solved with surgery (**Figure 2**). When intervention is considered, one should remember that it has been shown to result in about 20% of complications compared to 7% for nonsurgical treatment [87]. Clinical discretion should be used in all cases.

Foreign body removal: foreign body, e.g., bullet fragments, shrapnel, and intact bullets, is considered an absolute indication for removal in cases of incomplete SCI, definitely when it is progressive. When there is imaging evidence of cord compression, early intervention has been shown to be beneficial in many studies [47, 51, 88].

Removal of bullets in cases of complete and static SCI is not efficient and will not restore any neurological function [47, 62, 86].

Another possible indication for bullet removal from the spinal canal is the concern of fragment migration (**Figure 2**). This might happen early [89] or late [90, 91] in the course of injury, as shown in some sporadic cases. In both cases, neurologic deterioration had resolved following the surgery. That is why some surgeons suggest preventing this complication by surgically removing the foreign body, especially in cases with easy access and expectedly low complications.

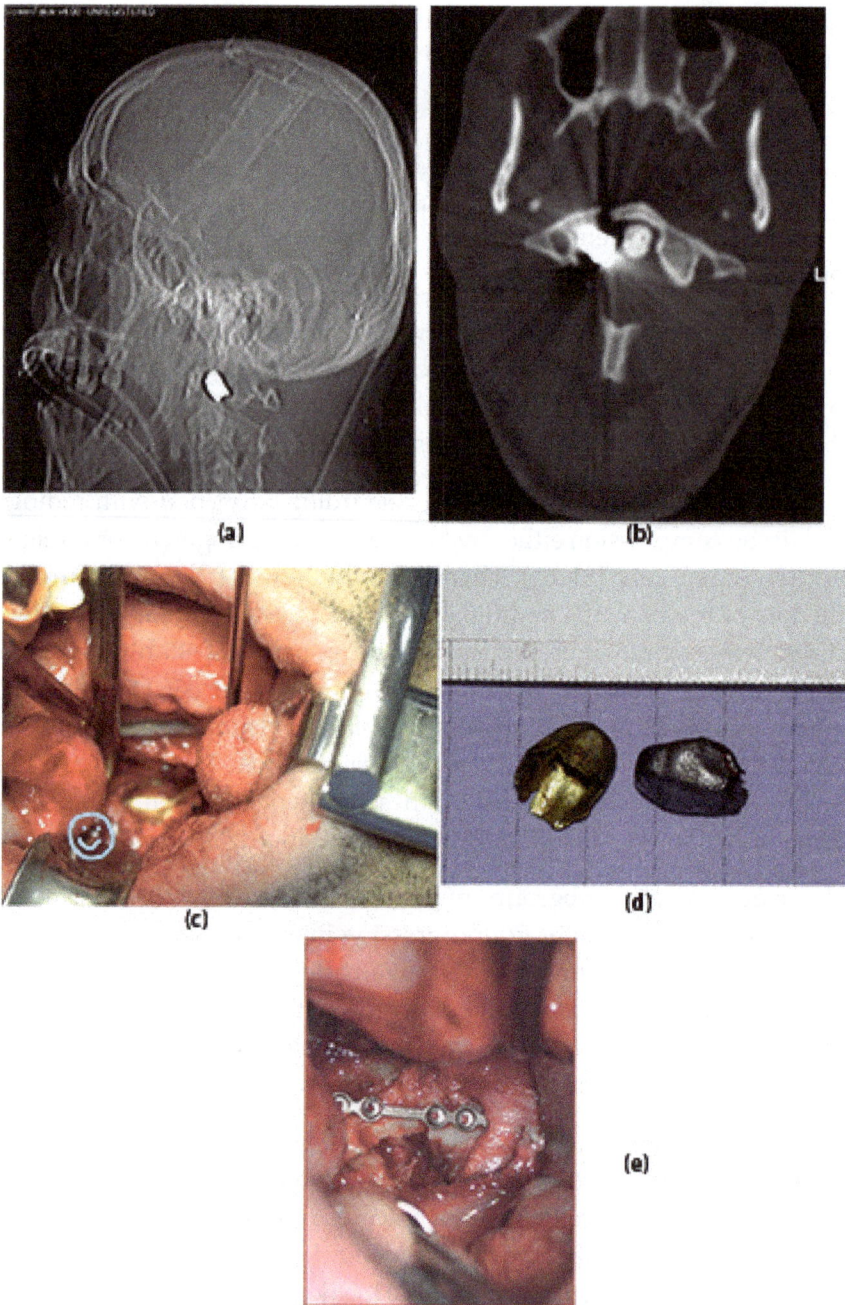

Figure 2. A 30-year-old patient, who sustained a low-velocity gunshot wound. He had a few entry wounds in his head and neck. He was conscious, alert, and hemodynamically stable with normal neurological status. The following images describe the evolution of events. (a) Plain radiograph showing the patient's skull with a bullet located at the center; (b) axial CT scan showing the broken arc of C1 with the bullet located next to the dens; (c) trans-oral approach to C1 vertebra with the bullet at the base of the surgical dissection. The smiley gives the orientation of the patient's face; (d) the bullet is shown outside of the patient's spine; (e) C1 ring following osteosynthesis.

The presence of foreign body inside the spinal canal was not shown to be associated with increased risk of infection, regardless of the previous path of the bullet, prior to its final location in the spinal canal [92, 93]. Thus, we do not consider bullet removal as an indication for surgery in order to prevent potential infection. Metal toxicity is usually not a concern since most materials used to manufacture bullets and shotgun pellets today are often made of copper or lead.

Lead toxicity or plumbism was shown to happen in cases of retained bullets in joint spaces and intervertebral disks [94, 95]. The symptoms can include anemia, abdominal pain, anorexia, nephropathy, lethargy, encephalopathy, and motor neuropathy, all of which can appear intermittently or continuously. Symptoms develop insidiously and can appear even 40 years after the exposure [96], making the diagnosis often challenging. Missiles retained in bone and soft tissues are usually asymptomatic.

Spinal instability: low-velocity spinal GSW involving the vertebral column are normally stable and do not mandate surgical stabilization. Risk of instability is higher with high-velocity injuries. Preventive stabilization should be considered if instability is anticipated following the surgery. There are reports claiming that stabilization may improve neurology [44], and other reports state that it may facilitate rehabilitation [37].

CSF leak: should bullet or other foreign bodies enter the spinal canal, durotomy is suspected. If a clinical presentation of post-LP syndrome (positional headaches, diplopia, photophobia, nausea, and neck stiffness) presents, surgical exploration should be considered. The preferable treatment is direct repair of the dural defect. This might prevent fistula formation, secondary meningitis, cord herniation, and neurologic impairment. If primary repair is not feasible, like in the ventral cervical and thoracic cord, fibrin glue combined with synthetic or local graft should be used. Submuscular drains are controversial. Position restrictions (upright for cervical injuries or reclining for lumbar) are not mandatory and case specific. Subarachnoid continuous drainage is optional as primary treatment for minor tears or as an adjuvant to surgical repair.

The optimal timing of surgery for any indication is debatable [97–99]. Early surgical intervention has been reported to have less complication, while late intervention (more than 2 weeks) was associated with a high rate of arachnoiditis and spinal abscess [83].

No significant benefit of steroids has been shown [3]. A Cochrane review that shows some neurologic improvement in SCI following steroid administration (up to 8 h of injury) excluded penetrating injuries [100].

Empiric Intravenous antibiotic should be given for a minimum of 3 days and up to 2 weeks, in most cases. The covered spectrum should be wide in order to treat Gram-positive, Gram-negative, and anaerobic bacteria. This treatment was shown to prevent most infections including trans-colonic and trans-oral injuries [41, 81].

4. Summary

This chapter is an overview of two relatively rare-penetrating spinal cord injuries, their epidemiology, mechanism of injury, initial evaluation, and emergency primary and late definitive treatment. We also reviewed the complication and prognosis of each injury.

	NMPSCI	MPSCI (high velocity)	MPSCI (low velocity)
Incidence	1.5% of SCI	17–21% of SCI	17–21% of SCI
Primary evaluation	ATLS Extracting the penetrating object must not be done on site	MTLS "scoop and run"	ATLS
Preferred primary imaging	CTA/X-ray	CTA	X-ray
Surgical treatment	OR/observation depending on neurological status and comorbidity	OR mandatory	ER/OR
Antibiotics	IV antibiotics (empiric)	IV antibiotics	PO antibiotics/observation
Steroids	No	No	No
Complication	CSF leak, infection(less than 1%), pneumo-/hemothorax, vascular (common)	Multiple organs-common. Spine instability, infection	Not common
Common incomplete SCI	Brown-Sequard syndrome	Any	Any, not common

Table 1. Summarized table comparing evaluation, treatment, and complications between NMPSCI and MPSCI.

In order to emphasize the differences between these entities, we present a summarized table that compares between them (**Table 1**).

Conflict of interest

The authors certify that they have NO affiliations with or involvement in any organization or entity with any financial interest (such as honoraria; educational grants; participation in speaker bureaus; membership, employment, consultancies, stock ownership, or other equity interests; and expert testimony or patent-licensing arrangements) or nonfinancial interest (such as personal or professional relationships, affiliations, knowledge, or beliefs) in the subject matter or materials discussed in this chapter.

Author details

Moti M. Kramer[1], Asaf Acker[2]* and Nissim Ohana[2]

*Address all correspondence to: ackerortho@gmail.com

1 Assuta Ashdod University Medical Center, Ashdod, Israel

2 Soroka University Medical Center, Beer-Sheva, Israel

References

[1] Conran J. Characteristics and outcomes of gunshot-acquired spinal cord injury in South Africa. South African Medical Journal. 2017;**107**(6):518-522

[2] McCaughey EJ, Purcell M, Barnett SC, Allan DB. Spinal cord injury caused by Stab Wounds: Incidence, natural history, and relevance for future research. Journal of Neurotrauma. 2016 Aug 1;**33**(15):1416-1421. DOI: 10.1089/neu.2015.4375. Epub 2016 Mar 18

[3] Sidhu GS et al. Civilian gunshot injuries of the spinal cord: A systematic review of the current literature. Clinical Orthopaedics and Related Research. 2013;**471**(12):3945-3955

[4] Wilkins RH. Neurosurgical Classics. 2nd ed. Park Ridge, Illinois: American Association of Neurological Surgeons. 1992. ISBN: 978-1-879284-09-8. LCCN: 2011293270

[5] Arthur John Brock (translator). Introduction. Galen. On the Natural Faculties. Edinburgh. 1916

[6] Lipschitz R, Block J. Stab wounds of the spinal cord. Lancet. 1962 Jul 28;**2**(7248):169-172

[7] Peacock WJ, Shrosbree RD, Key AG. A review of 450 stab wounds of the spinal cord. South African Medical Journal. 1977;**51**:961-964

[8] Velmahos GC, Degiannis E, Hart K, Souter I, Saadia R. Changing profiles in spinal cord injuries and risk factors influencing recovery after penetrating injuries. The Journal of Trauma. 1995;**38**:334-337

[9] Holtz A, Levi R. Spinal Cord Injury. New York: Oxford University Press; 2010

[10] Farmer JC, Vaccaro AR, Balderston RA, Albert TJ, Cotler J. The changing nature of admissions to a spinal cord injury center: Violence on the rise. Journal of Spinal Disorders. 1998;**11**:400-403

[11] Miyamoto S, Ide T, Takemura N. Risks and causes of cervical cord and medulla oblongata injuries due to acupuncture. World Neurosurgery. 2010 Jun;**73**(6):735-741

[12] Enicker B, Gonya S, Hardcastle TC. Spinal stab injury with retained knife blades: 51 consecutive patients managed at a regional referral unit. Injury. 2015 Sep;**46**(9):1726-1733. DOI: 10.1016/j.injury

[13] De Régloix SB, Baumont L, Daniel Y, Maurin O, Crambert A, Pons Y. Comparison of penetrating neck injury management in combat versus civilian trauma: A review of 55 cases. Military Medicine. 2016 Aug;**181**(8):935-940

[14] Sakar M, Dogrul R, Niftaliyev S, Bayri Y, Dagcınar A. Direct withdrawal of a knife lodged in the thoracic spinal canal in a patient with normal neurologic examination: Is it safe? Spinal Cord Series and Cases. 2016 Jul 7;**2**:1-3

[15] Johnson S, Jones M, Zumsteg J. Brown-Séquard syndrome without vascular injury associated with Horner's syndrome after a stab injury to the neck. The Journal of Spinal Cord Medicine; 2016;**39**(1):111-114

[16] Beer-Furlan AL, Paiva WS, Tavares WM, de Andrade AF, Teixeira MJ. Brown-Sequard syndrome associated with unusual spinal cord injury by a screwdriver stab wound. International Journal of Clinical and Experimental Medicine. 2014 Jan 15;7(1):316-319

[17] Brown-Séquard C-É. De la transmission croisée des impressions sensitives par la moelle épinière. Comptes rendus de la Société de Biologie. 1850;**1851**(2):33-44

[18] Young JS, Burns PE, Bowen AM, et al. Spinal Cord Injury Statistics: Experience of the Regional Spinal Cord Injury Systems. Phoenix, AZ: Good Samaritan Medical Center; 1982

[19] Stab wounds of the spinal cord. British Medical Journal. 1978 Apr 29;**1**(6120):1093-1094

[20] Brasel KJ, Chapleau W, Al-khatib J, Haskin D, leBlanc P, Cardenas G, et al. ATLS: The ninth edition. Subcommittee, American College of Surgeons Committee on Trauma, International ATLS

[21] Saito et al. Imaging of penetrating injuries of the head and neck: Current practice at a level I trauma Center in the United States. The Keio Journal of Medicine. 2014;**63**(2):23-33

[22] Jones FD, Woosley RE. Delayed myelopathy secondary to retained intraspinal metallic fragment. Case report. Journal of Neurosurgery. 1981;**55**(6):979-982

[23] Wolf SM. Delayed traumatic myelopathy following transfixion of the spinal cord by a knife blade. Case report. Journal of Neurosurgery. 1973;**38**:221-225

[24] Fung CF, Ng TH. Delayed myelopathy after a stab wound with a retained intraspinal foreign body: Case report. The Journal of Trauma. 1992;**32**:539-541

[25] Li et al. Stab injury to the spinal cord with no neurolgic deficit. Orthopedics. 2012;**35**(5): e770-e773

[26] Bracken MB, Shepard MJ, Holford TR, Leo-Summers L, Aldrich EF, Fazi M, et al. Administration of methylprednisolone for 24 or 48 hours or tirilazad mesylate for 48 hours in the treatment of acute spinal cord injury: Results of the Third National Acute Spinal Cord Injury Randomized Controlled Trial-National Acute Spinal Cord Injury Study. JAMA. 1997;**277**:1597-1604

[27] Levy ML, Gans W, Wijesinghe H, Soohoo WE, Adkins RH, Stillerman CB. Use of methyl-prednisolone as an adjunct in the management of patients with penetrating spinal cord injury: Outcome analysis. Neurosurgery. 1996;**39**:1141-1149

[28] Jones et al. Delayed myelopathy secondary to retained intraspinal metallic fragments. Journal of Neurosurgery. 1981;**55**:979-982

[29] Vinces FY, Newell MA, Cherry RA. Isolated contralateral vertebral artery injury in a stab wound to the neck. Journal of Vascular Surgery. 2004;**39**:462-464

[30] Karadag O, Gurelik M, Berkan O, Kars HZ. Stab wound of the cervical spinal cord and ipsilateral vertebral artery injury. British Journal of Neurosurgery. 2004;**18**:545-547

[31] Jakoi A et al. Gunshot injuries of the spine. The Spine Journal. 2015;**15**:2077-2085

[32] Pool JL. Gunshot wounds of the spine. Surgery, Gynecology & Obstetrics. 1945;**81**:617-622

[33] Yashon D, Jane JA, White RJ. Prognosis and management of spinal cord and cauda equina bullet injuries in sixty-five civilians. Journal of Neurosurgery. 1970;**32**:163-170

[34] Stauffer ES, Wood RW, Kelly EG. Gunshot wounds of the spine: The effects of laminectomy. The Journal of Bone and Joint Surgery. American Volume. 1979;**61**:389-392

[35] Heiden JS, Weiss MH, Rosenberg AW, Kurze T, Apuzzo ML. Penetrating gunshot wounds of the cervical spine in civilians. Review of 38 cases. Journal of Neurosurgery. 1975;**42**:575-579

[36] Miller CA. Penetrating wounds of the spine. In: Wilkins RH, Rengachary SS, editors. Neurosurgery. San Francisco: McGraw-Hill Book Co; 1985. pp. 1746-1748

[37] Beaty N, Slavin J, Diaz C, Zeleznick K, Ibrahimi D, Sansur CA. Cervical spine injury from gunshot wounds. Journal of Neurosurgery. Spine. 2014;**21**:442-449

[38] Aarabi B, Alibaii E, Taghipur M, Kamgarpur A. Comparative study of functional recovery for surgically explored and conservatively managed spinal cord missile injuries. Neurosurgery. 1996;**39**:1133-1140

[39] Chittiboina P, Banerjee AD, Zhang S, Caldito G, Nanda A, Willis BK. How bullet trajectory affects outcomes of civilian gunshot injury to the spine. Journal of Clinical Neuroscience. 2011;**18**:1630-1633

[40] Gentleman D, Harrington M. Penetrating injury of the spinal cord. Injury. 1984;**16**:7-8

[41] Lin SS, Vaccaro AR, Reisch S, Devine M, Cotler JM. Lowvelocity gunshot wounds to the spine with an associated transperitoneal injury. Journal of Spinal Disorders. 1995;**8**:136-144

[42] Buxton N. The military medical management of missile injury to the spine: A review of the literature and proposal of guidelines. Journal of the Royal Army Medical Corps. 2001;**147**:168-172

[43] DeMuth WE Jr. Bullet velocity as applied to military rifle wounding capacity. The Journal of Trauma. 1969;**9**:27-38

[44] Duz B, Cansever T, Secer HI, Kahraman S, Daneyemez MK, Gonul E. Evaluation of spinal missile injuries with respect to bullet trajectory, surgical indications and timing of surgical intervention: A new guideline. Spine. 2008;**33**:E746-E753

[45] Hammoud MA, Haddad FS, Moufarrij NA. Spinal cord missile injuries during the Lebanese civil war. Surgical Neurology. 1995;**43**:432-442

[46] Hanigan WC, Sloffer C. Nelson's wound: Treatment of spinal cord injury in 19th and early 20th century military conflicts. Neurosurgical Focus. 2004;**16**(1):E4

[47] Le Roux JC, Dunn RN. Gunshot injuries of the spine—A review of 49 cases managed at the Groote Schuur acute spinal cord injury unit. South African Journal of Surgery 2005;**43**:165-168

[48] Levy ML, Gans W, Wijesinghe HS, SooHoo WE, Adkins RH, Stillerman CB. Use of methylprednisolone as an adjunct in the management of patients with penetrating spinal cord injury: Outcome analysis. Neurosurgery. 1996;**39**:1141-1148

[49] Heary RF, Vaccaro AR, Mesa JJ, Northrup BE, Albert TJ, Balderston RA, et al. Steroids and gunshot wounds to the spine. Neurosurgery. 1997;**41**:576-583

[50] Ivey KM, White CE, Wallum TE, Aden JK, Cannon JW, Chung KK, McNeil JD, Cohn SM, Blackbourne LH. Thoracic injuries in US combat casualties: A 10-year review of operation enduring freedom and Iraqi freedom. Journal of Trauma and Acute Care Surgery. 2012;**73**(6 Suppl 5):S514-S519

[51] Robertson DP, Simpson RK, Narayan RK. Lumbar disc herniation from a gunshot wound to the spine: A report of two cases. Spine (Phila Pa 1976). 1991;**16**:994-995

[52] Meyer PR, Apple DF, Bohlman HH, Ferguson RL, Stauffer ES. Symposium: Management of fractures of the thoracolumbar spine. Contemporary Orthopaedics. 1988;**16**:57-86

[53] Hollerman JJ, Fackler ML, Coldwell DM, Ben-Menachem Y. Gunshot wounds: 1. Bullets, ballistics, and mechanisms of injury. American Journal of Roentgenology. 1990; **155**(4):685-690

[54] Coupland RM, Kneubuehl BP, Rowley DI, Bowyer GW. Wound ballistics, surgery and the law of war. Trauma. 2000;**2**(1):1-10

[55] Moss GM, Leeming DW, Farrar CL. Military Ballistics: A Basic Manual. London: Brassey's; 1995. pp. 9-22

[56] Jandial R, Reichwage B, Levy M, Duenas V, Sturdivan L. Ballistics for the neurosurgeon. Neurosurgery. 2008;**62**(2):472-480

[57] French RW, Callender GR. Ballistic characteristics of wounding agents. In: Beyer JC, editor. Wound Ballistics. Washington, DC: Office of the Surgeon General, Department of the Army; 1962. pp. 91-141

[58] Bellamy RF, Zajtchuk R. Conventional Warfare: Ballistic, Blast, and Burn Injuries. Washington, DC: Walter Reed Army Medical Center, Office of the Surgeon General; 1991. pp. 107-162

[59] Jaiswal M, Mittal RS. Concept of gunshot wound spine. Asian Spine Journal. 2013;**7**(4): 359-364

[60] Hopkinson DA, Marshall TK. Firearm injuries. The British Journal of Surgery. 1967;**54**(5): 344-353

[61] Tindel NL, Marcillo AE, Tay BK, Bunge RP, Eismont FJ. The effect of surgically implanted bullet fragments on the spinal cord in a rabbit model. The Journal of Bone and Joint Surgery. American Volume. 2001;**83**:884-890

[62] Kupcha PC, An HS, Cotler JM. Gunshot wounds to the cervical spine. Spine (Phila Pa 1976). 1990;**15**:1058-1063

[63] Mirovsky Y, Shalmon E, Blankstein A, Halperin N. Complete paraplegia following gunshot injury without direct trauma to the cord. Spine (Phila Pa 1976). 2005;**30**:2436-2438

[64] Gugala Z, Lindsey RW. Classification of gunshot injuries in civilians. Clinical Orthopaedics and Related Research. 2003;**408**:65-81

[65] Romanick PC, Smith TK, Kopaniky DR, Oldfield D. Infection about the spine associated with low-velocity-missile injury to the abdomen. The Journal of Bone and Joint Surgery. American Volume. 1985;**67**:1195-1201

[66] Haywood IR. Missile injury. Problems in General Surgery. 1989;**6**(2):330-347

[67] Medzon R, Rothenhaus T, Bono CM, Grindlinger G, Rathlev NK. Stability of cervical spine fractures after gunshot wounds to the head and neck. Spine (Phila Pa 1976). 2005;**30**:2274-2279

[68] DiMaio VJ. Gunshot Wounds: Practical Aspects of Firearms, Ballistics, and Forensic Techniques. 2nd ed. Boca Raton, FL: CRC Press; 1999

[69] Kneubuehl BP. General wound ballistics. In: Kneubuehl BP, Coupland RM, Rothschild MA, Thali MJ, editors. Wound Ballistics: Basics and Applications (Translation of the Revised 3rd German Edition). Berlin: Springer; 2011. pp. 87-161

[70] Stefanopoulos PK et al. Gunshot wounds: A review of ballistics related to penetrating trauma. Journal of Acute Disease. 2014:178-185

[71] American College of Surgeons Committee on Trauma. Advanced Trauma Life Support Program for Doctors. 9th ed. Chicago, IL: American College of Surgeons; 2012

[72] Inaba K, Barmparas G, Ibrahim D, Branco BC, Gruen P, Reddy S, et al. Clinical examination is highly sensitive for detecting clinically significant spinal injuries after gunshot wounds. The Journal of Trauma. 2011;**71**:523-527

[73] Fullen WD, Hunt J, Altemeier WA. Prophylactic antibiotics in penetrating wounds of the abdomen. The Journal of Trauma. 1972;**12**:282-289

[74] Brand M, Grieve A. Prophylactic antibiotics for penetrating abdominal trauma. Cochrane Database of Systematic Reviews. 2013;**11**:CD007370

[75] Teitelbaum GP, Yee CA, Van Horn DD, Kim HS, Colletti PM. Metallic ballistic fragments: MR imaging safety and artifacts. Radiology. 1990;**175**:855-859

[76] Bashir EF, Cybulski GR, Chaudhri K, Choudhury AR. Magnetic resonance imaging and computed tomography in the evaluation of penetrating gunshot injury of the spine. Case report. Spine. 1993;**18**:772-773

[77] Finitsis SN, Falcone S, Green BA. MR of the spine in the presence of metallic bullet fragments: Is the benefit worth the risk? AJNR. American Journal of Neuroradiology. 1999;**20**:354-356

[78] Hess U, Harms J, Schneider A, Schleef M, Ganter C, Hannig C. Assessment of gunshot bullet injuries with the use of magnetic resonance imaging. The Journal of Trauma. 2000;**49**:704-709

[79] Smugar SS, Schweitzer ME, Hume E. MRI in patients with intraspinal bullets. Journal of Magnetic Resonance Imaging. 1999;**9**:151-153

[80] Waters RL, Sie IH. Spinal cord injuries from gunshot wounds to the spine. Clinical Orthopaedics and Related Research. 2003;**408**:120-125

[81] Bono CM, Heary RF. Gunshot wounds to the spine. The Spine Journal. 2004;**4**:230-240

[82] Benzel EC, Hadden TA, Coleman JE. Civilian gunshot wounds to the spinal cord and cauda equina. Neurosurgery. 1987;**20**:281-285

[83] Cybulski GR, Stone JL, Kant R. Outcome of laminectomy for civilian gunshot injuries of the terminal spinal cord and cauda equina: Review of 88 cases. Neurosurgery. 1989; **24**:392-397

[84] Klimo P Jr, Ragel BT, Rosner M, Gluf W, McCafferty R. Can surgery improve neurological function in penetrating spinal injury? A review of the military and civilian literature and treatment recommendations for military neurosurgeons. Neurosurgical Focus. 2010;**28**:E4

[85] Kumar A, Pandey PN, Ghani A, Jaiswal G. Penetrating spinal injuries and their management. Journal of Craniovertebral Junction & Spine. 2011;**2**:57-61

[86] Waters RL, Adkins RH. The effects of removal of bullet fragments retained in the spinal canal. A collaborative study by the National Spinal Cord Injury Model Systems. Spine. 1991;**16**:934-939

[87] Venger BH, Simpson RK, Narayan RK. Neurosurgical intervention in penetrating spinal trauma with associated visceral injury. Journal of Neurosurgery. 1989;**70**:514-518

[88] Yoshida GM, Garland D, Waters RL. Gunshot wounds to the spine. The Orthopedic Clinics of North America. 1995;**26**:109-116

[89] Kafadar AM, Kemerdere R, Isler C, Hanci M. Intradural migration of a bullet following spinal gunshot injury. Spinal Cord. 2006;**44**:326-329

[90] Avci SB, Acikgoz B, Gundogdu S. Delayed neurological symptoms from the spontaneous migration of a bullet in the lumbosacral spinal canal. Case report. Paraplegia. 1995;**33**: 541-542

[91] Conway JE, Crofford TW, Terry AF, Protzman RR. Cauda equine syndrome occurring nine years after a gunshot injury to the spine. A case report. The Journal of Bone and Joint Surgery. American Volume. 1993;**75**:760-763

[92] Roffi RP, Waters RL, Adkins RH. Gunshot wounds to the spine associated with a perforated viscus. Spine. 1989;**14**:808-811

[93] Kihtir T, Ivatury RR, Simon R, Stahl WM. Management of transperitoneal gunshot wounds of the spine. The Journal of Trauma. 1991;**31**:1579-1583

[94] Bolanos AA, Demizio JP Jr, Vigorita VJ, Bryk E. Lead poisoning from an intra-articular shotgun pellet in the knee treated with arthroscopic extraction and chelation therapy. A case report. The Journal of Bone and Joint Surgery. American Volume. 1996;**78**:422-426

[95] Windler EC, SM RB, Bryan WJ, Woods GW. Lead intoxication and traumatic arthritis of the hip secondary to retained bullet fragments. A case report. The Journal of Bone and Joint Surgery. American Volume. 1978;**60**:254-255

[96] Dillman RO, Crumb CK, Lidsky MJ. Lead poisoning from a gunshot wound. Report of a case and review of the literature. American Journal of Medicine. 1979;**66**:509-514

[97] Vaccaro AR, Dougherty RJ, Sheehan TP, Dante SJ, Cotler JM, Balderston RJ, et al. Neurologic outcome of early versus late surgery for cervical spinal cord injury. Spine. 1997;**22**:2609-2613

[98] Fehlings MG, Perrin RG. The timing of surgical intervention in the treatment of spinal cord injury: A systematic review of recent clinical evidence. Spine. 2006;**31**:S28-S35

[99] Fehlings MD, Vaccaro A, Wilson JR, Singh AW, Cadotte D, Harrop JS, et al. Early versus delayed decompression for traumatic cervical spinal cord injury: Results of the surgical timing in acute spinal cord injury study (STASCIS). PLoS One. 2012;**7**:e32037

[100] Bracken MB. Steroids for acute spinal cord injury. Cochrane Database of Systematic Reviews. 2012 Jan 18;**1**:1-51. DOI: CD001046

Permissions

All chapters in this book were first published in ESCIM&RMFFSCI, by InTech Open; hereby published with permission under the Creative Commons Attribution License or equivalent. Every chapter published in this book has been scrutinized by our experts. Their significance has been extensively debated. The topics covered herein carry significant findings which will fuel the growth of the discipline. They may even be implemented as practical applications or may be referred to as a beginning point for another development.

The contributors of this book come from diverse backgrounds, making this book a truly international effort. This book will bring forth new frontiers with its revolutionizing research information and detailed analysis of the nascent developments around the world.

We would like to thank all the contributing authors for lending their expertise to make the book truly unique. They have played a crucial role in the development of this book. Without their invaluable contributions this book wouldn't have been possible. They have made vital efforts to compile up to date information on the varied aspects of this subject to make this book a valuable addition to the collection of many professionals and students.

This book was conceptualized with the vision of imparting up-to-date information and advanced data in this field. To ensure the same, a matchless editorial board was set up. Every individual on the board went through rigorous rounds of assessment to prove their worth. After which they invested a large part of their time researching and compiling the most relevant data for our readers.

The editorial board has been involved in producing this book since its inception. They have spent rigorous hours researching and exploring the diverse topics which have resulted in the successful publishing of this book. They have passed on their knowledge of decades through this book. To expedite this challenging task, the publisher supported the team at every step. A small team of assistant editors was also appointed to further simplify the editing procedure and attain best results for the readers.

Apart from the editorial board, the designing team has also invested a significant amount of their time in understanding the subject and creating the most relevant covers. They scrutinized every image to scout for the most suitable representation of the subject and create an appropriate cover for the book.

The publishing team has been an ardent support to the editorial, designing and production team. Their endless efforts to recruit the best for this project, has resulted in the accomplishment of this book. They are a veteran in the field of academics and their pool of knowledge is as vast as their experience in printing. Their expertise and guidance has proved useful at every step. Their uncompromising quality standards have made this book an exceptional effort. Their encouragement from time to time has been an inspiration for everyone.

The publisher and the editorial board hope that this book will prove to be a valuable piece of knowledge for researchers, students, practitioners and scholars across the globe.

List of Contributors

Aaron Z. Bailey, Hunter J. Fassett, Tea Lulic, Jenin El Sayes and Aimee J. Nelson
Department of Kinesiology, McMaster University, Hamilton, Ontario, Canada

Filipe Barroso
Department of Physiology, Feinberg School of Medicine – Northwestern University, Chicago, IL, USA
Neural Rehabilitation Group, Cajal Institute, Spanish National Research Council (CSIC), Madrid, Spain

Diego Torricelli and Juan C. Moreno
Neural Rehabilitation Group, Cajal Institute, Spanish National Research Council (CSIC), Madrid, Spain

Farhad Abbasi and Soolmaz Korooni
Bushehr University of Medical Sciences, Bushehr, Iran

Mengliang Zhang
Department of Neuroscience and Pharmacology, University of Copenhagen, Copenhagen, Denmark
Neuronano Research Center, Department of Experimental Medical Science, Lund University, Lund, Sweden

Sherif M. Amr
The Department of Orthopaedics and Traumatology, Cairo University, Cairo, Egypt

Irene Paterniti, Emanuela Esposito and Salvatore Cuzzocrea
Department of Chemical, Biological, Pharmaceutical and Environmental Sciences, University of Messina, Messina, Italy

Haruo Shimazaki
Division of Neurology, Department of Internal Medicine, Jichi Medical University, Tochigi, Japan

Paola Suárez-Meade
Faculty of Health Sciences, Anáhuac University, Universidad Anáhuac Av. Huixquilucan Edo. Mexico, Mexico

Antonio Ibarra
Faculty of Health Sciences, Anáhuac University, Universidad Anáhuac Av. Huixquilucan Edo. Mexico, Mexico
CAMINA Research Project A.C. Mexico City, Mexico

Moti M. Kramer
Assuta Ashdod University Medical Center, Ashdod, Israel

Asaf Acker and Nissim Ohana
Soroka University Medical Center, Beer-Sheva, Israel

Index

www.ingramcontent.com/pod-product-compliance
Lightning Source LLC
Chambersburg PA
CBHW061958190326
41458CB00009B/2908